de Launey and Land

Principles and Practice
of
Dermatology

THIRD EDITION

by

Harvey Rotstein MBBS, FRACP, FACD

Butterworth-Heinemann

Sydney   Oxford   Boston   London   Munich
New Delhi   Singapore   Tokyo   Toronto   Wellington
1993

BUTTERWORTH-HEINEMANN

AUSTRALIA   BUTTERWORTH-HEINEMANN 271–273 Lane Cove Road, North Ryde 2113
                 BUTTERWORTH-HEINEMANN 18 Salmon Street, Port Melbourne 3207

UNITED KINGDOM   BUTTERWORTH-HEINEMANN LTD   Oxford

USA   BUTTERWORTH-HEINEMANN Stoneham

National Library of Australia Cataloguing-in-Publication entry

---

De Launey, W. E. (Wallace E.).
  Principles and practice of dermatology.

  3rd ed.
  Includes index.
  ISBN 0 409 30259 7.

  1. Dermatology. 2. Skin - Diseases. I. Land, W.A. (William A.). II. Rotstein, Harvey. III. Title.

616.5

First published by Butterworths in 1978.
Second edition published by Butterworths in 1984.

Typeset in Baskerville and Aristocrat by Midland Typesetters, Maryborough, Victoria.

Printed in Australia by Star Printery Pty Ltd.

Contents

Preface to the third edition

When it first appeared, de Launey and Land's text *Principles and Practice of Dermatology* was enthusiastically accepted by medical students as essential reading. The reasons were obvious. Firstly the book demystified dermatology by explaining physical signs and management on the basis of pathophysiology. Secondly it was a pleasure to use. Details were comprehensive and concise, chapter division was clinically relevant and discussion was pertinent to Australian situations and conditions.

The third edition hopefully retains all these features. In addition, changes have been incorporated that clarify the text and make it even easier to read. At the beginning of each chapter a contents list has been presented, headings have been made clearer and new line drawings have been introduced. The chapters are now more even in length. A new chapter has been added to aid in the early diagnosis of melanoma, and extra sections encompass newly described yet relatively common conditions and the skin signs of infection with the human immunodeficiency virus. Where possible, the thought processes that go into making a diagnosis have been explained in greater detail.

However, at all times during this revision, whenever any alterations were made I was mindful of the need to preserve the innate character that has made this book an institution among Australian medical students.

Harvey Rotstein
1992

Preface to the first edition

There is a real need for a small, up-to-date textbook of dermatology, suitable for the Australian undergraduate and general practitioner. Cutaneous tumours and other diseases encountered more frequently in Australia, warrant greater emphasis than is provided in books written overseas. We have therefore designed this book to be sufficiently comprehensive for the undergraduate or family physician interested in dermatology, and have given priority to aspects of importance to Australian doctors. Where possible, we have related the clinical aspects to what is known of the mechanisms involved.

W E de Launey
W A Land
1978

Acknowledgments

The influence of my parents Hela and Alec, my original mentors John A Brenan and Denis M Clarke, and the Sisters of Charity at St Vincent's Hospital in Melbourne cannot be overemphasised, for they successfully provided an environment that enabled me to enjoy my chosen field.

This edition could not have been completed with the encouragement and invaluable research assistance supplied by my wife Eva. The necessary words that kept me going were provided by John Coxhill of Butterworths, John Wolf of Wolf, Klooger and Co, and my children, Andrew, Richard and Fiona.

Special thanks are due to Dianne Cameron, Evelyn Wilkins and Helena Christos who typed the manuscript; to Mario Cotela and Ross Servanis for photographic assistance, to Ben Elisha for the new line drawings, to Susan Auster for assistance with proof reading and to Graham Mason of Dorevitch Pathology for the transparencies used in preparing the cover art.

Table of line drawings

Table of colour plates

The colour plates appear, in groups of six, on unnumbered pages. These pages are printed on special art quality paper and are readily distinguished from the text pages.

Glossary

Macroscopic features

Alopecia
Loss of hair.

Annulus
A ring or ring-shaped structure.

Atrophy
Thinning of the skin, with diminution of normal skin markings.

Bulla
A circumscribed, elevated lesion which contains fluid, and is larger than 0.5 cm in diameter.

Crust ('scab')
The dried exudate from an erosion or ulcer.

Erosion
A superficial, circumscribed loss of epidermis, which heals without scarring.

Erythema
Redness due to vasodilatation.

Exanthem
The rash or eruption produced by the action of an organism or its toxins on the small blood vessels of the skin.

Excoriation
An area of skin denuded of epidermis by scratching. Excoriations may be linear or rounded and are a frequent accompaniment of itching dermatoses.

Lichenification
A response to rubbing and scratching of the skin that produces thickening together with accentuation of the normal skin markings.

Macule
A circumscribed area of altered skin colour. A macule may be of any size, but retains normal skin texture and is impalpable. The altered colour may be due to erythema, to increased or decreased melanin pigmentation, or to the presence of a non-melanin pigment, such as haemosiderin.

Nodule
A circumscribed, elevated area of skin, which is larger than 1 cm in diameter, and is usually rounded or dome-shaped. A nodule may result

from inflammation, from neoplasia, or from various deposits in the dermis or subcutis.

Papule
A circumscribed, elevated area of skin, which is less than 1 cm in diameter. Papules may have normal or altered colour, and may be produced by oedema, by epidermal hyperplasia, by cellular infiltrates, or by various deposits in the dermis.

Plaque
A circumscribed, palpable area of skin which is larger than 1 cm in diameter. The thickness of a plaque is small in relation to its breadth, and the lesion may be elevated or depressed.

Scale
An abnormal accumulation of keratin. Scaling may occur on normal skin if desquamation is impeded (as under a plaster cast) but more commonly forms on abnormal skin.

Sclerosis
Localised or diffuse hardening of the subcutaneous tissue, which may also involve the dermis.

Telangiectasis
A visible lesion composed of permanently dilated blood vessels.

Ulcer
A circumscribed area of tissue loss which varies in depth. An ulcer may involve skin only, or may extend to subcutaneous tissue, muscle and bone.

Vesicle
A circumscribed, elevated lesion which contains fluid and is less than 0.5 cm in diameter. Vesicles are usually multiple and frequently grouped.

Weal
An area of transient, localised oedema of the skin.

Microscopic appearances

Acanthosis
Increased thickness of the stratum spinosum.

Dyskeratosis
Abnormal keratinisation of individual cells in the epidermis.

Granuloma
A chronic proliferative change, characterised by the presence of mononuclear cells together with epithelioid cells, multinucleated giant cells, or both.

Hyperkeratosis
Increased thickness of the stratum corneum.

Parakeratosis
Abnormal maturation of cells in the epidermis, marked by incomplete keratinisation and retention of cell nuclei in the stratum corneum, and an absent stratum granulosum.

Spongiosis
Accumulation of fluid between cells of the epidermis, which results in a widening of the spaces between them.

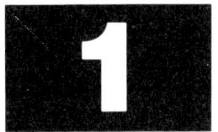

Structure and functions of the skin

1. Structure
    (a) epidermis
    (b) dermis
    (c) appendages
2. Functions
    (a) epidermis
    (b) dermis
    (c) appendages

The skin is a metabolically active interface between the environment and ourselves. It is thinly coated on the surface with a fluid lipid film, and, in most areas of the body, rests on an insulating layer of adipose tissue.

The skin is composed of a stratified squamous epithelium, the epidermis, which is firmly anchored to the underlying dermis—a meshwork of fibres embedded in a gelatinous ground substance. This basic architecture is modified by the presence of hair follicles and secretory glands, and by regional variations of its thickness.

The structure of the skin may be conveniently considered as comprising epidermis, dermis, and appendages (hair follicles, sebaceous glands, apocrine glands, eccrine glands, and nails).

Structure

Epidermis

The epidermis is a mosaic of epithelial cells which varies in depth from less than 0.1 mm thick on the eyelid to more than 1 mm thick on the sole. The lowermost cells constitute the *basal layer* which is only one cell thick. The division of epidermal cells normally occurs in the basal layer, where the rate of mitosis is just sufficient to replace cells lost from the surface.

Keratinocyte

This is the basic cell of the epidermis. It migrates upwards from the basal layer of the epidermis to form the surface keratin layer which is the barrier layer of the epidermis. A series of morphological changes occur as the cell moves upwards and finally arrives at the surface as

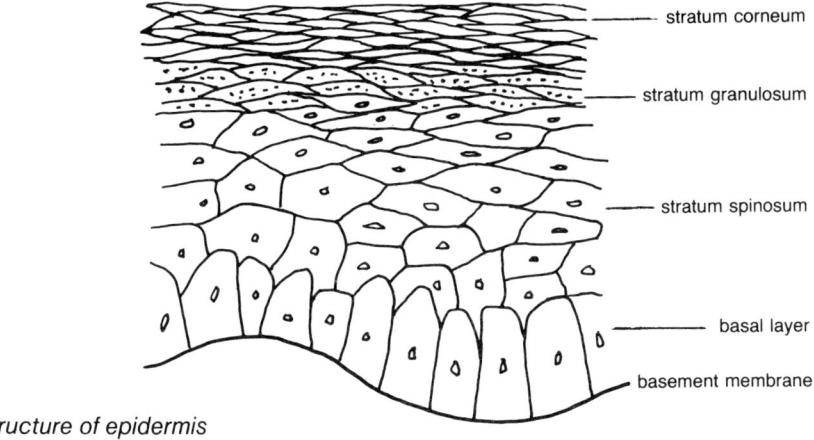

stratum corneum

stratum granulosum

stratum spinosum

basal layer

basement membrane

Structure of epidermis

a dead cell with homogeneous dense cytoplasm, a very thickened cell membrane, and no nucleus or organelles. Because all the cells in a normal epidermis move upwards at the same rate, they all undergo the same changes at roughly the same position within the epidermis, thereby giving the false impression that the various zones or layers occur when the cell crosses a certain line. That this is not so is clearly shown in disorders of differentiation such as Bowen's disease in which fully keratinised cells may be found near the basal layer and basaloid cells may be found near the surface. Also, in diseases where there is a very rapid transit from basal layer to the surface (such as psoriasis), the full series of changes may not have had time to take place and keratinised cells may still retain nuclei and other organelles.

The majority of basal cells are columnar, with a round or oval nucleus. The cytoplasm is traversed by bundles of fine filaments (***tonofilaments***), mostly aligned in a direction perpendicular to the skin surface. Between adjacent cells there are areas of adhesion which are visible with the light microscope as tiny points of intercellular attachment that resist the shrinkage of cells away from one another during fixation and in real life allow the cells to resist shearing forces. With the electron microscope, these areas of attachment (***desmosomes***) are seen as a series of dense plates which involve adjacent cell membranes, and to which tonofilaments are attached on the cytoplasmic side. Where basal cell membranes adjoin the dermis, the dense plates are modified to form 'half-desmosomes' (hemidesmosomes) which are peculiar to this site.

Above the basal layer, the cells of the ***stratum spinosum*** (Malpighian layer) are more polygonal. With electron microscopy the cell membranes appear ruffled and tortuous, being closely apposed only at desmosomes. Bundles of tonofilaments spread out from the region of the nucleus to attach to cell membranes at the desmosomal plates. The tonofilaments become more organised and prominent in upper regions of the layer and dominate the appearance of the most superficial cells. Cells of the stratum spinosum become progressively flatter until they arrive at a band of almost rhomboidal cells which are prominent by virtue of their coarse irregular granules—the ***stratum granulosum***. Superficial to the granular

2

layer there is an abrupt change to flat, dead cells which lack organelles and which are packed with coarse fibres of keratin. With ordinary stains, this layer appears to be a flat bundle of parallel wavy fibres, and is called the *stratum corneum*.

There is a steady migration of cells from the basal layer to the surface. During their passage, the cells are transformed from metabolically active, dividing basal cells to the shrunken, fully keratinised dead cells of the stratum corneum, and are ultimately shed from the surface as epidermal dust.

Melanocytes

Interspersed at intervals along the basal layer and, having neither tonofilaments nor desmosomes, melanocytes stand out from their neighbours as larger 'clear cells' with small round nuclei. With silver staining, melanocytes are seen as branched cells with five or six dendritic processes which divide and subdivide, sending branches between cells of the epidermis. Melanin granules (*melanosomes*) are transmitted by the tips of the dendritic processes and phagocytosed by the adjacent epidermal cells where they aggregate as a crescentic arrangement on the surface side of the nucleus. There appears to be an optimal size of particle for phagocytosis of melanin by the keratinocyte. Large melanosomes such as those of the Australian Aboriginals are taken up singly, whereas the smaller melanosomes of the caucasoids are arranged three to four in a membrane-bound organelle. Apparently these organelles contain substances that destroy melanosomes, because in caucasoids melanosomes have disappeared by the time keratinocytes form the granular cell layer, whereas in Aborigines melanosomes may be seen in cells of the keratin layer. Intercellular oedema fluid also influences melanosome phagocytosis by impairing melanocyte-to-keratinocyte transfer, producing post-inflammatory hypopigmentation.

Langerhans cells

These are also 'clear dendritic cells' and, like melanocytes, are argyrophilic. However, they lie more superficially in the epidermis and are bone marrow derived cells, which may be demonstrated by specific staining with antibodies to $CD1_a$ and MHC class II molecules.

Dermis

Dermo-epidermal junction

The epidermal surface of the dermis is thickly studded with conical projections, the *dermal papillae*. The epidermis overlies these projections and bulges down to fill the spaces between them, forming the *rete ridges*, so that in cross-section the interface between dermis and epidermis appears as an undulating line of ridges and troughs.

With a few exceptions, such as the face, the undulation is least developed where there is a lot of hair. This suggests that the undulating pattern acts to minimise the separation of epidermis and dermis when shearing forces are applied to regions where hairs cannot function as 'holding pins'.

Between dermis and epidermis there is a continuous **basement membrane**, rich in collagen and composed of a fine fibrillar material embedded in a dense matrix. Fine fibrils pass from the basement membrane towards the half-desmosomes of the basal cells, the 'anchoring fibrils'. On the dermal side, bundles of elastic fibrils emerge from the basement membrane to connect with dermal elastic tissue, presumably to reinforce stability of the dermo-epidermal junction.

Fibres

The **collagen fibres** are arranged in a criss-crossing mesh of bundles, seen in sections as wavy fibrous bands, or as rounded blocks when cut end-on. In the deeper (reticular) dermis, the bundles tend to lie parallel to the surface, but in the superficial (papillary) dermis the orientation is less organised. **Reticulin fibres** are visible with special stains as a fine network which surrounds collagen fibres, enmeshes hair follicles, sebaceous and sweat glands, and supports neurovascular bundles. Just below the dermo-epidermal junction, there is a condensation of fine elastic fibrils, while coarser **elastic fibres** are interspersed among collagen bundles throughout the dermis.

Ground substance

The ground substance of the dermis is a viscid gel, rich in mucopolysaccharides—a continuum in which are embedded fibres, vessels, nerves and cells. In normal skin, ground substance is scanty and difficult to demonstrate, the bulk of the dermis being formed by collagen.

Cells

The normal dermis has only a small cellular component, which is more apparent in its papillary part. Fibroblasts are sparsely scattered between bundles of collagen, and a few histiocytes and macrophages are visible, mainly around blood vessels. Mast cells are present in small numbers around capillaries, while occasional lymphocytes and other transient leucocytes may be identified.

Blood vessels

There is a variable but abundant network of dermal vessels, with a concentration at two levels. The deeper **subdermal plexus** lies close to the junction of dermis and subcutaneous tissue and communicates freely with the more superficial **subpapillary plexus**. From the subpapillary arteriolar plexus, loops pass in a candelabra-like pattern to course through the superficial dermis, giving off capillaries which supply the dermal papillae before draining into postcapillary venules. Capillary perfusion may be largely bypassed by more direct flow from arteriolar to venous segments of the subpapillary plexus—a shunt of considerable significance for thermoregulation.

Lymphatic drainage

In each dermal papilla there is a single lymphatic capillary, which begins as a dead-end vessel and drains into a subpapillary lymphatic plexus. There is a deeper plexus of valved vessels from which lymphatics pass

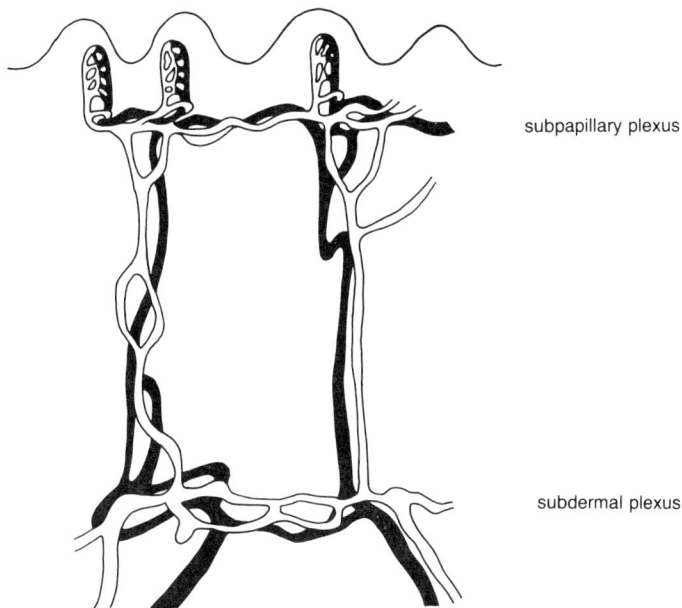

Vascular anastomoses of dermis

subpapillary plexus

subdermal plexus

centrally, following the path of the larger blood vessels and draining into regional lymph nodes.

Innervation

Bundles of nerve fibres enter the dermis from the underlying adipose layer and send branches toward the surface from a network deep in the dermis. Nerve fibres cross from one bundle to another and, although there is a tendency for fibres to follow the path of blood vessels, there is a very extensive net-like pattern of interlacing nerve fibres at all levels in the dermis. As part of this overall network, there is a condensation of fibres around hair follicles. Eventually all fibres end as terminal filaments, some of which are simply naked fibrils, while others appear to be modified into anatomical variants.

Innervation of the skin is both sensory and autonomic. The autonomic fibres are all postganglionic sympathetic fibres, but those supplying eccrine sweat glands are unique in that they liberate acetyl choline at their endings after stimulation; they are cholinergic sympathetic fibres.

Appendages

Hair follicles

Hair follicles occur all over the body, except on palms, soles and such mucocutaneous junctions as the glans penis and the vermilion border of the lip. In most areas, the hair is short and fine, as on the forearm of a child or the cheek of a normal woman (*vellus hair*). The longer hair on the scalp is broader in section and is usually pigmented (*terminal hair*). There is no clear distinction between vellus and terminal types.

In fact, the same follicle may change from terminal to vellus, as on the scalp of a man, or from vellus to terminal, as on the chin of a male adolescent.

The bulk of a hair is formed by the **cortex**, composed of elongated, keratinised cells which are cemented firmly together and contain a variable amount of melanin. The cortex of terminal hair may enclose a core of loosely cemented, incompletely keratinised cells (**medulla**). The cortex is surrounded by an adherent sheath of flat cells (**the cuticle**) which are arranged like roof tiles with each cell overlapped by the one below, the free edge directed upwards. Surrounding the hair with its cuticle is the **internal root sheath**, the innermost cells of which also form a cuticle. This layer interlocks with the cuticle of the hair so that the internal root sheath grows out, bound to the hair by its cuticle. On reaching the surface, the cells of the internal root sheath are shed. The hair outside the follicle has no covering sheath.

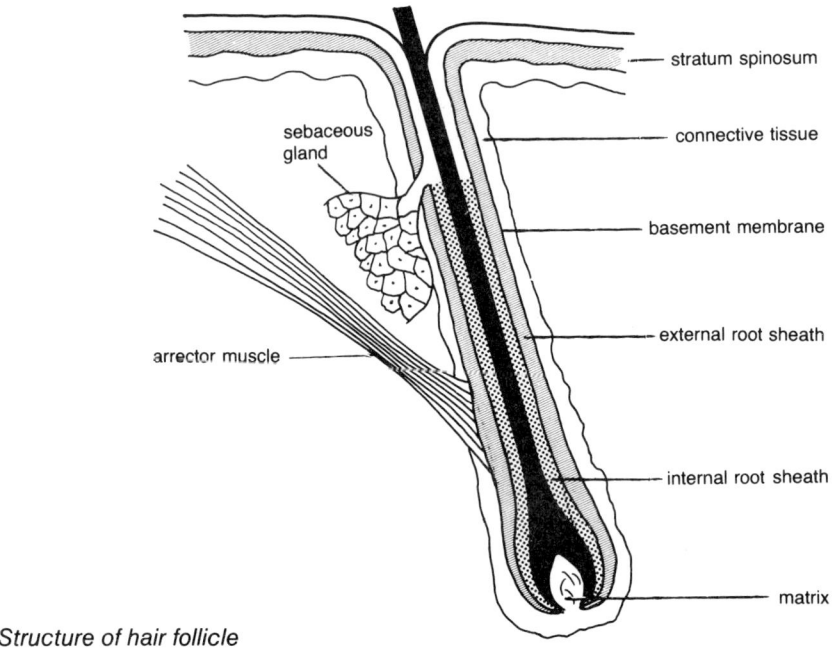

Structure of hair follicle

A layer of cells (**external root sheath**) surrounds the internal root sheath and is continuous above with the stratum spinosum. Around the external root sheath is a **basement membrane** which is continuous with that of the dermo-epidermal junction. The cells of the hair itself, and those of the internal and external root sheaths, are continuous below with a cluster of rapidly dividing cells (**matrix**) from which they are replaced.

Sebaceous glands

Sebaceous glands occur over the whole skin surface, except on palms and soles. They vary in size and number, but are largest and most numerous over the face, scalp and anogenital region. Each gland consists of a group of **lobules** which open into a common duct, and each lobule is a sac-like cluster of cells which is surrounded by a basement membrane. At the periphery of a lobule, cells are small and proliferating but, as they proceed towards the centre, they accumulate lipid droplets and enlarge, while the nuclei become smaller and eventually disappear.

At the centre of the lobule, cells rupture, and the lipid droplets together with the cellular debris are discharged into the short excretory duct as *sebum*. In most areas, the common duct of the gland opens into the pilosebaceous canal, but at such mucocutaneous junctions as the vermilion border of the lip the ducts open directly onto the surface.

Apocrine glands

In postnatal life, apocrine glands are mainly found in the axillae, in the pubic region and around the areolae. Each gland consists of a tubular secretory portion which is arranged in coils in the subcutaneous tissue and is connected by a short duct to the upper part of the pilosebaceous canal. Secretion is produced by small portions of the secretory cells budding off into the lumen.

Eccrine glands

Eccrine glands are found over the whole skin surface, but with considerable regional variation in the density of distribution, being most numerous over the palms, soles and axillae. Each gland has a coiled, tubular secretory portion deep in the dermis of adjoining subcutaneous tissue.

The secretory coils, which are smaller than those of apocrine glands, are connected to a relatively long and thin ductal portion which passes through dermis and epidermis to open onto the surface of the skin

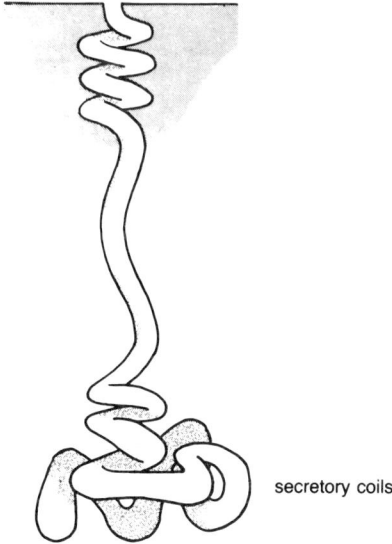

secretory coils

Eccrine gland

independently of the pilosebaceous ducts. Sweat is transported via intercellular cannaliculi from cells into the lumen.

Nails

The nail itself, the **nail plate**, is composed of firmly adherent, keratinised cells which are derived from a rapidly dividing matrix. Most of the matrix is hidden by the skin proximal to the nail plate, but its most distal portion is visible through the nail as a pale, semilunar area, the **lunula**. The nail plate is surrounded on three sides by the nail folds and rests on the **nail bed**. Although it is a keratinising epithelium, the bed contributes little to the keratin of the nail plate. A small, thin extension of the epidermis of the proximal nail fold projects for a short distance over the nail as the **cuticle**, sealing off the potential space between nail and nail fold.

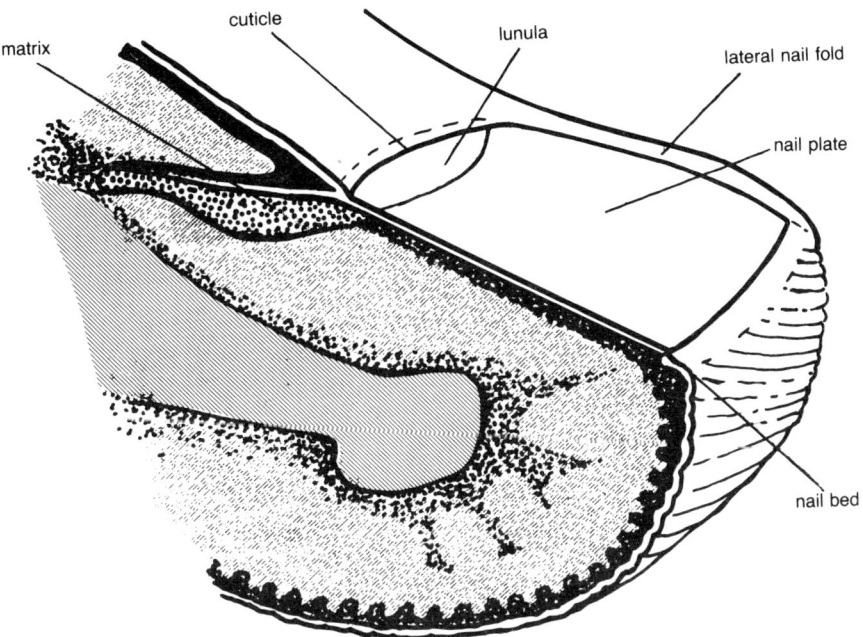

Sagittal section through distal phalanx

Functions

Epidermis

Chemical barrier

Normal epidermis provides an effective barrier to the passage of substances into or out of the skin. It reduces the loss of water and electrolytes through the skin, and impedes the penetration of substances from the exterior. When large areas of skin are altered, for example by acute dermatitis, the barrier function of the skin may be so altered that the loss of water, protein and electrolytes becomes important.

At the same time, damage allows greater penetration from the exterior, which may explain the increased liability of inflamed skin to contact dermatitis. The barrier may be temporarily impaired by overhydration, as occurs in areas of skin occluded by plastic sheeting—a condition which may be utilised to enhance penetration of corticosteroids.

The acid pH surface of the skin allows it to withstand acids much better than alkalis. The fact that the cells of the keratin layer are dead and keratin chemically very inert is ideally suited to the stratum corneum's function as the main barrier layer of the epidermis.

Mechanical barrier

The skin is a useful mechanical barrier and withstands considerable deformation without permanent damage. The skin is resilient, and tends to resume its previous shape after deformation; however, this resilience is decreased by the excess water content of oedematous skin.

Immunological barrier

The Langerhans cells within the epidermis, like other cells bearing MHC class II molecules, function as macrophages that present antigens to effector T lymphocytes. The Langerhans cells play an important role in allergic contact dermatitis and graft rejection.

Endocrine organ

The cutaneous synthesis of vitamin D_3 is the most important source of this vitamin in humans. Ultraviolet light of wavelength 290 nm to 300 nm reacts with 7-dehydrocholesterol (provitamin D) cleaving the bond between carbons 9 and 10 to form previtamin D_3, which is a thermally unstable molecule that undergoes internal isomerisation of its double bonds to form vitamin D_3. This is then transported into the dermal capillaries, is hydroxylated in the liver and then hydroxylated in the kidney to form the metabolically active form of vitamin D_3 (1, 25 dihydroxycholecalciferol). The transfer of vitamin D_3 into the dermal capillaries is the rate limiting process and causes a build up of previtamin D_3 which is further acted on by ultraviolet light to form non-active metabolites, so preventing toxic buildup of circulating vitamin D_3.

As well as controlling calcium and phosphate metabolism, vitamin D_3 influences keratinocyte differentiation and proliferation.

Defence against micro-organisms

The skin surface is never sterile. There is a permanent resident flora, which, although variable from site to site and from person to person, consistently includes micrococci, coagulase-negative staphylococci, Corynebacteria, and saprophytic yeasts. There is considerable evidence that, far from being harmful, the presence of these relatively innocuous strains inhibits the growth of more virulent organisms arriving at the skin surface from the environment.

Bacteria are constantly being shed from the skin with desquamating cells, but a more active antibacterial mechanism is provided by the thin coating of lipid which covers the skin surface. This lipid film contains unsaturated fatty acids with a significant bactericidal action. Though more effective against streptococci than staphylococci, the surface lipids are active against both. Surface lipids derived from sebaceous glands also have activity against the fungi that produce tinea, and this is probably the reason why some varieties of tinea capitis are almost never seen in those who have passed puberty.

The skin is a relatively dry surface. Some organisms, especially the coliform bacilli, are intolerant of desiccation, dying off in a matter of hours. If, however, the skin is kept moist, as with hands inside rubber gloves, these bacteria survive and multiply. On the normal skin of healthy individuals, Gram-negative bacteria occur only as transients and in small numbers. Although desiccation is a factor, some Gram-negative bacteria die more quickly on the skin than on an inert surface, which indicates the effect of physiological mechanisms, the nature of which remains to be explained.

Defence against ultraviolet light

For skin unprotected by hair or clothing, the only significant defence against the damaging effects of ultraviolet light is the presence of melanin within the epidermis. Without melanin, the epidermis is little more than a thin transparent membrane which gives virtually no protection against ultraviolet radiation. Within epidermal cells melanin is distributed as a crescent between the incident radiation and the nucleus. Melanin provides important protection by absorption and scattering of radiation, and by trapping electrons and free radicals released by the dissipation of radiant energy.

Melanin is a dense, insoluble compound of high molecular weight, formed from tyrosine under the influence of enzyme tyrosinase. Much remains to be learned of the mechanisms involved in the regulation of melanogenesis, but it is likely that free radicals, released in tissue after exposure to ultraviolet light, diminish inhibitory controls on the enzyme. Tyrosinase is produced within melanocytes and packaged with a protein matrix inside small cytoplasmic organelles, the *melanosomes*. Melanin is deposited on the inner matrix of these organelles until, with increasing deposition of melanin, the melanosome is ultimately converted into a dense, opaque particle with no visible internal structure.

Melanocytes are scattered along the basal layer, where they are uniquely adapted to produce and deliver melanin to the cells of the epidermis. There is no significant difference in melanocyte populations in the skin of different racial groups, skin colour depending on melanin production and distribution, and not on numbers of melanocytes. Pale-skinned people who tan poorly have only a few lightly melanised melanosomes which, after transfer to epidermal cells, are arranged in groups surrounded by a membrane.

In Australian Aboriginals and other dark-skinned races, the transferred melanosomes are larger granules that are individually dispersed in the cytoplasm, in contrast to the membrane-bound melanosome complex of caucasoid skin. As epidermal cells approach the surface, progressive degradation of melanosomes converts the melanin particles to an inconspicuous amorphous form.

Dermis

Support

The ground substance acts to hold in place the vessels, nerves and appendages. The nature and arrangement of collagen and elastic fibres in the dermis put the skin under tension, so that the edges retract when skin is cut. When the dermis becomes degenerate, as in aged or atrophic skin, the normal tension of skin is reduced, the skin is unable to resist shearing forces and therefore allows damage to blood vessels resulting in purpura, or actually tears and breaks off as a flap.

Thermoregulation

The metabolic processes of the body continually produce heat, which must be dissipated if a stable body temperature is to be maintained. At a comfortable environmental temperature, a person at rest easily maintains thermal balance merely by hypothalamic adjustment of cutaneous vasomotor control. The variability of cutaneous blood flow is remarkable, flow increasing as much as a hundredfold from maximal vasoconstriction to marked vasodilation, with proportional variation of heat loss. When vasodilation is inadequate to provide necessary heat loss, further cooling is achieved by evaporation of sweat. To be effective, sweating must be accompanied by evaporation and is therefore most efficent in dry, moving air.

In acute inflammatory skin diseases, vasodilation is accompanied by an increase of cutaneous blood flow with increased heat loss, which explains the 'chills' without fever in patients with generalised acute dermatitis. Such patients are unable to respond to low environmental temperature with cutaneous vasoconstriction, which makes effective thermoregulation difficult.

Sensory organ

The skin is richly supplied with nerve endings and provides an effective sensory defence against potentially harmful agents. Cutaneous stimuli are interpreted centrally as one or more of a broad range of qualities (of which the four 'primary sensations', heat, cold, touch and pain, are probably no more than arbitrary examples) which are commonly experienced.

Specific areas of skin are supplied by sensory nerves derived from single dorsal nerve roots (sensory dermatomes). There is considerable overlap of dermatomes, so that section of a single dorsal root produces little impairment of sensation. However, when a single dorsal root is isolated by section of those above and below, the segmental dermatome can be demonstrated as a spared island in intact sensation.

Appendages

Hair

During foetal life, most of the body is covered by soft, fine hair. Before birth, this silky 'lanugo' is replaced by vellus hair, except for the scalp, eyebrows and eyelashes, where coarser terminal hair develops. This first

11

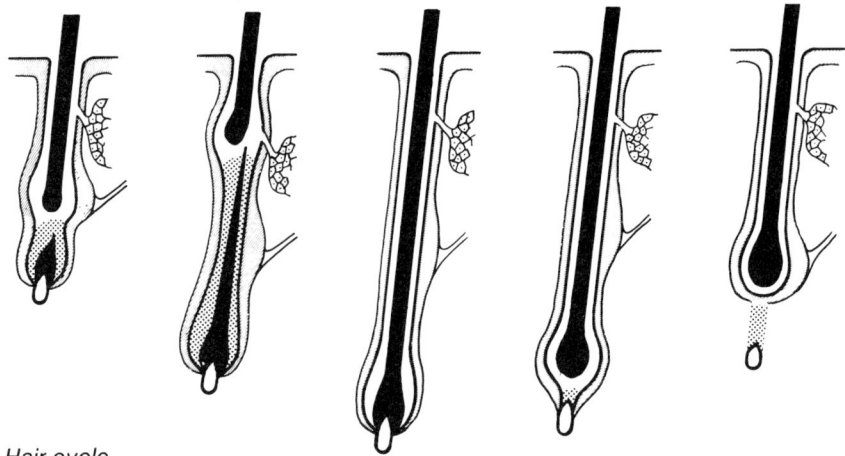

Hair cycle

crop of terminal hair is shed and replaced in the first few months after birth. Thereafter, individual follicles behave independently, with a cycle of growth and regression uncoordinated with similar cycles in other follicles.

There are three distinct phases of the hair cycle—a phase of hair growth (***anagen***), a phase of regression (***catagen***) and a resting phase (***telogen***). The duration of each phase varies considerably in different body regions, but the sequence of anagen followed by catagen, followed in turn by telogen, does not alter. On the scalp, anagen usually lasts two to six years, catagen about two weeks, and telogen for about three months. Eyebrow follicles have an anagen phase lasting only ten weeks, with a telogen of nine weeks.

During anagen, rapid division of matrix cells results in continuous hair growth. With the onset of catagen, mitoses cease in the matrix and the cells become keratinised. The lower part of the follicle shrinks and comes to lie at the level of the arrector muscle. During telogen, the hair, which is no longer growing, rests within the shrunken follicle, its lower end rounded to the shape of a club. As anagen recommences, there is a downgrowth of follicular epithelium, followed by the resumption of mitoses in the again active matrix. With growth of a new hair, the old club hair is pushed to one side and is soon removed by minor trauma.

At puberty, pubic and axillary hair growth occurs in both males and females as a result of vellus hairs being transformed to terminal hairs. In males there is also growth of beard and moustache hair, and increased growth of hair over the limbs and trunk, especially the front of the chest. The mechanisms which restrict the areas of response to these regions are unknown. Although these events are definitely androgen-dependent, different processes are involved in each region. The appearance of facial and body hair requires high levels of testosterone and target tissues must be capable of transforming it to dihydrotestosterone using the enzyme 5-alpha-reductase. However, pubic and axillary hair growth requires only low androgen levels and is not dependant upon 5-alpha-reductase. It is seemingly paradoxical that testosterone, which stimulates the pubertal conversion of follicles, is necessary for the development of male-pattern baldness. Men castrated before puberty do not develop male-pattern baldness, but may do so if treated with testosterone.

Sebaceous glands

Sebum is a complex mixture of lipids discharged onto the skin surface through the pilosebaceous canal. It is not synonymous with the skin surface lipid, which contains an admixture from the epidermis. Sebaceous glands in children are small, and sebum production remains very low until puberty when the glands enlarge and become productive. The amount of sebum produced is directly related to gland size, which is influenced by androgen levels.

There is good evidence for a limited antibacterial and antifungal action of surface lipids, and substantial experimental evidence that the pliability and normal barrier function of the stratum corneum is closely related to its lipid content.

Eccrine and apocrine sweat glands

The evaporation of sweat secreted by eccrine glands is crucial to thermoregulation in hot environments, but apocrine secretion has no known function in the human. Eccrine glands begin to function within a few days of birth, but apocrine glands do not secrete in children. Their functional development at puberty is believed to be endocrine-influenced.

Apocrine secretion is protein rich, viscid and scanty. It is odourless when secreted, but its bacterial decomposition products have a distinctive odour. Apocrine secretion is probably continuous but delivery to the surface tends to occur at times of emotional stress or excitement.

Eccrine sweat is secreted nearly isotonic to plasma and is modified by the resorption of sodium and bicarbonate during its movement through the ductual portion. Resorption is less efficient with higher rates of flow. Secretion is continuous but is modified by mostly cholinergic nerves that are controlled by a complex interaction of skin and central body temperatures.

Nails

The nails serve to protect the terminal phalanges of fingers and toes. The palmar and distal surfaces of fingers play an important part in the sensation of fine touch. The fingernails aid in picking up objects, and their loss creates a real disability. However, most patients seeking advice about their nails (like those seeking advice about their hair) do so for cosmetic reasons.

2

Principles of diagnosis

1. History
2. Examination
3. Special procedures

Many patients, and a few physicians, wrongly assume that the visibility of cutaneous lesions obviates the need for more than a glance at the skin to arrive at an accurate diagnosis. Although a brief preliminary examination will often indicate the line of questioning likely to prove most helpful, it does not obviate the need for logical progression from an adequate history and systematic examination to consideration of the differential diagnosis and, when necessary, appropriate investigation.

History

The patient should be encouraged to outline the course of the disorder, describing its onset and the evolution of abnormal changes. The necessary details of the history will vary from one patient to another, but will often include the following.

Pruritus and pain

Pruritus is so common in cutaneous diseases that its presence is usually not of great diagnostic help. However, the timing or, occasionally, the lack of pruritus may be of considerable significance.

Examples
■ Episodes of a dermatitis at the back of the neck may be noted to follow the wearing of a necklace with a nickel-plated clasp, which suggests contact allergy to nickel.
■ The patient with a leg ulcer may be aware of increased itch around the ulcer after application of a particular ointment, which suggests sensitivity to a component of the ointment.
■ A patient with scabies may complain of the nocturnal aggravation which is characteristic of the disease.
■ Lack of pruritus is a frequent feature of the skin lesions of secondary syphilis, but virtually excludes such notoriously itchy dermatoses as atopic dermatitis or dermatitis herpetiformis.
■ Pain is an uncommon symptom in dermatology, but may suggest the diagnosis, for example, in early stages of herpes zoster, or of an ischaemic

ulcer of the leg. Lack of pain may also have diagnostic significance, as with a neurotrophic ulcer on the sole of a diabetic.

Primary lesion

The nature and site of the initial lesion may be of considerable importance, and should be sought by careful questioning. By the time a patient seeks advice, the original condition may be obscured by such secondary factors as trauma and infection, which make recognition difficult.

Examples
■ The appearance of crusted erosions on the lower lip may be non-specific, but the knowledge that they developed from clusters of small vesicles on an erythematous base a few days previously would make herpes simplex the likely diagnosis.
■ Widespread impetigo which began on the itchy scalp of a child would necessitate a search for head lice, whereas recurrent impetigo which always begins about the nostrils of a child would suggest nose-picking, or a chronic nasal discharge as possible factors.

Evolution and course

Having established the nature of the primary lesion, the rate and mode of subsequent changes should be determined. The speed and pattern of extension may provide valuable diagnostic clues.

Examples
■ The clinical distinction between keratoacanthoma and squamous cell carcinoma can be very difficult, but rapid evolution over a few weeks would favour the diagnosis of keratoacanthoma.
■ The history of a solitary pink macule on the trunk, followed a week later by the appearance of multiple smaller pink macules limited to the trunk and proximal areas of the limbs, would suggest pityriasis rosea. A similar rash, beginning over the presternal region and slowly spreading over the trunk, might result from seborrhoeic dermatitis.

Systemic symptoms

Diseases which involve the skin are not always diseases of the skin alone. Constitutional features and associations are not rare and should not be overlooked. The ability to detect an inner malfunction from surface changes provides a most interesting and challenging facet of dermatology.

Examples
■ Productive cough and weight loss in an adult with dermatomyositis would necessitate exclusion of lung cancer.
■ For a patient with malaise, hoarseness, headache and an asymptomatic red rash, serological tests for syphilis would be mandatory.
■ Weight loss and night sweats, in a patient with increasing dryness and itching of the skin, should arouse the suspicion of Hodgkin's disease.

Therapy

Specific inquiry should be made about systemic and topical therapy. The patient should be asked not only about prescribed drugs, but also of the many compounds such as analgesics, laxatives and antihistamines, not regarded as 'drugs' by most patients. All recently used applications should be noted, bearing in mind that self-treatment is very common and may obscure the clinical picture.

Example
■ The diagnosis of tinea is not difficult in most patients. However, when the typical features have been masked by prolonged treatment with corticosteroids, confident clinical diagnosis may be impossible.

Psychological assessment

Emotional factors influence the course of many common dermatoses. The patient should be questioned about possible psychological stresses, but an objective assessment should also be made when the history is being taken. It is an error, however, to presume an emotional cause for the disease simply because no other aetiological factors have been discovered.

Past history

This should encompass cutaneous and systemic diseases, operations, and other forms of therapy.

Examples
■ A woman might seek advice about excessive hair loss, which is sufficient to produce objective thinning over the scalp. A history of parturition three months previously, or a recent course of anticoagulants, would explain her alopecia.
■ A patient might present with a painless red nodule on one ear. A history of previous nephrectomy for hypernephroma would raise the possibility of the nodule being a metastasis.

Family history

The family history may provide information which will be relevant, not only to genetically influenced disease, but to some acquired disorders.

Examples
■ A close family history of asthma and hay fever would add weight to the suspicion of atopic dermatitis in an infant.
■ A history of nocturnal pruritus in family contacts would suggest scabies as a possible cause of impetigo in a child.

Occupation

A wide variety of chemical irritants and allergens may be present in the work environment.

Examples
■ Hand dermatitis and inflammation of nail folds are common in cleaners and barmaids.
■ An acne-like folliculitis of the forearms is common in workers handling machine oil.
■ Even past occupations may be relevant, as with the patient who develops skin cancers years after the absorption of arsenic from industrial exposure.

Leisure

Hobbies and sports are a source of many potentially harmful agents.
Examples
■ Contact allergy to rhus may produce severe acute dermatitis in the home gardener.
■ An intensely itchy eruption may develop on the legs of fishermen after wading in lakes infested with the parasite responsible for 'swimmer's itch'.

Travel

Overseas travel is undertaken by an increasing proportion of the population. Some diseases which were very seldom encountered in Australia are no longer to be considered rare. The large migrant intake over the past 40 years also accounts for some cases of hitherto exotic diseases.

Example
■ A crusted ulcer on the cheek might be non-specific in itself, but its occurrence two months after a holiday in the Middle East would warrant exclusion of cutaneous leishmaniasis.

Ancestry

Some diseases are more common or more severe in particular racial groups.
Examples
■ Pemphigus vulgaris is more common in Jews.
■ Sarcoidosis tends to be more severe in American Negroes.
■ Lupus erythematosus is more common in the Chinese.

Examination

To reach a final diagnosis an examination is conducted to achieve the following goals:

Confirm the history
In addition to confirming that the distribution and arrangement of the rash are as claimed by the patient, examination can support details of patient-given history that a non-medical person would have to accept without question.

Examples
■ Pruritus can be confirmed by the finding of excoriations, lichenification and prurigo nodules.
■ Treatment with dithranol leaves a characteristic pattern of staining of the skin.
■ Scaling on the palms that began as vesicles shows characteristic circles of scale formed as the roof of the vesicles is broken and the fluid resorbed.

Correct the history
Patients may be mistaken in giving a history either because of confusion regarding terminology or because of a lack of symptoms.

Examples
- A rash said to have healed to leave 'scars' is seen, in reality, to have faded to leave post-inflammatory hypopigmentation. 'Blisters', 'scars' and 'pimples' are terms often used by patients to describe changes quite different to the correct meanings.
- The id eruption of tinea suddenly appearing on the hands will cause more patient concern than the tinea pedis that the patient has had for many years and forgotten about because it was not regarded as a problem.

Test the history-based diagnosis

While listening to the patient, diagnoses may come to mind and suggest specific questions, the answers to which will elicit more details. Examination can further refine these details.

Examples
- Dermatomal distribution can be confirmed when the history suggests herpes zoster.
- The history of tender pinkish nodules on the anterior lower legs can be confirmed as erythema nodosum by examination revealing the nodules as deep and poorly defined with a bruised tinge.

Demonstrate discriminatory local signs

A close examination in good light, often with the aid of magnification, can provide valuable information that has been missed by those who have taken only a cursory glance.

Examples
- The observation that papules are distributed around hair follicles in a febrile patient can distinguish between miliaria and folliculitis.
- Irregularities in outline caused by small areas of loss in pigmentation due to scarring would indicate that a pigmented lesion is likely to be a melanoma.

Seek distant confirmatory signs

Initial examination will often suggest a diagnosis that cannot be confirmed because local signs are not fully developed. In this situation the doctor should draw on medical knowledge to look for signs on the skin, buccal mucosa and other keratinising structures that will help to confirm the diagnosis.

Examples
- Pitting and onycholysis of fingernails, in a patient with a groin rash that is a glazed red colour, suggest that the flexural rash is psoriasis.
- Lacy white lines on the buccal mucosa of a patient with blotchy pigmentation of the skin indicate that lichen planus is the cause of the skin signs.
- The suspicion that patchy scaling in the scalp is due to psoriasis is strengthened by the finding of psoriasis on the knees.

Redirect the history

Examination may often reveal signs that cast doubt on the first thoughts the doctor may have had, or that suggest a diagnosis quite different from the one made on the basis of the patient's history. In this situation further information obtained from direct questions asked of the patient is very helpful.

Examples

■ The history given is of recurrent episodes of blisters on the glans of the penis that heal over in 10 to 14 days. The provisional diagnosis is herpes simplex, but examination reveals intense pigmentation localised to the previously blistered region, suggesting fixed drug eruption. The direct question regarding ingestion of laxatives stirs the patient's memory and a temporal association between laxative intake and appearance of rash is confirmed.

■ An 18-year-old complains of vesicles and crusts over the trunk. As there is no history of varicella during childhood, this is the initial diagnosis. However, examination reveals urticarial papules sumounted by a vesicle with lesions arising in crops elsewhere. The direct question regarding onset of new crops reveals that episodes appeared after evenings spent watering the garden, which incriminates insect bites as the cause.

Implicate systemic disease

A wide range of disease processes involving all organ systems can manifest as skin changes. In these cases skin signs will indicate that examination beyond the skin and mucosae is required to complete the physical examination.

Examples

■ Plum-coloured, horseshoe-shaped dermal infiltrates can lead to the discovery of enlarged spleen and lymph nodes of a lymphoma.

■ Diffuse alopecia and pale dry skin may reveal reflexes with the slow relaxation phase of hypothyroidism.

■ Acne and hirsutism appearing in a 30-year-old female with irregular menses would indicate the need for abdominal examination that could reveal an androgen-secreting ovarian tumour.

Formulate local pathology

A definite diagnosis often cannot be made with certainty following an examination, and tests are required. To decide which ones to perform, and to help the pathologist know what to look for, it is important to consider what type of process is causing the signs, what part of the skin is involved, and what are the possible causative diseases.

Examples

■ Pustules on the face could be caused by bacterial folliculitis, herpes simplex, tinea, acne, rosacea and ingrown hairs.

■ Scaling with no induration indicates that changes predominantly involve the epidermis. Superficial induration suggests changes within the dermis. Poorly defined deep nodules indicate changes within the fat.

■ Blisters that are subepidermal are usually tense, stable, contain blood-tinged fluid and heal to leave a base that is re-epithelialised rapidly. Intra-epidermal blisters, by contrast, contain clear fluid, are flaccid, and break readily to leave a raw area.

Special procedures

Diascopy

Pressure from a glass slide is used to blanch the skin, so that some features become more apparent when viewed through the glass. The technique is useful, for example, in distinguishing true erythema from extravasation of red cells into the dermis, or for visualising the dermal granulomas of sarcoidosis.

Wood's lamp

Designed to transmit ultraviolet light, mainly of wave-lengths around 350 nm to 365 nm, Wood's lamp is particularly helpful in the diagnosis of some types of tinea of the scalp and, in a few other diseases, to demonstrate the presence of fluorescent material on the skin. The contrast between white and surrounding skin is enhanced by Wood's light, making the detection of white macules easier. Wood's light makes melanin within the epidermis appear much darker, whereas melanin in the dermis becomes a little harder to distinguish from surrounding skin colour.

Skin scrapings

Microscopic examination of skin scrapings is routine in all lesions suspected of being fungal in origin. For the identification of species, culture on special media is necessary.

Cytodiagnosis

A clinical diagnosis of basal cell carcinoma may be confirmed by cytodiagnosis, which may also be helpful in suspected viral infections. A sample is taken from the superficial part of a lesion, spread on a slide, stained, and examined microscopically.

Biopsy

This simple procedure is of great value in dermatological diagnosis. The specimen may be removed with a biopsy punch or by scalpel excision. Circular punches, up to a centimetre in diameter, are designed for rapid removal of a plug of skin down to the subcutis, suitable for microscopic examination. However, an ellipse of skin removed with a scalpel more easily provides a wedge of tissue showing the gradation from normal skin through the edge of a lesion to the abnormal area. The resulting scar is also much more acceptable than the circular depressed area which follows healing of the unsutured punch biopsy.

The specimen is usually placed in 10 per cent solution of formalin but, when culture for bacteria or fungi is required, normal saline solution is used. Special techniques, such as lipid staining, require other fixatives, and immunofluorescence or immunoperoxidase testing is best performed on fresh unfixed tissue.

Serological tests

To demonstrate the presence of antibodies, especially those produced in response to infection, serological tests are performed. For example, syphilis serology may be required in the case of the 'difficult' rash; HIV serology when unusual infections are present; Antistreptolysin-O in the investigation of a cause for erythema nodosum.

Patch testing

In an attempt to confirm allergic contact dermatitis, patch testing may be done on a small area of skin, usually on the back. The test substance is applied to the skin on a small square of lint, which is covered with an inert occlusive material. It is then removed and read at 48 hours, because contact allergy is a type IV (cell-mediated) allergic reaction. By trial and error, suitable concentrations and vehicles have been formulated for most relevant substances. These factors are very important in obtaining accurate results.

Patch testing should be conducted only by those with a special knowledge of the procedure and its pitfalls.

Immunofluorescence

This technique is used particularly for the demonstration of immunoglobulin and complement in tissue sections, or of serum antibodies after fixation to slides of normal tissue. The method provides a valuable diagnostic tool for investigation of bullous and connective tissue diseases.

Monoclonal antibodies

Differentiation between similar-looking disorders that cannot be identified with certainty using normal stains (eg spindle cell tumours) can be achieved with the use of monoclonal antibodies. These highly specific antibodies, which react in a very selective manner with just one of the many antigens in a larger complex structure, are stained in tissue sections, using immunoperoxidase techniques.

3

Dermatitis and eczema

    1. Exogenous dermatitis
    2. Endogenous eczema
    3. Dermatitis of more complex aetiology
    4. Erythroderma

Nature

Dermatitis is a pattern of cutaneous inflammation, which may follow contact with an injurious substance (exogenous), or which may develop without apparent external cause (endogenous). Some dermatologists use the word 'dermatitis' when the cause is exogenous and the word 'eczema' for the endogenous variety. However, the pathologic process is the same, and the terms are interchangeable.

Evolution

Acute dermatitis

When acute dermatitis follows a single exposure to an irritating chemical, the injured area becomes erythematous, and somewhat swollen. If the injury is not severe, there may be no progression, and the inflammation will subside as the skin returns to normal. With greater damage, vesicles and sometimes bullae develop, which after rupture are succeeded by oozing and crusting. The crusts dry and separate, and the surface develops light scaling as the skin heals.

    The sequence of erythema, oedema, vesiculation, crusting, and scaling is characteristic of acute dermatitis of any type, but there is considerable overlap of these phases, even in a single lesion. There may be scaling in one part, while new vesicles are still forming in another. With repeated injury the sequence may be blurred, with one phase tending to dominate the clinical picture. In some patients vesicular and crusted lesions predominate, while in others a prolonged scaling phase develops with little prior oozing.

Histology

The characteristic microscopic feature is an intra-epidermal vesicle formed by accumulation of fluid between cells of the stratum spinosum. Intercellular attachments are stretched by increasing intercellular oedema until some are ruptured, forming clefts. As more fluid accumulates, the clefts enlarge to form small vesicles separated by thin septa of resisting

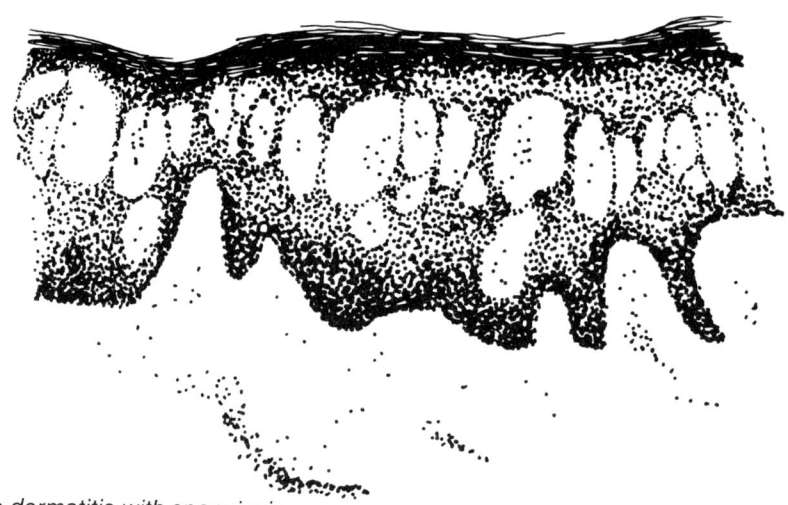

Acute dermatitis with spongiosis

cells. The distinctive honeycombed appearance is called 'spongiosis'. Vesicles may enlarge or coalesce to form bullae.

The stratum corneum often shows parakeratosis. In the dermis, there is vasodilatation, and a perivascular infiltrate of lymphocytes and polymorphs.

Chronic dermatitis

Skin which is affected for weeks by dermatitis is apt to develop additional changes. The skin tends to thicken and become more deeply pigmented. Itch is almost invariably present, and scratching may lead to excoriations or small surface elevations (scratch papules). Crusting is uncommon, except over excoriations, and vesicles are seen only during acute exacerbations. With persistent rubbing and scratching the thickening

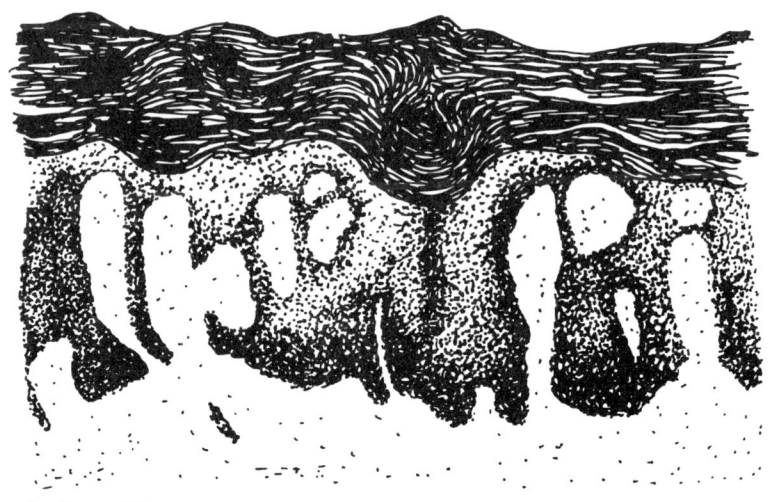

Chronic dermatitis

becomes more pronounced and the normal skin lines become exaggerated and more readily seen (lichenification).

Histology

Acanthosis is accompanied by elongation and broadening of the rete ridges, usually with hyperkeratosis, although there may be areas of parakeratosis. There may be intercellular oedema, but frank spongiosis is not a feature. The dermal infiltrate is predominantly perivascular and lymphocytic.

Complications of acute and chronic dermatitis

■ *Secondary infection*, either by bacteria or by *Candida*, easily develops in skin damaged by dermatitis.

■ *Secondary contact dermatitis* is readily produced by inappropriate therapy in the presence of an impaired epidermal barrier.

■ *Sweat retention* caused by poral occlusion leads to aggravation of pruritus, and scratching.

Types

Dermatitis which develops in response to contact with a foreign substance is called exogenous or contact dermatitis. Inflammation of the skin that occurs for internal reasons is called endogenous eczema.

Exogenous dermatitis

1. Irritant
   (a) primary irritant
   (b) phototoxic

2. Allergic
   (a) allergic eczematoid
   (b) photoallergic

Irritant contact dermatitis

■ *Primary irritants* are substances which induce inflammation in the skin of any person, provided that the concentration and duration of exposure are sufficient. There is no allergic mechanism involved, and injury results from direct chemical damage. Powerful primary irritants, such as strong acids or alkalis, may cause necrosis at the site of contact, while less damaging agents produce the changes of acute dermatitis. Weak irritants, such as detergents and solvents, require repeated or prolonged exposure to produce overt damage, usually manifested as dryness, fissuring, and chronic dermatitis. Irritant contact dermatitis remains more or less confined to the area of actual contact, unlike the allergic type which tends to spread into surrounding skin.

■ *Phototoxic substances* are those capable of inducing dermatitis in virtually any person, but only if sufficient contact is accompanied by exposure to ultraviolet light (in practice, sunlight). Phototoxic dermatitis closely resembles sunburn, and is followed by hyperpigmentation. Phototoxins are present in creosote and other derivatives of coal tar, and in such plants as celery, parsley and limes. One group of phototoxic chemicals, the psoralens, is used therapeutically to promote repigmentation in the treatment of vitiligo.

Allergic contact dermatitis

Contact allergens are generally relatively simple chemicals which are handled by most people without ill effect. The capacity of various substances to act as contact sensitisers varies widely, but most contact allergens are low molecular weight substances of considerable chemical reactivity. Being small molecules, they penetrate the stratum corneum and are conjugated with epidermal protein to form an antigen able to provoke an allergic reaction in some individuals.

The allergic response is mediated by thymus-influenced lymphocytes (T-cells) after preliminary involvement of monocytic macrophages and Langerhans cells. Following initial sensitisation there is a latent period, after which further contact anywhere on the skin triggers an inflammatory response at the site of contact. Allergic contact dermatitis is typically acute and eczematous but, with prolonged or repeated exposure, chronic dermatitis may develop.

■ **Photocontact allergens** are substances which sensitise a minority of those people who are exposed, so that subsequent contact induces eczematous dermatitis, but only when it is combined with exposure to ultraviolet light. The dermatitis is indistinguishable from the more common allergic eczematoid contact dermatitis, except that the lesions are confined to areas of contact which are unprotected from exposure to light.

Diagnosis of exogenous dermatitis

Neither acute nor chronic contact dermatitis is in itself distinctive, but may be suggested by:

1. History
2. Pattern of distribution
3. Morphology of individual lesions.

■ **History.** Strong primary irritants produce damage so quickly that the patient is in no doubt as to the cause. In fact, the effect of these destructive chemicals is so well known that, occasionally, a calculating or mentally disturbed patient will use such agents to produce artefactual lesions. Weak irritants may be unsuspected by the patient, who usually presents with chronic dermatitis of the hands. Although more damaging to sensitive or previously inflamed skin, primary irritants are harmful to any skin. The handling of even weak irritants for prolonged periods implies at least secondary involvement in any dermatitis of the hands and forearms.

The patient with phototoxic or photoallergic dermatitis *may* notice precipitation or aggravation by sunlight, but usually does not. Generally, the pattern of distribution is more helpful than history in the recognition of photosensitivity.

The time between exposure and onset of allergic contact dermatitis varies considerably, but is usually between 12 and 48 hours. Because of the time lag, patients are less likely to recognise the relationship than is the case with acute irritant dermatitis. However, patients may volunteer the information that a wound became itchy or 'infected' after application of a cream, or that a hand dermatitis was aggravated by a particular hand lotion. Questioning may remind the patient of a related episode, sometimes years before. A woman with contact allergy to nickel may have had attacks of earlobe dermatitis from earrings, or an itchy patch on the back of the neck from the clasp of a necklace. A man with acute hand dermatitis from dichromate in a spackling compound may have previously had 'cement dermatitis', also due to dichromate.

The course of contact dermatitis may be suggestive. Dermatitis which progresses from Monday to Friday, with improvement at weekends, is likely to be caused or aggravated by the patient's employment. Sometimes the reverse occurs, with weekend aggravation from leisure activities or a weekend job. Most endogenous dermatitis is recurrent or chronic; the sudden eruption of typically eczematous dermatitis in an adult with no previous skin problems should in itself arouse suspicion of an exogenous cause.

■ *Pattern of distribution.* Most forms of endogenous dermatitis are bilateral and roughly symmetrical. This may also be the pattern of exogenous dermatitis, but in many cases contact dermatitis is localised, asymmetrical and distinctive in distribution. A patient sensitised to a constituent of rubber may, for example, develop dermatitis which approximates the area covered by a fingerstall, a pair of rubber gloves, or the elastic waistband of underpants. A band of dermatitis across the forehead corresponding to a leather hatband, or patches behind the ears at the site of contact with spectacle frames are just two of many suggestive patterns.

Being confined to light-exposed areas, photosensitive dermatitis spares areas protected by hair and clothing, and shows relative sparing of the eyelids, retro-auricular folds and the shaded triangle below the chin. Dermatitis caused by such airborne contactants as sprays and pollens may resemble photosensitivity, but does not spare the eyelids.

Irritant dermatitis is confined to areas of obvious contact, but allergic dermatitis may spread to apparently unexposed areas. When a patient is sensitised, for example, to an ingredient of an ointment, dermatitis develops not only on and around the area of known application, but may spread to the face, hands, anogenital and other areas to which small amounts of the ointment are inadvertently carried by the fingers. When multiple sites are involved, the areas of greatest contact are usually affected first and most severely.

There is considerable regional variation of susceptibility to allergic contact dermatitis. In general, areas with a very thin keratin layer, such as the eyelids and anogenital region, are very susceptible, while the palms and soles are rarely involved because of the protective effect of the thick keratin layer.

■ *Morphology of individual lesion.* Lesions of endogenous dermatitis tend to be round or oval, quite unlike the linear, square, or triangular patterns often seen with contact dermatitis. The streaky, vesicular lesions caused by plants scratching over the skin of a forearm or leg are never reproduced by endogenous dermatitis; nor are the lines of dermatitis which may occur in the patient sensitive to nail lacquer who scratches the side of her neck.

26

Precise cause of exogenous dermatitis

The agent responsible for acute irritant dermatitis is generally obvious. In chronic irritant dermatitis, careful questioning will usually reveal the irritants, often multiple, which are relevant. The patient with allergic contact dermatitis is frequently unaware of the cause, and even a careful history and examination is likely to reveal only a range of possibilities.

It is inadequate, for example, to recognise shoe dermatitis without then determining the precise cause. A patient with contact dermatitis caused by shoes may be sensitive to any of a number of components, including chromate, formaldehyde, dyes, adhesives, antimildew chemicals, and the various constituents of rubbers. It is important, where possible, to identify the precise allergen, not only to enable the purchase of shoes free of the offending chemical, but also to avoid contact with the chemical in other ways. A patient sensitive to formaldehyde would be prone to develop dermatitis from contact with certain textiles, commercial nail-hardeners, some antiperspirants and some industrial adhesives.

The precise cause can usually be determined by patch testing, using the appropriate range of possible allergens for the particular patient. Although they may not necessarily duplicate clinical conditions, correctly applied and interpreted patch tests are of great value in the management of allergic contact dermatitis, but are never performed with known primary irritants.

Common causes of allergic contact dermatitis

A comprehensive list of potential sensitisers would be enormous, but a surprisingly large number of cases of contact dermatitis are produced by a relatively small group of substances.

- **Chromates.** Most chromate-sensitive patients are sensitised by contact with cement but, once sensitised, the patient may react to chromate in paints, varnishes, leather, fur dyes and electroplating solutions.

- **Nickel.** Nickel is present on many electroplated metal objects. However, nickel sensitisation is usually induced by objects worn close to the skin, such as watches, earrings, brassière clips, zippers and cheap jewellery, and is therefore more frequent in women than men. *(Colour plate 1)*

- **Rhus.** The rhus tree is a close relative of the poison ivy of North America and, in this country, its leaves are a very common cause of severe acute dermatitis.

- **Rubber compounds.** Natural rubber rarely sensitises, but the vulcanisers, anti-oxidants, accelerators and peptizers which are used in the manufacture of rubber are common causes of contact dermatitis.

- **Paraphenylenediamine** (PPD). Paraphenylenediamine is still widely used as a hair dye in this country. It is also employed in fur dyeing and in the processing of leather. People sensitised by PPD may cross-react with other chemicals of similar structure, including procaine, benzocaine and sulphonamides.

- **Formaldehyde.** Finishes containing formaldehyde are sometimes used to provide crease-resistance or to add bulk to cheap fabrics. Although less frequently used than previously, formaldehyde remains a common

27

cause of textile dermatitis. Formaldehyde is encountered also in some polishes and glues, and as a preservative in cosmetics and shampoos.

■ *Cosmetics.* Contant dermatitis caused by cosmetics is most often due to the perfume, but sensitisation may develop to the preservatives, organic dyes, antibacterial agents and fillers. However, in relation to the quantities used, cosmetics are a very uncommon cause of contact dermatitis.

■ *Therapeutic applications.* Neomycin, benzocaine, clioquinol and several antihistamines are relatively frequent contact sensitisers.

Common causes of allergic contact dermatitis in different regions

■ Hands and forearms: rubber, chromate, nickel, hand creams, lanolin, plants.
■ Face: cosmetics, hair sprays and dyes, sunscreens, airborne dusts and pollens.
■ Eyelids: cosmetics, nail lacquer, or any other sensitiser carried on the hands.
■ Lips: lipstick, oranges, toothpaste.
■ Ears: earrings, perfume, spectacle frames, hair sprays and dyes.
■ Perianal region: benzocaine, hydroxyquinolines and other ingredients of suppositories, preservatives, perfumes, and antibiotics in creams and ointments.

Treatment of acute exogenous dermatitis

The treatment of acute contact dermatitis is based on the following measures:

1. Removal of the cause
2. Consideration of systemic corticosteroid therapy
3. Topical therapy
4. General measures
5. Prevention of recurrences

■ *Removal of the cause.* Primary irritants strong enough to cause acute dermatitis are not difficult to identify and avoid. Phototoxic agents are less obvious, but can usually be detected by careful questioning. Allergens and photoallergens may be harder to identify. Patch testing should not be performed until the dermatitis has healed, or misleading results may be obtained. It is necessary to treat the dermatitis symptomatically, excluding contact with all suspected allergens, until the inflammation has resolved and accurate patch testing is possible.

■ *Systemic corticosteroids.* With avoidance of the cause, acute contact dermatitis is self-healing within two or three weeks. Systemic corticosteroid therapy should not be used for mild cases of dermatitis, and should be avoided when possible in the presence of such contra-indications as active peptic ulcer. For the badly affected, healthy patient, systemic corticosteroids are effective and desirable, provided that the diagnosis is clear. With prednisone, an appropriate schedule would be 40 mg daily for two days, 30 mg daily for five days, and 20 mg daily for a week, with gradual withdrawal during the third week. A more rapid rate of reduction in dosage may sometimes be associated with a dramatic return of the dermatitis.

■ *Topical therapy.* The aims are to relieve discomfort, to minimise the risk of infection, to protect the injured skin, and to settle the inflammation.

Early oedematous, vesicular and weeping lesions are best treated with cold wet applications. Compresses, soaks or baths may be chosen, depending on the area involved. Of the many liquids employed, normal saline is quite satisfactory, or an aqueous solution of potassium permanganate may be used, provided that a concentration of 1 in 10,000 (sufficient to colour the water light pink) is not exceeded. Vesicular and oozing lesions will usually dry out within two or three days of such treatment.

When oozing is not marked, or when crusting predominates, 5 per cent aluminium acetate emulsion (Burow's emulsion) is effective when applied four times daily. As crusts separate and scaling begins, a cream or ointment is substituted. At this stage, corticosteroids are most effective.

On the face and scalp, compresses are impractical and a corticosteroid lotion may be used early, to be replaced by a cream or gel as the crusted phase passes.

Details of these applications and others outlined elsewhere in the text are discussed more fully in Chapter 25.

■ *General measures.* The patient with severe, widespread dermatitis should be at rest in bed, preferably in an airconditioned hospital ward. The environment should be comfortably cool, and bed clothes not too warm. A severely inflamed hand or forearm should be supported by a sling. A badly affected leg should be rested and elevated to the level of the hip. For those confined to bed, a bed cradle is desirable. Sedatives will allow the itchy patient to sleep, and a systemic antibiotic may be necessary for secondary bacterial infection. As with all itching dermatoses, the patient with dermatitis should be encouraged to avoid the damage added by scratching and rubbing.

■ *Prevention of recurrences.* Every effort must be made to determine the precise agent which is responsible. For allergic dermatitis, this may involve patch testing with the full range of suspected allergens. The patient should be told which chemical is responsible for his or her dermatitis, and should be given a written list of all commonly encountered materials which contain the allergen, and of any substances with which cross-reaction may occur.

Treatment of chronic exogenous dermatitis

The treatment of chronic contact dermatitis should be conducted on the following lines:
1. Removal of the cause and general management
2. Topical therapy
3. Prevention of recurrences

■ *Removal of the cause and general management.* Successful management necessitates an understanding by the patient of the nature of the disease and the rationale of therapy. Chronic irritant dermatitis is usually occupational; it affects the hands of most patients, and the forearms of many. The disease is most common in housewives, in professional cleaners, and in those handling lipid solvents, or such common irritants as kerosene and turpentine. Onset may be related to the vigorous scrubbing, often with abrasive soaps, which is necessary for the removal of such adherent materials as paint or tar. Other workers may initiate their dermatitis by the repeated use of petrol or kerosene for the rapid removal of oil and grease.

Among housewives, the principal cause is overexposure to soaps and detergents. Prolonged immersion in soapy water, inadequate rinsing and a failure to clean away soap adhering to rings are frequent contributing factors. As dermatitis develops, rubber gloves are often used for protection, but the gloved hands working in hot water soon become macerated and itchy, with aggravation from scratching. The patient may become sensitised to a component of rubber or to an ingredient of a hand cream, which will superimpose an allergic contact dermatitis. As the skin becomes more vulnerable, such common substances as fruit and vegetable juice, polishes, window-cleaning liquids and the baby's soiled napkins add to the list of aggravating factors.

These details need to be explained to the patient, together with practical methods for their avoidance. Simple bar soaps should be substituted for powerful detergents, and the hands should be thoroughly rinsed after washing up. Long-handled scrapers rather than steel wool should be used for cleaning pots and pans. Tongs or a stout stick can be used to lift wet clothing from the washing machine into a laundry basket for wheeling to the clothes line. Frozen and canned vegetables obviate the need for peeling and dicing, and spray-on polishes should supplant liquid furniture polish. Rubber gloves should not be worn for longer than 10 minutes at a time, and should be loose-fitting with cotton gloves inside. Cotton gloves, worn for dusting and sweeping, reduce trauma to dry, easily fissured hands. Barrier creams do little to protect the hands from contact with sensitising chemicals. Application of a suitable barrier cream before work does, however, facilitate removal of adherent compounds without recourse to solvents or vigorous scrubbing.

Appropriate patch testing is necessary when an allergic basis is suspected, or when any chronic dermatitis does not respond to conventional therapy.

■ *Topical therapy.* Applications are chosen which have a low potential for allergic sensitisation. Fluorinated corticosteroids are the most effective treatment, and are better prescribed without the addition of neomycin, hydroxyquinolines and similar agents incorporated into some proprietary preparations. For many patients an ointment base is best, but during hot, humid weather, a cream may be preferable. If improvement is slow, the ointment may be used with a plastic occlusive dressing overnight to enhance penetration.

For stubborn cases, a tar paste is helpful, a good combination being betamethasone ointment applied four times during the day, and liquor picis carbonis 4 per cent in zinc paste applied at bed time. Intradermal injection of hydrocortisone or triamcinolone is occasionally necessary for persistent lichenified plaques.

■ *Prevention of recurrences.* Skin which has recently healed from chronic dermatitis remains abnormally sensitive for months afterwards. A return to careless work habits may result in prompt recurrence of dermatitis.

Many patients with chronic hand dermatitis have genetically predisposed skin which is unable to tolerate even mild chemical insults.

Regular use of a bland emollient cream, such as hydrophilic cream, may help to prevent recurrences, but for some, lifelong protection from irritants becomes necessary.

In general, allergic contact dermatitis can be prevented if the allergen is known. However, some types of allergic contact dermatitis share a very poor long-term prognosis even if the allergen is avoided. Chromate allergy is one such example; also, some photoallergens permanently bind to the skin to produce patients called 'persistent light reactors'. Other allergens, such as nickel and lanoline, because of the ubiquitous presence in our environment, will cause frequent exacerbations in those sensitised, despite best attempts at avoidance.

Endogenous eczema

The principal recognisable forms are classified as:
1. Atopic eczema
2. Discoid eczema (nummular dermatitis)
3. Pompholyx (dyshidrotic eczema)
4. Seborrhoeic eczema
5. Asteatotic eczema
6. Stasis eczema
7. Pityriasis alba
8. Juvenile forefoot eczema (juvenile plantar dermatitis)
9. Lichen simplex chronicus

Atopic eczema

There is an unexplained association of asthma, hay fever and a characteristic pattern of dermatitis in some families, which is presumed to be genetically transmitted. The association is called 'atopy', and the dermatitis 'atopic'.

Aetiology

About 3 per cent of all infants develop atopic dermatitis, and in 70 per cent of these there is a close family history of atopic diseases. The atopic diathesis is associated with altered responses to some physiological stimuli, but it is not known whether these altered responses are aetiologically related to the dermatitis. There are altered dermal vascular reactions, with increased vasoconstriction in response to cold and to catecholamines. The reaction to firm stroking or to intradermally injected acetyl choline is changed, the erythematous phase being quickly replaced by sustained pallor.

As a group, atopic individuals display an exaggerated capacity to synthesise specific IgE antibodies to many common ingested and inhaled antigens, but a significant role for these antibodies in the pathogenesis of atopic dermatitis seems unlikely. Elevated serum levels of IgE are common, but are neither necessary for the disease to develop nor sufficient to cause it. Impaired cell-mediated immunity can be demonstrated in several ways, but appears to be the result, not the cause, of the dermatitis.

The role of psychological factors is controversial. Many atopics are anxious, restless people, who respond to stress by scratching. Trauma

31

aggravates and perpetuates atopic dermatitis, and periods of exacerbation are often related to emotional upsets. On the other hand, the personality of most people would be considerably modified by an itchy and often disfiguring skin disease.

Clinical features *(Colour plate 2)*

The essential feature of atopic skin is a low itch threshold. The skin is generally dry (atopic xeroderma) and somewhat pale, but many of the objective changes are the result of rubbing and scratching. Stimuli which pass unnoticed by others may provoke intense pruritus in the atopic. Sweating and sudden changes of temperature are sufficient to trigger scratching, and the atopic is especially sensitive to contact with irritating fibres, such as wool, nylon and satin. The earliest lesions are usually small oedematous papules, but the typical lesions are a variable mixture of erythema, oozing, scaling and lichenification. Almost any site can be affected at any age, but distribution tends to follow distinct patterns during infancy, childhood and adult life.

■ *In infancy,* oedematous, reddish or weeping crusted areas develop on the face, particularly the cheeks, and less often on the buttocks, neck and scalp. As the child begins to crawl, the skin over the knees and ankles tends to thicken, and excoriated papules are common. Onset may be at any age, but in 75 per cent of sufferers it begins between two and six months. In about half of these the dermatitis clears by the third year, but in many it recurs later. In those with persisting disease, the course is chronic and fluctuating, with a tendency to improvement during school life.

■ *During childhood,* the dermatitis tends to settle in the popliteal and antecubital fossae, and around the wrists and ankles, with variable involvement of other areas. Lichenification and hyperpigmentation are often marked, but there may be residual hypopigmentation in chronically affected sites. The face and neck tend to improve, but dermatitis may persist around the eyes and behind the ears. At this stage, there are often periods of patchy dissemination, and secondary infection is more common.

■ *During adolescence,* dermatitis frequently returns to the face and neck, and the upper trunk is also commonly involved. Persistence in the flexures of elbows and knees is the rule but, by the fourth decade, the disease usually subsides, persisting in some as chronic dermatitis of the hands or feet. In a few patients, the dermatitis continues unabated throughout life.

Complications and associations

■ *Asthma and hay fever* occur in more than one-third of patients.

■ *Secondary bacterial infection* is very common, particularly in children.

■ *Generalised herpes simplex* is a serious but infrequent complication.

■ *Conjunctivitis* is common. Keratoconus and atopic cataract affect less than 5 per cent of patients.

■ *Anaphylactic reactions* to drugs and insect bites are very uncommon, but more frequent than among non-atopics.

■ *Pompholyx and nummular dermatitis.* There is an increased incidence of these conditions.

Prognosis

A chronic and recurring disease, with a tendency to improve during childhood and adult life.

Diagnosis

▶   **Suspect** the diagnosis of atopic eczema in all infants presenting with dermatitis, and in any patient with facial and/or flexural dermatitis.

▶   **Consider and exclude**

■ *Seborrhoeic dermatitis*, which is an eczema that involves the scalp, major flexures, interscapular and presternal areas and has a marked tendency to spare the distal parts of the limbs. Itch is not severe, unlike atopic dermatitis, in which pruritus is invariable. Often there is a fine greasy surface scale which is a pinkish yellow.

■ *Napkin dermatitis* does not involve the face, but may complicate the infantile phase of atopic dermatitis.

■ *Contact dermatitis* is distinguished by the history, distribution and pattern of dermatitis. Chronic hand dermatitis of the primary irritant type is a common complication of atopic dermatitis.

■ *Systemic diseases* such as phenylketonuria, ataxia telangiectasia, and Wiskott–Aldrich syndrome may present with dermatitis indistinguishable from that of the atopic. Only an awareness of the cutaneous presentation of these diseases allows their exclusion.

▶   **Confirmation.** There is no specific criterion by which atopic eczema can be diagnosed with certainty. However, consideration of the mode of onset, personal and family history, and an examination of the skin allow a confident diagnosis to be made in most cases.

Treatment

As with any other chronic dermatosis, the nature of the disease, and the aims and limitations of therapy should be carefully explained. Patients should be reassured that available methods of treatment, while not curative, provide good relief for the great majority.
1. General management.
2. Topical therapy.
3. Systemic therapy.
4. Inadvisable forms of therapy.

■ *General management.* The patient should be advised of the consequences of rubbing and scratching, and urged to exercise as much self-control as can be mustered. For infants and young children, protective clothing and sedation are better than physical restraints. Known precipitants of pruritus should be avoided. Rough-textured clothing, particularly wool, should not be worn in contact with the skin. Water for bathing should be tepid and the shower jet not too forceful. During winter, undressing should be in a warmed room, and during the summer an air-conditioned bedroom is desirable. Vigorous sports which promote sweating are unsuitable for the severely affected atopic.

The vulnerable atopic skin is less tolerant of solvents, soaps and other irritants—factors of importance in the choice of occupation. Bricklaying, joinery, hairdressing, nursing and many factory jobs are unsuitable.

Most patients benefit from common-sense reassurance and support; occasionally, more formal psychotherapy is necessary.

■ *Topical therapy.* Acute weeping dermatitis is treated with wet compresses until sufficient drying prepares the skin for a corticosteroid ointment or cream. An ointment base is usually better, but individual preference may indicate a non-greasy preparation. Hydrocortisone acetate is often sufficient; but when a more powerful steroid is necessary, the dangers of prolonged use should not be forgotten. Particularly with young children or when large areas are being treated, the weaker concentration should be prescribed.

For many patients, such simple applications as hydrophilic or sorbolene cream are effective, corticosteroids being reserved for exacerbations. Regular application of simple emollients considerably modifies the xeroderma which underlies at least some of the irritability of atopic skin. For chronic areas of low-grade dermatitis or lichenified plaques, tar preparations, such as 2 to 3 per cent crude coal tar in sorbolene cream, or 2 to 4 per cent ichthammol in zinc ointment, are of considerable value.

■ *Systemic therapy.* Sedatives such as antihistamines and diazepam raise the itch threshold and decrease the psychological impact of the disease. Nocturnal sedation may be invaluable.

Systemic corticosteroids should be prescribed only after consideration of the special risks of their administration to the atopic patient. Although sometimes permissible for short periods during severe exacerbations, long-term use of systemic corticosteroids is rarely justified. Withdrawal is often followed by a severe rebound of dermatitis, and doses which are necessary for prolonged suppression are usually unacceptably high. Nevertheless, there are rare patients with dermatitis of life-ruining severity for whom the risks of incomplete suppression with doses of 5 mg to 7.5 mg of prednisone daily may be preferable to an otherwise miserable existence.

■ *Inadvisable forms of therapy.* Atopic dermatitis is not improved by dietary restrictions nor by hyposensitisation to the ingested or inhaled allergens demonstrable by skin-testing.

Discoid eczema (nummular dermatitis)

It is likely that the coin-shaped ('nummular') plaques of discoid eczema represent a pattern of dermatitis that is produced by a number of causes, rather than a specific disease entity. A nummular pattern may be a manifestation of atopic dermatitis in children, or of the dermatitis sometimes seen in the dry skin of elderly people. Some adults suffer repeated recurrences at times of worry and stress, but with many patients no cause is found.

Clinical features

The onset is often very abrupt, as multiple discrete lesions erupt suddenly on apparently normal skin. Individual plaques, from 1 cm to 5 cm in diameter, are formed by intensely itchy clusters of papules and papulovesicles on an erythematous, slightly thickened base. Oozing and crusting soon follow, with little tendency to peripheral extension or central clearing. Lesions may persist for weeks or months, and are notorious for recurring at previously affected sites.

The distribution of plaques is roughly symmetrical, most often over the dorsum of hands and forearms, the lower legs and feet. If the trunk is involved, it is predominantly the limb girdle regions.

Complications

Bacterial infection is common.

Prognosis

Although therapy is effective in clearing lesions, recurrences are the rule, the skin remaining clear in some patients only for as long as treatment is continued.

Diagnosis

▶ **Consider and exclude**

■ *Tinea*, which is distinguished by the asymmetry of distribution, centrifugally spreading margins which are frequently vesicular and, when necessary, by examination of scrapings.

■ *Impetigo* may resemble discoid eczema, and impetiginised eczema is not uncommon. The distribution of impetigo is unlikely to be symmetrical, and does not conform to the pattern of discoid eczema.

■ *Contact dermatitis* may produce individual lesions resembling those of discoid eczema, but differs in distribution.

Treatment

Early plaques may be treated with topical corticosteroid from the outset, or aluminium acetate emulsion may be applied initially, until oozing is controlled. Half-strength Castellani's paint, applied twice daily for four days, is useful for very acute, weeping lesions. The response to topical steroids is usually good but occasionally, patients with more chronic lesions respond poorly. For these, 2 per cent crude coal tar in equal parts of Lassar's paste and soft paraffin is sometimes very effective.

Secondary infection is common and, in such cases, the administration of systemic antibiotics is frequently necessary. Patients with an underlying xeroderma should be managed with restricted bathing and regular applications of triethanolamine aqueous cream or a similar emollient. Sedation helps many patients with recurrent attacks, but systemic corticosteroid therapy is very rarely indicated.

Pompholyx (dyshidrotic eczema)

Pompholyx is a distinctive, vesicular dermatitis of the palms, soles and interdigital skin.

Aetiology

Although there is no convincing evidence for eccrine involvement in the pathogenesis, hyperhidrosis is a frequent association. Recurrences are more common during warm, humid weather or at times of emotional upset—circumstances which aggravate the hyperhidrosis. However, as with all eczema and dermatitis, the vesicles are due to intercellular oedema between epidermal cells—not sweat. The vesicles probably become macroscopic in pompholyx due to the thickness of the keratin layer giving the microscopic vesicles time to coalesce.

The disease is very uncommon in children and has its highest incidence in young adults.

Clinical features (Colour plate 3)

■ *The blisters* which characterise pompholyx erupt suddenly, with itch, but without accompanying erythema. Vesicles may be only a millimetre or two in diameter, or may coalesce to form bullae several centimetres across. The eruption differs from vesicular dermatitis of other areas in the absence of erythema and also in that vesicular fluid is reabsorbed without rupture onto the surface. Scaling follows vesiculation, but may be accompanied by further waves of blistering.

■ *Distribution* is usually bilateral and symmetrical, but of variable extent. Only interdigital skin may be affected, or there may be involvement of palms or soles or both. Virtually the whole surface of palms and soles may be studded with vesicles of various sizes, or there may be small circumscribed areas which remain active for months. Occasionally pompholyx is unilateral.

Course

This is unpredictable, but frequently prolonged. In some patients recurrences are confined to the summer months, or occur only during periods of anxiety. In others, recurrences follow one another for years, with healing and eruption of new lesions proceeding concurrently.

Complications

■ *Secondary bacterial infection* is common.

■ *Secondary irritant dermatitis* is also a common complication and, with pompholyx, a frequent contributor to the chronicity of hand dermatitis.

Diagnosis

▶   Consider and exclude

■ *Tinea of the palms* typically involves only one hand, and close inspection will usually reveal increased inflammation around the periphery. However, when both hands are involved, appearances may be very similar.

■ *Tinea pedis* may not only resemble pompholyx of the feet but, when acute, may produce a sterile vesicular reaction on the palms (id reaction) which resembles pompholyx of the hands.

■ *Exogenous dermatitis* between the fingers may be vesicular and scaling, but is accompanied by erythema. With allergic contact dermatitis, there is also involvement on the dorsum of the hands. Irritant dermatitis severe enough to induce vesiculation is recalled by the patient.

Treatment

Severe acute pompholyx is best treated initially by cool soaks for 10 minutes every two hours, using saline solution or a weak solution of potassium permanganate. Less acute disease may be treated with a fluorinated steroid cream, the penetration of hydrocortisone acetate being inadequate for the thick palmar and plantar skin. Systemic steroids are occasionally necessary to suppress very severe attacks, but should be used only for short periods.

General measures include protection of involved skin from physical and chemical trauma, systemic antibiotic therapy for secondary infection, sedation when indicated, and avoidance of occlusive gloves and footwear.

Seborrhoeic eczema (seborrhoeic dermatitis)

Aetiology

The precise cause is unknown. Sebum secretion seems to play an as yet undefined role. Affected skin frequently has a rather greasy appearance, but many people have a very oily skin without ever suffering from dermatitis. The disease is more common in patients with rosacea and acne and, apart from during the first few months of life, does not occur until adolescence. In people with Parkinsonism and other diseases of basal ganglia, sebum excretion is increased. The prevalence of seborrhoeic eczema is increased among these patients and, in those with unilateral increase in sebum production, the dermatitis is more severe on the affected side. Some studies suggest that this eczema is a reaction to increased numbers of the pityrosporum yeasts already present on the skin of all humans. Patients with HIV infection often have severe extensive seborrhoeic eczema and usually increased numbers of these yeasts, but patients with normal skin may also show increased colonisation. Psoriasis will not uncommonly be found years later in other parts of the body in those diagnosed as having seborrhoeic eczema.

Clinical features

There are four characteristic regions of involvement, although in the severely affected patient, distribution may be more generalised.

1. Hair-covered areas
2. Face
3. Body folds and flexures
4. Trunk

■ *Hair-covered areas.* The scalp is usually the first and often the only affected site. Small, ill-defined areas of redness and light scaling develop around individual hairs. With increasing size and coalescence, larger areas form which may extend to cover the entire scalp and are associated with mild to moderate itching. The dermatitis may involve the sideburns, and extend from the scalp onto adjoining areas of the forehead, neck and skin around the ears. Scaling is rather diffuse but, when marked, may heap up around the base of hairs to form a soggy white or yellowish white collarette.

Similar changes may develop in the eyebrows, and extend to the skin at the base of the nose. In men, the presternal and the unshaved beard or moustache areas are also common sites.

■ *Face.* The face tends to be oily and shiny. The lid margins are often red, and sometimes scaly. Typically there is dermatitis of the nasolabial folds, sometimes with moderate, soft, yellowish scaling. In severe cases there may be a reddish scaly band across the forehead, just below the frontal hair line. The ears may be affected on either surface, but the dermatitis is often localised around the auditory meati.

■ *Folds and flexures.* The large flexures are common sites, particularly in obese patients. In these areas, the dermatitis is more clearly demarcated, the colour is deeper red to reddish-brown, and the scaling is soft, moist, and less abundant. The axillae, groins, natal cleft, folds of the neck, umbilicus, and submammary folds of women are all frequently affected. In the retro-auricular folds, scale tends to accumulate, and fissuring with secondary infection may supervene.

■ *Trunk.* Over the presternal and interscapular regions, early lesions are often small, reddish pink, perifollicular papules. When larger areas result from coalescence, lesions are macular, well-demarcated, scaly, and reddish brown. Discrete round or oval patches may develop on other parts of the trunk and occasionally on the proximal areas of the limbs.

Seborrhoeic dermatitis of infants resembles that of adults in distribution, but with a greater tendency to flexural involvement, especially of the napkin area.

Complications

Seborrhoeic dermatitis, like any other form of dermatitis, may be complicated by sweat retention, secondary infection, and secondary contact dermatitis. In addition, there are complications to which patients with seborrhoeic dermatitis are especially vulnerable.

■ *Fissuring* may occur at any site of flexural involvement, but is particularly common in the retro-auricular folds.

■ *Bacterial infection* may complicate fissuring, but the patient with seborrhoeic dermatitis appears more prone to other cutaneous infections, including impetigo.

■ *Secondary candidiasis* is very common, especially in the infant, and in the groins, natal cleft, and beneath the pendulous breasts of affected women. *(Colour plate 4)*

■ *Blepharitis.* Involvement of the eyelid margins may occasionally be the only manifestation of seborrhoeic eczema. In severe cases, adherent scale and crusts form. When these are detached, erosions remain which can result in loss of eyelashes.

■ *Folliculitis* is an uncommon complication, but, when severe, may lead to destruction of follicles by secondary bacterial infection, with permanent loss of hair. This rare complication usually affects the beard of unshaven men.

■ *Generalised exfoliative dermatitis* is a rare complication.

- **Psoriasis.** The relationship between seborrhoeic dermatitis and psoriasis is unexplained, but the association is not uncommon.

Prognosis

The infant with seborrhoeic dermatitis responds well to treatment and, even with severe disease, permanent resolution within a few months is almost invariable. The adult is very prone to chronicity and recurrence.

Diagnosis

▶ **Consider and exclude**

- **Intertrigo,** which is caused by maceration and friction, and is strictly confined to apposing skin surfaces.
- **Candidiasis** is suggested by flat, flaccid white pustules, a festooned border and satellite lesions around the margins.
- **Napkin dermatitis** is really a primary irritant dermatitis caused by the irritant products of urine and faeces. The major areas of involvement are therefore the convex surfaces in contact with the napkin, with relative sparing of the skin deep in the folds of the groins and natal cleft.
- **Atopic eczema,** unlike seborrhoeic eczema, is rare before eight weeks of age and is very itchy. The forehead and cheeks are affected rather than the scalp, and the elbow and knee flexures rather than the groins and axillae. _sometimes pruinans follows seb. derm. (Sebo-psoriasis)_
- **Psoriasis** on the scalp is sharply demarcated, with much adherent scaling. On the trunk and limbs, psoriatic plaques are palpably thickened, _pits in nails_ bright reddish pink and covered with silvery white scale. Flexural psoriasis has less scaling, but retains the ham-red colour of psoriasis elsewhere.
- **Lichen simplex chronicus** on the scalp is a sharply demarcated, intensely itchy, palpably thickened plaque.
- **Pityriasis versicolor** may produce scaly reddish-brown macules in the interscapular and presternal regions but the face and scalp are spared and scrapings will show stubby hyphae and spores.
- **Tinea** seldom duplicates the distribution of seborrhoeic dermatitis, but in doubtful cases is distinguished by microscopic examination of scrapings.

Treatment

Hydrocortisone 1 per cent cream is a safe effective treatment for all areas of the body in most patients. However, tachyphylaxis is not uncommon. Alternatives include topical imidazoles and a cream containing 2 to 3 per cent of sulphur and salicylic acid. Stubborn facial involvement may require the more expensive aclometasone 0.05 per cent cream. Away from the face and flexures, a more potent topical steroid can be used. Regular control of the scalp helps to minimise recurrences not only in this zone, but also in other regions. Shampoos containing tar or zinc pyridinethione or selenium sulphide help in this regard.

For acute weeping dermatitis of the large flexures, the patient should be confined to bed and treated with wet compresses for two or three days, after which a steroid cream is used. Secondary bacterial infection

Daktacort or Econacort

For scalp rotate Efalith (lithium based), a myconazole (like) and a tar based product the to prevent resistance from building up. If extensive Itraconazole 200g daily for 7 days (check feminine)

may necessitate the administration of a systemic antibiotic, and secondary candidiasis, which is very common in flexural lesions, is treated with topical anticandida agents.

Asteatotic eczema ('winter itch')

Aetiology

The normal texture and resilience of the skin depends upon its water content, which is related to the presence of surface lipid. Decreasing surface lipid in the skin of elderly people renders the skin more vulnerable to changes of atmospheric humidity, especially during the drier months of winter. Excess drying is followed by splitting of the stratum corneum, which curls away from the crack. Underlying skin becomes red and irritable, and may progress to frank dermatitis.

The dermatitis is predominantly a disease of middle-aged and elderly people, and is more common in men. A constitutionally dry skin predisposes to the disease, which may be precipitated by scratching, electric blankets, diuretics, excessive use of soap, and low-humidity heating systems.

Clinical features (Colour plate 5)

The legs are the usual site, but the buttocks, trunk and arms may also be involved. At first the legs are involved only during the winter months, with remission in the more humid months of summer. Recurrences tend to persist longer during succeeding winters and, with increasing severity, may persist throughout the year.

Affected areas may present a crazy-paving pattern of reddish splits in dry, scaling skin, with a variable amount of surrounding inflammation. Itching is severe and scratching adds excoriations and further inflammation. Some patients develop a nummular pattern of dermatitis, which may be frankly vesicular or less acute, with dry scaling discoid lesions.

Prognosis

The disease reponds well to simple measures, and recurrences can be prevented by attention to the underlying xeroderma.

Diagnosis

▶ **Consider and exclude**

■ *Myxoedema*, which is more widespread and is distinguished by the presence of other features of hypothyroidism.

■ *Discoid eczema* may be a pattern of asteatotic eczema but arises on apparently normal skin.

■ *Acquired xeroderma* may be the presenting feature of a lymphoma, particularly Hodgkin's disease. Onset of xeroderma in adult life always requires exclusion of a systemic cause.

■ *Xeroderma* may be a component of drug eruptions and may complicate diuretic therapy or the use of lipid-lowering agents.

Treatment

- ■ *Reduction of xeroderma.* For the first week or two, bathing should be infrequent and restricted to tepid water and the sparing use of a bland soap. Almost any greasy application relieves xeroderma, but useful emollients for dry itchy skin are equal parts of hydrophilic cream and soft paraffin, or 10 per cent glycerin in sorbolene cream, applied once or twice daily.

- ■ *Symptomatic relief.* With attention to the xeroderma, the application of corticosteroids is usually unnecessary, but is effective if required. Pruritus from xeroderma is worse at night, and for the first week of treatment sedation may be required.

- ■ *Prevention of recurrences.* Recurrences can usually be avoided by minimising the use of soap and, during the cooler months, regularly using a moisturising cream such as aqueous cream or 10 per cent urea cream.

Stasis eczema

Stasis eczema occurs on the lower leg in the presence of inadequate venous drainage, usually as a late complication of deep vein thrombosis.

Aetiology

After deep vein thrombosis, recanalisation with re-establishment of patency is the rule, but venous contractility remains compromised and destroyed valves are not replaced. Venous return is assisted by the pumping action of muscular contraction squeezing blood along the veins. With incompetent valves, blood is as easily forced away from the heart as towards it. The rise in venous pressure is transmitted to capillaries, resulting in oedema. With increased intraluminal pressure, the capillaries develop endothelial thickening and become more tortuous. Greater capillary permeability increases viscosity and reduces blood flow. Delivery of oxygen is impaired and tissue viability is further endangered by thrombosis of small vessels.

Capillary damage allows the escape of erythrocytes, with haemosiderin staining of the dermis. Protein-rich oedema fluid is eventually invaded by fibroblasts, producing a woody fibrosis which impedes lymphatic drainage. Lymphoedema develops and increases the liability to cellulitis in the tissue.

Clinical features

Oedema of the lower leg is a frequent but not invariable manifestation. Swelling increases during the day, to disappear overnight with elevation of the limb. Rust-coloured deposits of haemosiderin are almost always present, beginning on the medial side of the leg just above the malleolus. The spotty brownish discolouration may become quite extensive over the lower third of the leg, sometimes with small white areas of atrophy. A chronic dermatitis, with scaling and thickening, slowly develops; episodes of more acute dermatitis, with oozing and sometimes secondary infection, may supervene.

In longstanding cases, a brawny low-grade cellulitis is characteristic, and progressive fibrosis may produce a woody narrowing of the lower third of the leg. The affected area is irritable and very prone to secondary inflammation by primary irritants, and to allergic contact dermatitis.

Complications

■ *Ulceration* is an important and frequent complication of the stasis syndrome. The ulcer may develop suddenly, but is usually preceded by an itchy, dusky erythema. It may be precipitated by trauma from scratching, chemical irritation from ill-advised therapy, or an episode of cellulitis or acute dermatitis.

■ *Recurrent cellulitis*

■ *Lymphoedema*

■ *Subcutaneous calcification* may be a late sequel.

■ *Secondary thrombophlebitis*

■ *Contact dermatitis.* Stasis eczema is particularly prone to the development of allergic contact dermatitis and, therefore, whenever possible, the topical treatment should be restricted to agents with low sensitising potential.

■ *Squamous cell carcinoma* may rarely develop in a chronic ulcer.

Prognosis

Many of the changes are irreversible and management is mainly directed to the prevention of complications. Recent ulceration can usually be encouraged to heal, but longstanding ulcers may be intractable. In such patients, it is sometimes necessary to concentrate on function and mobility rather than on complete healing of the ulcer.

Diagnosis

▶ **Consider and exclude**

■ *Capillaritis* (pigmented purpuric dermatoses), which may cause rusty brown patches with punctate haemorrhages, but the distribution is more widespread over the legs, and there is no oedema.

■ *Atopic eczema* is usually located over the dorsal aspects of the ankles and changes are also present away from the leg.

■ *Lichen planus* pigmentation is a darker brown, the characteristic violaceous flat-topped papules are present elsewhere, and the buccal mucosa may be involved.

■ *Tinea* shows increased inflammation around the periphery and, in this location, is often pustular.

■ *Kaposi's sarcoma* begins on the sole and dorsum of the foot first. Pigmented areas are usually plaques, but oedema may be a feature.

■ *Vasculitis* producing ulceration is usually very severe and shows more typical palpable purpura.

■ *Other leg ulcers*

Ischaemic ulcers are more tender and painful, especially in bed at night, and are more often on the lateral side of the ankle. However, ischaemia is an important factor contributing to many stasis ulcers.

Basal cell carcinoma (BCC) is uncommon on the leg, may retain the raised 'pearly' border of the BCC at other sites, and can be distinguished with certainty by biopsy.

Artefacts produced by chemical or physical trauma often have a peculiar geometrical or bizarre shape, and lack the oedema and other features of the stasis syndrome.

Ulcers due to tertiary syphilis are more punched-out, tend to form a scalloped border and occur anywhere on the leg.

Squamous cell carcinoma is a rare complication of chronic stasis ulcers. Malignant change should be suspected with a persistent, heaped-up nodule of reddish, granulation-like tissue in one area of the ulcer. Biopsy should be performed on doubtful lesions.

Treatment

1. Prevention
2. Arrest of progression
3. Prevention and treatment of complications
4. Surgical procedures

■ *Prevention.* Much morbidity can be avoided by the prevention of thrombophlebitis and deep vein thrombosis. When thrombosis has occurred, early and energetic treatment substantially reduces the risk of early and late complications.

■ *Arrest of progression.* The untreated stasis syndrome is progressive, but can to a large extent be halted by relatively simple measures. Prolonged standing should be avoided. When possible, the patient should rest with the leg elevated for an hour in the afternoon and early evening. Mobility is maintained and venous return is assisted by well-fitted elastic stockings or firm elastic bandaging which is applied immediately after rising, before oedema has begun to accumulate.

For severe stasis, proprietary bandages of the zinc-gelatin type are satisfactory when supported by elastocrepe bandaging. They may be used in the presence of ulceration, provided that oozing is not excessive. They are applied over paraffin gauze dressings to the ulcer or area of dermatitis, and can be left in place for one to two weeks. Inflatable plastic boots extending almost to the knee are comfortable and effective, but are expensive and ugly.

■ *Prevention and treatment of complications.* The patient should be made to understand that the crucial factor is venous return, not ointments or creams and should be warned against the dangers of trauma and self-prescribed treatment. The skin affected by stasis is unduly sensitive, and potential irritants and sensitisers must be avoided. For acute weeping dermatitis, a few days of bed rest and wet compresses should precede ambulant treatment. Normal saline solution or weak permanganate solution are suitable for this purpose. More chronic dermatitis may be relieved by the application of a corticosteroid ointment.

If an ulcer has already developed, wet packs of eusol, diluted one in sixteen, are useful when marked exudation precludes compressive bandaging. The ulcer which is rapidly extending, with marked surrounding inflammation and a purulent exudate, is likely to need systemic antibiotic therapy. However, this is uncommon and antibiotics are of little use in most cases. When exudate has been reduced, paraffin gauze may be used to cover the ulcer, with zinc oil as a soothing application for surrounding skin. A one way stretch elastic bandage is firmly applied from the base of the toes to just below the knee, and removed only at bedtime.

The ulcer often overlies an incompetent perforating vein, and a disc of sponge rubber provides useful compression beneath the elastic bandage. The disc should be larger than the ulcer and sloping at the edges to avoid annular compression. Associated systemic diseases, such as cardiac failure, anaemia and diabetes, should not be overlooked. After healing of the ulcer, the patient will need to continue to wear elastic stockings or to use compressive bandaging.

■ *Surgical procedures.* Particularly when recognised early, the stasis syndrome is frequently amenable to relief by surgical procedures. The advice of a surgeon experienced in the treatment of peripheral vascular disease is of great assistance.

Pityriasis alba

This very common pattern of mild eczema occurs mainly in children and adolescents. The cause is unknown, but the disease is more common in atopics and seems to be aggravated by an excessive use of soap.

Clinical features

Lesions begin as lightly scaling, circular or oval, pink areas, a centimetre or more in size. The erythema fades and is replaced by residual hypopigmentation, which may persist for months. During summer, when surrounding skin becomes tanned, the contrasting pale areas are more conspicuous.

There may be only two or three lesions, or there may be dozens. The face is the most common site, especially around the mouth, but the neck, upper limbs and, less often, the trunk may be affected. The course is usually prolonged, repigmentation of one area occurring as new lesions develop. However, there is little or no discomfort, and disfigurement is minor and temporary.

Diagnosis

▶ **Consider and exclude**

■ *Vitiligo*, which has no scaling, is a stark white rather than of faint pallor, and differs in distribution.

■ *Tinea* is very sharply demarcated, has a well defined inflamed margin, produces coarser, more marked scaling and slowly increases in size.

■ *Discoid eczema* has a different distribution, is very itchy as plaques develop, and has a crusted phase.

Treatment

Pityriasis alba is such a minor disorder that reassurance is usually the only necessary treatment. Hydrocortisone acetate ointment may be prescribed, but improvement is unlikely to be dramatic. Simple emollients and restricted use of soap are frequently just as effective as corticosteroids.

Juvenile forefoot eczema (Juvenile plantar dermatitis)

This characteristic pattern of eczema that occurs in children first began appearing in the late 1960s to early 1970s.

Aetiology

The exact cause is complex but maceration, sweat retention and friction seem important prerequisites for its development, and these are the conditions created by the constant wearing of track shoes, a fashion introduced around the time this disorder began appearing. In Europe, winter is the time of peak incidence but, in Australia, the condition is more common during the summer months and often in children who wear no shoes or only open sandals. There is commonly a family history of atopy but affected patients rarely have atopic eczema elsewhere. It is not understood why the condition is confined to children.

Clinical features

Both feet are involved. The plantar aspect of the distal sole and toes is red, and fissured. Pain is the predominant symptom, rather than itch. The heels, dorsum of feet and between the toes are spared, as are the hands. After undergoing exacerbations and remissions around the same time each year, spontaneous resolution occurs and results in perfectly normal skin.

Diagnosis

▶ Consider and exclude

■ *Tinea pedis* (rare in this age group), which is unilateral in children, interdigital when the toes are involved, and shows increased inflammation around the periphery. Scrapings will confirm the diagnosis.

■ *Allergic contact dermatitis* to components of footwear occurs on the dorsum of the toes, the instep and around the sides of the heel.

■ *Psoriasis* has a thicker scale and is usually evident elsewhere as well.

Treatment

Treatment with topical steroids is often disappointing even though the histology is that of eczema. All children, including those who habitually wear sandals, should be advised to wear cotton socks and leather shoes with leather soles. The use of urea-containing cream will usually minimise fissuring and relieve pain. The painting of splits with collodin or tincture of benzoin compound will induce healing of cracks by minimising their expansion. In severe cases, bed rest may be required. The condition eventually resolves.

Lichen simplex chronicus

This term is used to describe circumscribed areas of lichenification arising in predisposed people as a response to repeated rubbing and scratching of previously normal skin.

Aetiology

Lichenification may develop from scratching any itchy lesion, but the term 'lichen simplex' implies the absence of a pre-existing cause for pruritus. The scratching in lichen simplex begins as an unconscious movement of the fingers to an accessible area, as an inappropriate reaction to stress. Habitual rubbing promotes pruritus which then provokes conscious scratching, and the itch–scratch–itch cycle becomes self-perpetuating.

The incidence of lichen simplex is higher in women and among oriental races, but the disease is rare in children.

Clinical features

In most patients, typical lesions develop at characteristic sites and, in all patients, itching is severe.

The typical lesion is a rather well-defined, thickened plaque, surmounted by an adherent scale. There is a surrounding zone of increased skin markings and hyperpigmentation, and scratch papules may be distinguished towards the periphery. Lichen simplex may develop on any accessible area, but characteristic sites are the occipital region in women and the lower legs or ankles in men. Other common sites are the side of the neck, the forearms, thighs, vulva, scrotum and palm.

Severe itch is an invariable complaint, but usually disappears, when the patient is occupied, only to recur during periods of idleness. The pruritus is spasmodic and promotes vigorous scratching, which is usually continued until itch is replaced by pain.

Prognosis

If the condition has arisen merely from habit, careful explanation combined with topical therapy will often produce permanent cure. If, as occasionally happens, the disease is an expression of serious emotional disturbance, cure of the skin lesion will be difficult and sometimes undesirable without skilled psychiatric assistance.

Diagnosis

▶ **Consider and exclude**

■ *Psoriasis* of the scalp, which may be almost indistinguishable clinically, but lesions in other areas are likely to be present.

■ *Lichenification of any underlying dermatosis* such as contact dermatitis, lichen planus, or atopic dermatitis should be excluded by evaluation of the history and careful examination of other areas.

Treatment

If the patient understands the cause and is able to refrain from scratching, cure is certain. However, systemic benzodiazepines are often required as an aid to minimise scratching. Resolution is accelerated and symptomatic relief is obtained from the application of a fluorinated steroid ointment, which may be combined with plastic occlusion. If resolution is slow, clearing can be achieved with the intralesional injection of betamethasone or triamcinolone.

Dermatitis of more complex aetiology

The forms of dermatitis already described are those in which either a definite exogenous cause is known, or in which the pattern is sufficiently distinctive to allow clear separation. However, dermatitis is often caused by a number of factors acting in combination.

Intertrigo is produced in this way, but is discussed in relation to disorders of sweating. Other examples are:

1. Otitis externa
2. Dermatitis of the napkin area
3. Dermatitis of the anogenital region
4. Infective eczematoid dermatitis

Otitis externa

The external auditory canal is the only blind cul-de-sac in the body which is lined by stratified squamous epithelium. It is often tortuous, hairy, and may be partially or completely occluded by cerumen, which makes drainage of exudate and evaporation of moisture more difficult. Inflammatory swelling narrows the canal, and drying after swimming or showering is often hurried and inadequate. The moist environment and the presence of cerumen or epithelial debris provide favourable conditions for the growth of yeasts and Gram-negative bacteria.

At this site, so prone to maceration and overgrowth of micro-organisms, dermatoses may develop as on any other area of skin. Psoriasis, atopic and seborrhoeic eczema are common at the external meatus, usually as part of more generalised disease, but sometimes with little or no involvement elsewhere. Scratching adds further damage and may introduce infection. Secondary contact dermatitis may result from nail lacquer or from the many objects which are used to scratch the auditory canal. There may be sensitivity to nickel from hair pins, chromate from matches, and, not infrequently, to neomycin and other agents used in topical therapy.

Management

Treatment will vary according to the aetiological factors involved in the individual patient. Cleaning and drying the ear canal is relevant to most, as is the avoidance of scratching. Fungi, particularly aspergillus, and bacteria are more often colonists than pathogens, but chemotherapy is necessary for some patients. However, syringing away of debris, followed by careful drying, is usually more important than the application of antibiotics.

A solution of 8 per cent aluminium acetate applied on a gauze wick, or 3 per cent acetic acid in isopropyl alcohol will promote drying and relieve pruritus. Corticosteroids may be used as ear drops, or applied as a gel.

Dermatitis of the napkin area *(Colour plate 6)*

Repeated and prolonged exposure of an infant's napkin area to the irritant components of urine and faeces easily leads to an irritant dermatitis. Initially, the dermatitis tends to develop over the buttocks, but may spread to involve the whole area in contact with napkins, sparing only the skin deep in the groins and natal cleft. Some degree of sweat retention invariably follows the dermatitis, but is markedly increased if plastic or rubber pants are worn over the napkin.

The area is a common site for atopic and seborrhoeic eczema often with secondary candidiasis. The folds are difficult to clean gently, and provide a nidus for the accumulation of soap and water after inadequate rinsing and drying. Frequent apposition of skin folds reduces evaporation of sweat and leads to maceration of the skin. Particularly when applied to moist skin, an excess of baby powder easily becomes caked in the folds and adds a source of mechanical trauma.

Management
Napkins should be changed as frequently as possible, and the area should be gently cleansed with water and a bland soap, then carefully rinsed and gently dried after washing. Powder is helpful only if applied sparingly to dry skin, and only a fine unscented powder should be used. Busy mothers should be warned against using a corner of the napkin to clean faeces from the baby's buttocks, and the drawbacks of rubber or plastic pants should be emphasised. Candidiasis may be treated with nystatin or imidazole cream, whereas gentian violet 0.25 per cent aqueous solution has the added benefit of aiding in the resolution of oozing eczematous skin. Underlying atopic eczema, seborrhoeic eczema or irritant dermatitis may be treated with hydrocortisone 1 per cent cream.

Dermatitis of the anogenital area

The perineum is easily kept moist by obesity, sweating, occlusive clothing, and vaginal or anal discharge. It is a frequent site of involvement by many common dermatoses, including intertrigo, seborrhoeic eczema, psoriasis and tinea. The skin of the anogenital region is more susceptible to irritant dermatitis than most other areas, and aggravation by unsuitable topical therapy is common. Threadworms in children and maceration with secondary candidiasis are frequent causes of pruritus.

The area has a special erotic significance, and psychological factors are very often involved in habitual scratching of the area, which sometimes leads to lichen simplex chronicus.

Management
Management is often difficult, but always requires a careful assessment of the causative factors involved, especially the psychological ones which are so frequently relevant. The presence of candidiasis warrants the exclusion of diabetes.

Infective eczematoid dermatitis *(Colour plate 7)*

Apart from causing problems by direct infection, bacteria may also induce dermatitis as a result of an irritant or allergic reaction to the organisms

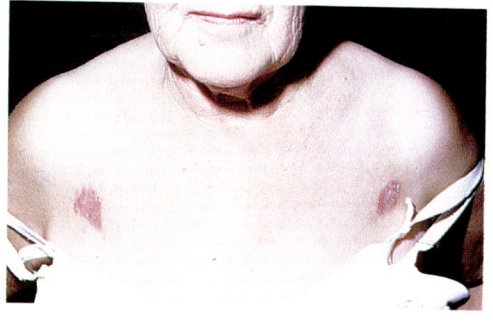

1. Allergic contact dermatitis due to nickel

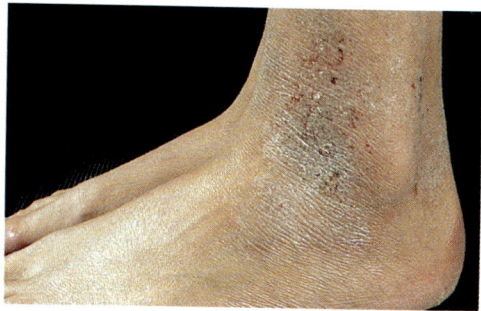

2. Lichenified plaque in patient with atopic dermatitis

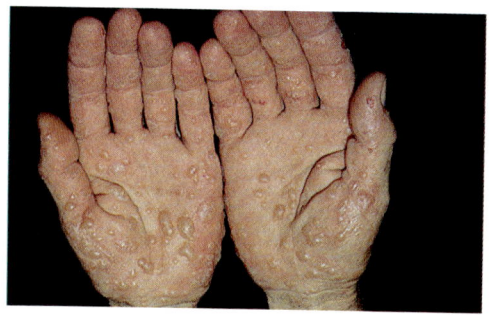

3. Severe pompholyx

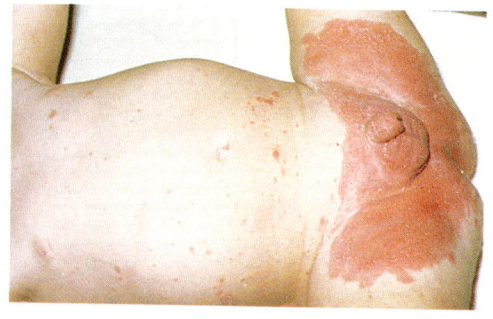

4. Seborrhoeic dermatitis with secondary candidiasis

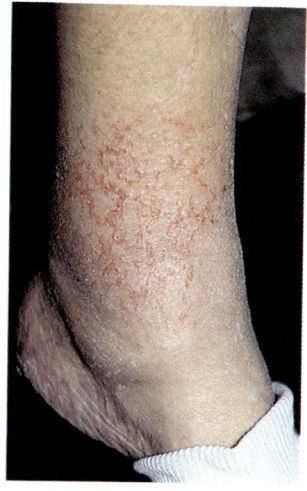

5. Asteatotic eczema

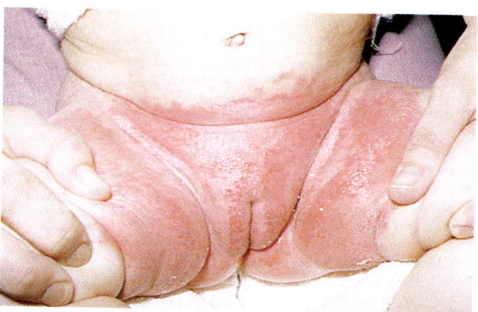

6. Napkin dermatitis with sparing of skin deep in flexures

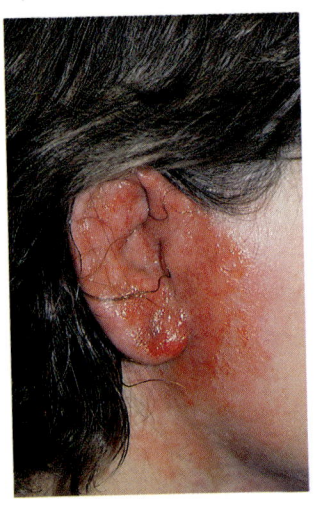

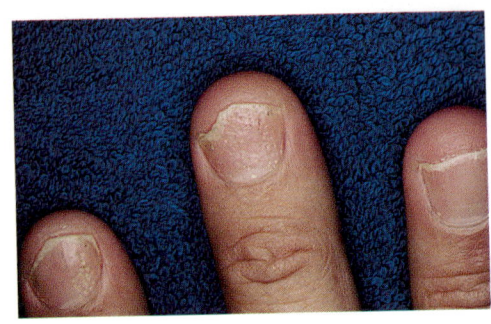

8. Psoriasis

7. Infective eczematoid dermatitis

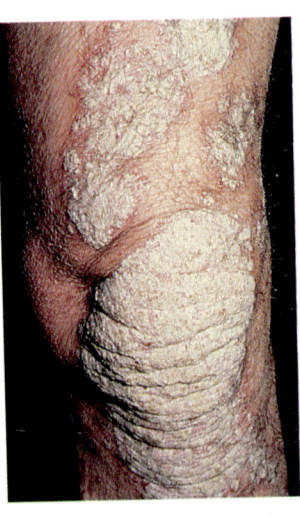

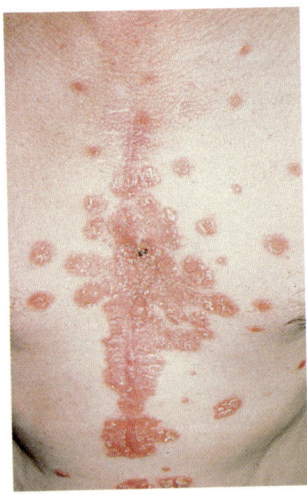

9. Psoriasis at typical site over the knee

10. Psoriasis at site of recent scar (Koebner phenomenon)

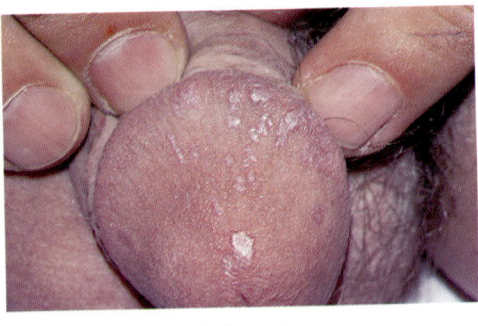

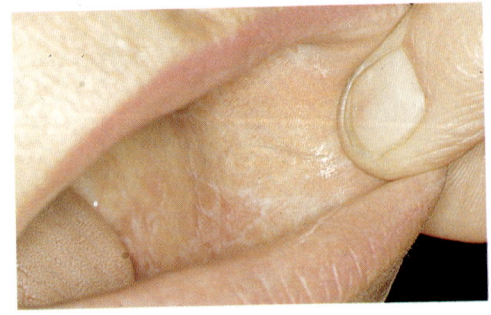

11. Lichen planus

12. Lichen planus in buccal mucosa

or products produced by them. The skin is often further inflamed as a result of oozing, which is usually present and has served to provide a favorable environment for bacterial growth. Contact dermatitis, either irritant or allergic, due to treatment applied to treat the infection, further exacerbates the process. This pattern is usually seen around discharging wounds, sinuses and fistulae, mucocutaneous junctions, flexures such as the inguinal and inframammary fold, the retro-auricular fold and around the external auditory meatus. Widespread dissemination is common.

Management

Following bacterial culture, treatment is commenced with an appropriate systemic antibiotic. Topical treatments that have been used are withdrawn and wet dressings used to induce resolution of the oozing. Topical corticosteroid cream can then be applied. Any underlying cause is corrected and patch testing may be necessary. In patients with extensive dissemination, oral prednisolone 30 mg per day causes dramatic resolution and can be withdrawn within one week, provided the correct antibiotic has been given and adequate topical treatment has cleared the primary site.

Erythroderma (generalised exfoliative dermatitis)

When dermatitis involves all, or almost all, of the skin surface, the terms 'erythroderma' or 'generalised exfoliative dermatitis' are applied. Each term emphasises one of the two major changes in the skin—erythema and scaling. Erythrodermic patients usually require hospital admission because of the profound systemic effects secondary to changes taking place in the skin.

Aetiology

Although the term 'generalised exfoliative dermatitis' is used, erythroderma is often due to a condition that is not really a dermatitis.

In about one-third of cases, the condtion is caused by a pre-existing dermatitis or eczema that has extended.

In the very young and the very old, seborrhoeic eczema is the type most often responsible. Atopic eczema may become generalised at any age, while nummular eczema, allergic contact dermatitis and asteatotic eczema are less frequent causes.

Psoriasis is the preceding dermatosis in about one-quarter of cases. Erythroderma most often complicates the pustular or unstable eruptive phases of the disease. Drug eruptions and underlying lymphoma or leukaemia each account for about 10 per cent of cases. Less common causes include pityriasis rubra pilaris, pemphigus foliaceus, Norwegian scabies, and ichthyosiform dermatoses. Erythroderma is always secondary to some primary disorder, but careful investigation fails to reveal the cause in about 15 per cent of patients.

Clinical features

When erythroderma follows extension of a preceding dermatitis, onset is usually gradual, but with widespread exposure to contact allergen the onset tends to be more abrupt. An acute course is also common when the cause is a drug, leukaemia, or lymphoma.

With an acute onset, there may be rigors and the patient feels cold, although the skin is hot to the touch. Itch is sometimes severe, and the skin is red and thickened, with a fine branny scaling. When the onset is more gradual, erythema tends to be less marked and the scaling varies from a fine desquamation to abundant flat flakes a centimetre or more across.

Fever is common, but the fixed vasodilatation impedes adequate thermoregulation and hypothermia may develop. There is malaise and often weakness, and substantial quantities of water and protein are lost from the surface. Cardiovascular changes may lead to high output failure.

Over a few weeks, scalp and body hair becomes scanty, and gynaecomastia may develop in men. There is subungual hyperkeratosis, the nails become dystrophic and may be shed. Without treatment, the patient becomes weaker and prone to pneumonia or other intercurrent infection. Even with careful management, there is still a significant mortality.

Complications

■ *Dehydration* is surprisingly uncommon.

■ *Hypoproteinaemia* may develop, although plasma estimations can be misleading because of haemodilution secondary to circulatory changes.

■ *Electrolyte abnormalities* occur due to loss through the skin, malabsorption, low protein, or haemodilution.

■ *Hypothermia*

■ *Intestinal malabsorption* is most commonly a biochemical steatorrhoea and recovers quickly when the erythroderma resolves.

■ *Anaemia* occurs in chronic cases and is normochromic, normocytic, with low serum iron but high iron stores.

■ *Pneumonia*

■ *Circulatory failure*

Diagnosis

The diagnosis of erythroderma presents no difficulty, the important diagnosis being that of the cause. This is not always possible, but the past history and a careful examination often allow at least a strong suspicion of the cause.

■ *Psoriatic erythroderma* often has more marked changes in the regions normally affected by psoriasis. Small flaccid pustules may be present in early cases.

■ *Seborrhoeic eczema* evolves slowly to erythroderma, and the previous history is usually suggestive.

■ *Atopic erythroderma* is preceded by a long history of dermatitis and the erythroderma is usually extremely itchy.

■ *Allergic contact dermatitis* is eczematoid. In the early stages of the eruption, vesicular dermatitis is suggestive.

50

■ **Leukaemia** is confirmed by blood and bone marrow examinations, but lymphomas may be difficult to detect in the erythrodermic stage. Skin and lymph node biopsy may be helpful.

■ **Drug-induced erythroderma** has no distinctive features apart from the history, symmetry of the early eruption, and the acute onset.

■ **Pityriasis rubra pilaris** is suggested by marked scaling from the scalp, severe facial involvement, often with ectropion, and follicular papules over the elbows, knees, fingers, and toes.

■ **Pemphigus foliaceus** may be suspected from detection of a few flaccid vesicles, and confirmed by biopsy.

■ **Norwegian scabies** is easily confirmed by examination of scrapings in which the mite abounds.

Treatment

1. General management
2. Drug therapy
3. Topical therapy

■ **General management.** The patient is admitted to hospital, where regular monitoring of temperature, cardiovascular function, and water and electrolyte balance is necessary. Temperature should be recorded with a low-reading rectal thermometer. When the erythroderma has been caused by a drug reaction or contact dermatitis, the relevant drug or application is withdrawn. Enforced rest in bed usually has a profound beneficial effect.

■ **Drug therapy.** Systemic corticosteroid therapy is necessary for most patients. Administration of prednisone in doses of 30 to 40 mg daily is generally sufficient for rapid suppression. For erythroderma which has evolved from psoriasis or pityriasis rubra pilaris, treatment with parenteral methotrexate may be preferable. When a leukaemia or lymphoma is involved, the advice of a haematologist should be obtained. Antibiotic therapy may be necessary for intercurrent infection.

■ **Topical therapy.** The patient is made more comfortable by the use of an application that has moisturising and emollient properties. This should be bland and non-irritating. Glycerine 10 per cent in sorbolene cream, or liquid paraffin 50 per cent and soft white paraffin 50 per cent are suitable. Tepid oatmeal baths are permissible and soothing, but soap is better avoided, at least for the first week.

4

Psoriasis, psoriasiform eruptions and lichen planus

1. Psoriasis
   (a) psoriasis vulgaris
   (b) pustular psoriasis
   (c) psoriatic arthropathy
2. Psoriasiform eruptions
   (a) Reiter's syndrome
   (b) pityriasis rubra pilaris
   (c) napkin psoriasis
   (d) acrokeratosis paraneoplastica
   (e) parapsoriasis en plaques
3. Lichen planus

Psoriasis

This common dermatosis is characterised by circumscribed areas of thickened, scaly skin. Psoriasis is never vesicular unless it is complicated by dermatitis, but in its very acute forms may be pustular.

Aetiology

More than 2 per cent of the population have recognisable psoriasis and nearly one-third of those affected are aware of having relatives with the disease. The pattern of inheritance is polygenic and the genes appear to be located close to the major histocompatibility complex on the short arm of chromosone 6. However, environmental factors that in most cases are not yet recognised seem to be required to induce clinical expression of the disease.

The following factors are known to precipate psoriasis.

■ *Trauma* is the most common precipitating factor. This probably accounts for localisation of psoriasis to the elbows and knees.

As a result of observing the lesions that appear at the site of an operation scar or other recalled injury, it is known that it takes seven to 14 days after the injury for psoriasis to appear. Picking and rubbing the skin may extend old lesions or precipitate new ones and a similar Koebner effect may complicate sunburn or add psoriasis to areas of lichen planus, seborrhoeic and other forms of dermatitis.

■ *Streptococcal upper respiratory tract infection* precipitates an acute guttate pattern of psoriasis. As with trauma, it takes about seven to 14 days after the onset of infection for clinical signs of guttate psoriasis to appear. Treatment of the infection may not prevent psoriasis appearing.

■ *Medications* such as lithium, various antimalarials, beta adrenergic blocking drugs, some non-steroidal anti-inflammatory drugs may precipitate or worsen psoriasis. The exact mechanisms by which these drugs exert their effect on psoriasis are not known and many patients may take these without any effect on their psoriasis. Lesions may develop as a Koebner reaction complicating drug eruptions caused, for example, by sulphonamides, while severe acute psoriasis has been reported as a rare complication of gold therapy. The administration of systemic corticosteroids is freqently followed by a curious rebound aggravation on withdrawal which is often pustular, and even the abrupt cessation of topical steroid therapy may lead to a rebound flare.

■ *Stress* and periods of worry are often blamed by patients for exacerbations, but the impact of emotional factors has probably been exaggerated.

Histology

There is diminished maturation of epidermal cells, with disordered keratinisation, so that early lesions show parakeratosis with an absent granular layer. The number of mitoses is increased and cell turnover accelerated.

The epidermis is irregularly thickened, with club shaped elongation of the rete ridges. Dermal papillae are correspondingly lengthened, with thinning of the overlying epidermis. The elongated papillae contain tortuous dilated capillaries and an infiltrate of lymphocytes and histiocytes. In early lesions, neutrophils are also visible between epidermal cells and may accumulate to sizeable clusters below the stratum corneum (*micro-abscesses*). In very acute lesions, the micro-abscesses may be large enough to form macroscopic pustules (*pustular psoriasis*). In older, resolving or partially treated plaques there may be reformation of the granular layer and loss of parakeratosis.

Clinical features *(Colour plates 8, 9)*

■ *Morphology* of a typical lesion is of indolent scaling plaques which are neither itchy nor tender. The individual plaque is sharply circumscribed and raised above the level of surrounding skin. The underlying colour is deep pink or bright red, but is partially masked in most areas by adherent, silvery white scale. The amount of scaling varies from a barely visible powdery desquamation to a grossly thickened mound of parakeratosis. When lightly scratched the scaly surface becomes more opaque, while more vigorous scratching produces tiny bleeding points as the scale is removed, elongated dermal papillae are denuded of epidermis, and the tortuous capillaries traumatised.

■ *The primary lesion* is a small reddish plaque or papule, sometimes perifollicular. With extension and coalescence, typical plaques develop, but in a few patients discrete perifollicular papules persist (*follicular psoriasis*). Particularly in children, psoriasis may erupt suddenly with multiple, rounded, reddish areas of thickening, up to a centimetre in size, scattered widely over the trunk and limbs (***guttate psoriasis***). Scaling is less marked and the prognosis for complete recovery is better than in patients with the more typical evolution of plaques.

■ ***Distribution*** of the lesions is most often over the extensor surfaces of the elbows and knees, the scalp, lumbosacral region and the legs. Any area may be involved, but the face is usually spared except where the skin adjoins the hairline. In the flexures, especially the groins and natal cleft, scaling is less apparent, lesions appearing as sharply demarcated, glazed red plaques. On the scalp, palms and soles, scaling is more prominent and tends to disguise the underlying colour. On the palms and soles, psoriasis often takes on a yellowish hue and on the legs may be purplish red, but at other sites the typical rich red colour is usually retained.

■ ***The nails*** are frequently affected, and nail involvement may precede all other manifestations. The nail plate may be pitted with small surface depressions, or discoloured yellowish white with distal separation from the bed (***onycholysis***). Subungual accumulations of keratin may accompany or follow separation, and secondary colonisation by yeasts and bacteria may alter the colour to yellowish green. The nail may become friable and crumbly, with loss of its distal part.

Course

The course for individual patients is unpredictable, although the guttate form is less likely to persist. Onset in preschool children is very uncommon, the peak age of onset being in young adults. For most patients, psoriasis is a chronic indolent disease, with unexplained periods of exacerbation and of partial remission. Slow extension may occur, but many patients have plaques restricted to a few areas which remain more or less unchanged for years.

■ ***Unstable phase.*** With more acute onset, developing lesions are often irritable and tender (unstable psoriasis), and even chronic psoriasis may enter an unstable phase of extension and eruption of new lesions. In the unstable phase, psoriasis is very prone to the Koebner response and to aggravation by irritating applications. *(Colour plate 10)*

At this stage, agents suitable for chronic lesions may provoke severe widespread disease, which readily progresses to erythroderma and its complications (see Chapter 3) or sometimes pustular psoriasis.

Diagnosis

▶ **Look for:**
■ plaques that are sharply defined, have a rich red colour and are covered with a silvery scale;
■ distribution involving extensor elbows and knees and scalp margins;
■ nail changes.

▶ **Consider and exclude:**
■ ***Seborrhoeic dermatitis,*** which may precede or coexist with psoriasis. It is not always possible to make a sharp distinction. Typical psoriasis

is not likely to be confused with typical seborrhoeic dermatitis, but there is considerable clinical and histological overlap.

■ *Tinea,* which is usually distinguishable by its raised border, less thickening, asymmetry and peripheral spread. This diagnosis may be confirmed microscopically, and by culture.

■ *Intertrigo,* which may resemble flexural psoriasis, but is strictly confined to flexural skin and lacks the scalp, nail and other changes associated with psoriasis.

■ *Pityriasis rosea,* which lacks the thickness of typical plaques of psoriasis, and has a finer, less adherent scale, and a suggestive distribution.

■ *Secondary syphilis,* which may be psoriasiform, but is accompanied by positive serological tests, and lacks the typical silver-on-red appearance of psoriasis.

▶ *Confirmatory tests* are usually not required because the majority of cases are typical. However, biopsy may be needed if the disease is localised to a region where the classic signs are not fully expressed (for example, flexures or palms), and there are no confirmatory features elsewhere on the body.

Treatment

1. General management
2. Topical therapy
3. Systemic therapy

■ *General management.* The patient with psoriasis, even more than most other patients, should be given a clear understanding of the disorder. The benign course, rarity of serious complications, the benefits of sun and surf for most psoriatics, and the deleterious effects of sunburn and mechanical trauma, should all be explained. Sedation is of doubtful value, but the depressed patient adjusts better to the disease after treatment of the depression. The time and inconvenience of applying ointments three or four times a day to large areas over long periods can be tedious and depressing. The doctor, as well as the patient, should keep the disease in perspective, so that treatment is never allowed to become more irksome than the disease itself.

■ *Topical therapy*

— *Tar* preparations are effective for chronic lesions but should be used with caution, if at all, during the unstable phase. An ointment containing from 1 to 5 per cent crude coal tar or from 3 to 8 per cent liquor picis carbonis (LPC) may be adequate, but from 2 to 4 per cent salicylic acid can be incorporated if necessary. Tar therapy is enhanced by irradiation with ultraviolet light in the UV-B range (290 nm to 320 nm), administered two hours after application of the ointment. The duration of irradiation should be just sufficient to produce minimal erythema. The ointment should be wiped off just prior to irradiation to allow maximum transmission of light. Tar therapy is effective and has a good safety record, but is messy and most useful in hospital or in psoriasis day care centres. Remissions induced by tars with or without ultraviolet light are longer lasting than psoriasis-free times induced by other treatment methods.

▬ *Dithranol* is used for indolent plaques, and may be effectively combined with tar baths (50 mL LPC in 90 litres of water) and irradiation with ultraviolet light. Irritation is common and there is occasional hypersensitivity but, with adequate supervision, dithranol is a safe and effective application. As a paste or ointment, initial concentrations of from 0.05 to 0.1 per cent are gradually increased to 1 per cent, depending on response and tolerance. Much the same results can be achieved by using stronger preparations for shorter periods. A 1 to 3 per cent ointment can be applied initially for 30 minutes before being washed off. The period of application is increased daily to a maximum of two hours. Many patients find the method preferable to the practical problems associated with more prolonged application.

Dithranol is relatively unstable and should be combined with 1 per cent salicylic acid, particularly when prescribed as a paste, to impede inactivation and enhance its shelf life. Dithranol temporarily stains the skin surrounding treated areas purplish-brown, while garments and bedclothes are discoloured by contact. When used as a paste, the application should be lightly dusted with talcum powder, and separated from clothing by stockinet. Dithranol is unsuitable for use on the face or in the flexures. If used on the scalp, it stains light-coloured hair.

▬ *Corticosteroid applications.* Hydrocortisone acetate is relatively ineffective in psoriasis, but stronger steroids give good initial results. However, recurrences follow more quickly than after treatment with dithranol, and repeat treatment is less effective. The effect of steroids is enhanced by plastic occlusive dressings, as are the undesirable accompaniments of steroid therapy. The local side effects of topical corticosteroids are well recognised, and the more potent preparations carry a greater risk of pituitary-adrenal suppression. Corticosteroids give best results when used on the scalp, genital or flexural areas, or for small plaques on the trunk and limbs.

However, LPC and salicylic acid cream is cheap and effective for most patients with scalp psoriasis. Small resistant plaques may be infiltrated with corticosteroid by intradermal injection, but clearing is unlikely to be well sustained.

For acute unstable psoriasis, applications should be bland and non-irritating. Tars are unsuitable, but corticosteroids may be used until the acute phase has passed. The patient with widespread acute psoriasis should be at rest in bed and is more easily managed in hospital.

■ *Systemic therapy*

▬ *Systemic corticosteroid therapy* is occasionally necessary when life is threatened by either psoriatic erythroderma or generalised pustular psoriasis, but is otherwise contra-indicated. Rebound aggravation after withdrawal is the rule, and suppression is not usually maintained with acceptable doses. Psoriasis is a common disease and may be associated with unrelated visceral disorders for which the administration of systemic steroids would be considered. In such patients, the steroid should be prescribed only after consideration of the possible consequences to the psoriatic patient.

▬ *Cytotoxic drugs,* mainly methotrexate, are occasionally used for severe life-threatening or life-ruining psoriasis. Generalised pustular psoriasis or disabling psoriatic arthropathy may be valid indications. However, early and late side effects are a serious hazard, and the drug is contra-indicated for women of child-bearing age unless conception is specifically excluded. Methotrexate therapy of psoriasis should be undertaken only by those with a special knowledge of the drug, after dermatological consultation to confirm the diagnosis and indication.

— *Photochemotherapy* of psoriasis combines the phototoxic effect of a psoralen, most often 8-methoxypsoralen, with a measured dose of UV-A from a high-output source. The combination ('PUVA') has an inhibitory effect on DNA synthesis, which is the probable basis for its influence on psoriasis. With two or three PUVA treatments a week, 85 per cent of patients achieve a substantial improvement within two months and some clear completely. Recurrences are the rule, but long remissions may be maintained with interval therapy. The potential risks of PUVA, particularly to the eyes, haematopoietic system and to the skin itself, are minimised by eye protection on treatment days and by excluding patients who have had past exposure to carcinogens such as oral arsenic or past X-ray therapy; but it will still be many years until the treatment has been in use for long enough to be considered free of serious toxic effects.

— *Oral retinoids.* These synthetic derivatives of vitamin A modify the growth and differentiation of epidermal cells. The aromatic retinoid, etretinate, is effective in some patients with psoriasis, particularly those with erythrodermic and pustular psoriasis, and in combination with PUVA for less acute forms of the disease. However, side effects are frequent and troublesome. Retinoids are teratogenic and have a very long half-life. In the case of etretinate, pregnancy should be avoided for two years after medication has been ceased, which is a stage that may never be reached because psoriasis is controlled rather than cured.

Pustular psoriasis

Pustular psoriasis is the appearance of sterile pustules which are a macroscopic manifestation of the accumulation of polymorphonuclear leucocytes into aggregates within the upper portion of the epidermis or the keratin layer, commonly seen as a microscopic feature in psoriasis.

The chemotactic factors responsible for this polymorph accumulation are complement components, in particular C5a, which are activated by the reaction of antikeratin antibody, present in every human, with changed keratin of psoriasis.

■ *Generalised pustular psoriasis* is a rare but life-threatening disease which may develop as a complication of longstanding psoriasis, often after previous corticosteroid therapy, or following an unstable phase.

Clinically, the disease may present as an acute illness with fever, severe toxaemia, neutrophilia, hypo-albuminaemia and a related hypocalcaemia. Broad areas of tender inflamed skin are studded with crops of small pustules which coalesce to form yellowish green lakes. Exacerbations occur approximately every seven days.

With a less acute onset, there may be localised or widespread annular patches of erythema, with pustules scattered at the periphery. An uncommon presentation is the development of pustules towards the edge of longstanding plaques, especially on the legs.

Treatment of the acute form seems to require strict bed rest for resolution. However, correction of fluid and electrolyte imbalance, especially hypocalcaemia, is also needed and only bland topical agents are used until the disease has stabilised. Should oral treatment be required, oral aromatic retinoids seem to be the most effective.

■ *Impetigo herpetiformis* is a rare pustular eruption, which clinically and histologically resembles generalised pustular psoriasis. The disease usually begins in the last few months of pregnancy with the development of tender areas of erythema which spread out from the large flexures. dotted with tiny sterile pustules, particularly at the extending margins.

Constitutional disturbance is severe, with fever, vomiting, diarrhoea, and hypocalcaemia. Delirium, convulsions, and tetany may follow. The high maternal morbidity is reduced by adequate doses of prednisolone and correction of the hypocalcaemia. Foetal mortality is also high, but may be decreased by careful antepartum monitoring of the foetal heart rate patterns and, when necessary, premature delivery of the child.

■ *Pustular psoriasis of the palms and soles* refers to an uncommon group of pustular eruptions of the hands and feet which have been variously classified on the basis of distribution, minor variations of morphology, and an alleged association, or otherwise with a focus of infection at other sites. The pustules are sterile, the eruption persistent and resistant to therapy. The lesions frequently occur in patients who have, or who later develop, typical psoriasis elsewhere; and may reasonably be considered a variant of psoriasis.

There may be fairly well circumscribed patches of pustules involving the palms, soles, or both. There may be involvement of only one palm or the sole of one foot, or there may be pustules scattered diffusely over the palms and soles on both sides, often with extension around the nail folds. The insteps and margins of the heels are common sites, but occasionally the disease begins around the nail of one or more fingers or toes, and slowly evolves to scaling or crusted erythematous areas. The disease is often chronic and intractable, although remissions and even permanent resolution may occur.

The lesions may become generalised and are then indistinguishable from generalised pustular psoriasis.

Psoriatic arthropathy

Arthropathy is clinically evident in between 2 and 5 per cent of psoriatics and is more frequent in patients with pronounced nail changes or in those with pustular psoriasis. However, arthropathy may be present for years before any skin signs appear. Minor changes, involving particularly the sacro-iliac joints, are radiologically demonstrable in more than 90 per cent of patients. Arthropathy with negative tests for rheumatoid factor affects psoriatics in five ways.

■ An asymmetric oligo-arthritis involving only a few large joints, fingers or toes. This is the commonest pattern of arthropathy accounting for about 80 per cent of patients with arthropathy. When the proximal interphalyngeal joints are involved with this pattern, the distal interphalyngeal joints are also affected, which is quite unlike rheumatoid arthritis.

▪ Diffuse involvement of only the distal interphalyngeal joints. Psoriatic nail changes are almost invariably present and severe.

▪ A destructive arthritis may involve the hands, feet, sacro-iliac and other joints. The phalanges subluxate, producing apparent shortening of the digits.

▪ Typical or atypical spondylitis.

▪ Arthritis clinically and radiologically indistinguishable from rheumatoid arthritis.

Psoriasiform eruptions

Reiter's syndrome

Reiter's disease is a multisystem disorder, characterised by the association of seronegative arthritis with urethritis and/or cervicitis. It is predominantly a disease of young men and is very often accompanied by conjunctivitis. Cutaneous lesions develop in more than half the patients, and have clinical and histological features in common with psoriasis.

The cutaneous eruption is largely confined to the palms, soles and penis, but a few scattered lesions are not uncommon at other sites. Rarely, the eruption becomes generalised. On the palms and soles, the primary lesion is a firm pustule arising on a reddish base. The pustules harden and form keratinous papules which coalesce to produce an irregular, patchy or diffuse thickening. There may be painless inflammation of the nail folds, followed by subungual hyperkeratosis and shedding of one or more nails.

Superficial circinate erosions often develop on the glans and around the corona. In circumcised men, the erosions may evolve to crusted and hyperkeratotic papules, resembling lesions at other sites. Painless erosions are common in the mouth and pharynx, and the tongue may shed papillae in a patchy pattern reminiscent of 'geographical tongue'.

Pityriasis rubra pilaris

This rare disease usually begins with diffuse scaling of the scalp, and extends onto the face and ears in a pattern resembling seborrhoeic dermatitis. Thick, yellowish hyperkeratosis of the palms and soles, and often the elbows and knees, adds a psoriasiform appearance. The early resemblance to psoriasis is enhanced when the nails thicken and are lifted by subungual hyperkeratosis. The clinical picture is completed by the eruption of reddish, keratinous, acuminate perifollicular papules. Often beginning on the back of the fingers and hands, the papules become more widespread and in many areas coalesce to form large scaling plaques which may extend to cover much of the body surface, leaving only islands of unaffected skin.

Napkin psoriasis

Although psoriasis does rarely appear during infancy, the term 'napkin psoriasis' is used to describe an irritant napkin dermatitis that shows psoriasiform features. In many cases, candida seems to be implicated, which suggests an inherent tendency to react to this infection in this way, but follow-up and HLA studies indicate that these children probably have no greater risk of psoriasis in later life.

Acrokeratosis paraneoplastica

This rare syndrome produces psoriasiform plaques on the hands, feet, ears and nose. The nails become thickened and crumbly. Patients have an associated neoplasm of the pharynx or upper respiratory tract. Almost all cases are males.

Parapsoriasis en plaques

Despite the title, the disease is in no way related to psoriasis, although lesions may bear a superficial resemblance. The histological appearance of early lesions resembles dermatitis rather than psoriasis, and the 'plaques' are, in fact, macules. Onset is usually during middle age, more commonly in men. In a small proportion of patients the disease progresses to lymphoma, but for most it is merely a persistent rash which is unresponsive to treatment and causes little or no discomfort. Parapsoriasis en plaques is arbitrarily divided into benign and premalignant types.

The benign form is suggested by round, oval or digitate macules, from 2 to 4 cm across, yellowish brown to pink, with a fine superficial scale and a slightly wrinkled surface. Lesions are rather poorly defined at the edges, and are more or less symmetrically scattered over the trunk, with variable extension on the limbs. Itch is slight or absent and, although temporary clearing may follow the application of topical corticosteroids or exposure to sunlight, persistence is the rule.

The premalignant form is suggested by larger lesions with areas of mottled pigmentation and atrophy, most often located over the buttocks or breasts, or spreading out from the major flexures. The patches may remain confined to portions of the trunk and limbs, or may extend and coalesce, involving much of the skin below the neck. The premalignant phase may persist for many years, but the development of increasing pruritus and areas of thickening should warn of evolution towards mycosis fungoides (cutaneous T-cell lymphoma).

Lichen planus

Lichen planus is a relatively common skin disease, characterised by a papular eruption, usually of distinctive appearance and distribution. Onset may be at any age, but is rare in the very young and very old.

Aetiology

A papular eruption closely resembling lichen planus may develop as a reaction to some drugs. The disease may also be mimicked by contact sensitivity to derivatives of paraphenylenediamine used in colour film developers. In these patients the eruption begins as an allergic contact dermatitis, and gradually evolves to a papular eruption with the clinical and histological features of lichen planus. A similar sequence occurs in some cases of chronic graft-versus-host reaction in which an early eczematoid dermatitis gradually assumes a lichenoid pattern.

Whether these lichenoid reactions are really lichen planus, or merely resemble it, is not known, but no cause is discovered for the overwhelming majority of cases of lichen planus. It may be that the disease is merely a pattern of cutaneous reaction to a number of causes at present largely unknown.

Histology

A biopsy specimen provides diagnostic features in most patients. There is hyperkeratosis with prominent stratum granulosum and irregular acanthosis. The rete ridges are lengthened, and in older lesions become pointed downwards in a sawtooth fashion. Liquefaction degeneration of the basal layer is an early and characteristic feature, as is a dense, band-like infiltrate, composed mainly of T-lymphocytes, just below the epidermis.

Because of changes to the basal cells, later lesions show a basal layer composed of squamous rather than columnar cells and the lymphocytic infiltrate also contains macrophages filled with melanin granules.

Clinical features *(Colour plates 11, 12)*

■ *The primary lesion* is a flat polygonal reddish-pink papule, often with a central depression. Usually between 2 and 4 mm across, papules may be smaller or larger, but are of fairly uniform size in the same patient. The surface is smooth, shiny and, with magnification, may show

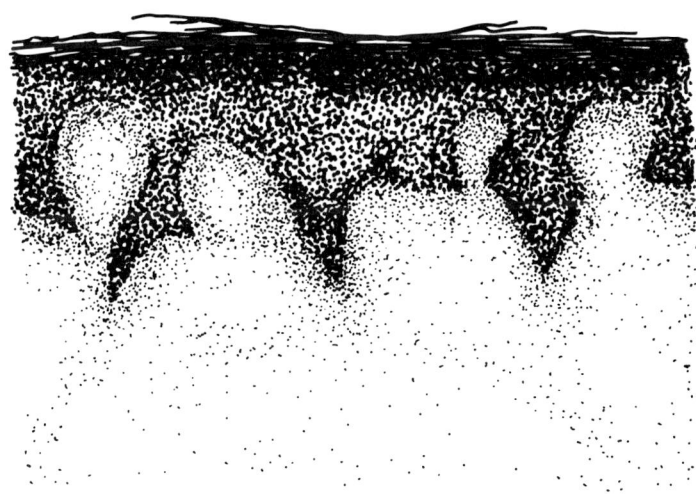

Lichen planus

61

fine grey lines or small puncta. Itch is common and may be severe, but excoriations are seldom a feature. The colour deepens to brown or purplish as individual papules persist, often for months, before slowly resolving. Slight residual atrophy and variable hyperpigmentation are common sequelae.

━ *Distribution* is typically to flexor surfaces, the front of the wrists being a particularly characteristic site. The ventral aspect of the forearms, the lumbosacral region, ankles, front of the legs and the genitalia are also frequently affected. Any area may be involved, but the face, palms and the soles are very uncommon sites. When mucosal surfaces are involved, the normal mucosal pattern of parakeratosis is replaced by hyperkeratosis which, like chronically moist keratin elsewhere, becomes white. This produces a white filigree of tiny white papules, typically in a lacy network. About one-third of patients have the buccal mucosa involved. The anal and genital mucosae may be similarly affected.

━ *The scalp* is a very rare site for the typical papules, but patchy hair loss may occur and is permanent. The alopecia is due to inflammatory destruction of hair follicles, and may extend after resolution of lesions in other areas.

━ *The nails* are usually unaffected but may become thin and brittle, and are occasionally shed. In rare cases, the cuticle adheres to the nail plate, grows over it, and eventually destroys the nail.

━ *Mucosal lesions* tend to persist longer and may occur in the absence of lesions elsewhere. Virtually all mucosae may be affected, including the vaginal, rectal and gastric.

Course

This is variable. An acute onset is uncommon, and papules usually evolve insidiously over weeks or months. Individual papules may persist for several months and resolve as others continue to appear. The disease clears completely within a year in many patients, and within two years in most, but recurrences are not uncommon.

Variants of lichen planus

▪ *Plaques, annular or linear lesions* may be formed by coalescence of papules as the disorder readily shows the Koebner phenomenon. Plaques are relatively common on the legs, where they may become hypertrophic and persist for years.

▪ *Lichen planus actinicus* is a variant in which lesions are confined to light-exposed areas.

▪ *Lichen planopilaris* produces lesions which are small acuminate follicular papules that often heal with scarring and destruction of the hair follicles.

▪ *Ulcerative lichen planus* is a rare entity in which chronic, painful ulcers of the soles, and often of the mouth and other mucosae, are associated with the scalp and nail changes of lichen planus.

▪ *Vesiculobullous lesions* are very uncommon. Papules may become vesicular and eroded, but frankly bullous lesions are rare. Very occasionally, patients develop large bullae on apparently normal skin, in the presence of typical papular lesions at other sites. There is an association of this variety of lichen planus with nasopharyngeal carcinoma.

Complications

Squamous cell carcinoma has been reported as an uncommon complication of longstanding mouth lesions and of chronic ulcerative lichen planus at other sites.

Diagnosis

▶ **Look for:**

■ violaceous flat-topped polygonal itchy papules that evolve to pigmented macules.
■ lacy white lines on buccal mucosa.

▶ **Consider and exclude**

■ *Lichen simplex chronicus* which, when on an ankle or leg, may closely resemble hypertrophic plaques of lichen planus. However, there are no papules in other areas, no mucosal changes and the histological features are different.

■ *Granuloma annulare* which may imitate the annular lesion of lichen planus, but is not itchy, lacks the characteristic papules elsewhere and is distinguishable histologically.

■ *Oral lesions* of leukoplakia, lupus erythematosus and secondary syphilis which may present white mucosal areas but do not develop the typical lacy pattern of lichen planus.

■ *Lesions of secondary syphilis* which are not generally itchy, often involve the palms and soles and may be confirmed serologically.

■ *Lichen nitidus,* the large lesions of which may mimic lichen planus. However, the more typical skin-coloured pinhead size papules arranged in groups are usually present and histology is confirmatory.

■ *Lichenoid drug eruptions.* These may be clinically and histologically indistinguishable. Although the distinction may not be jusitified, on biopsy there may be parakeratosis, a perivascular rather than bandlike infiltrate or eosinophils included in the infiltrate.

▶ **Special tests.** Biopsy is usually not required because the typical lesions are diagnostic but histology may confirm drug-induced lichen planus or may be required if unusual forms of lichen planus are suspected and typical papules are not present—for example, annular and hypertrophic lichen planus.

Treatment

The mainstay of therapy is with corticosteroids in one form or another. When lesions are few and cause little disturbance, reassurance may be sufficient. With more troublesome lesions, a topical fluorinated steroid often provides adequate relief. Hypertrophic areas may respond to the application of corticosteroids under plastic occlusion, or may need intralesional injections of triamcinolone or betamethasone.

Systemic steroids are suppressive, and may be necessary for severe, widespread disease which is unrelieved by topical therapy. Starting with 30 mg of prednisone daily, the dose should be rapidly reduced to the smallest amount adequate to maintain suppression. After six to eight weeks the drug should be gradually withdrawn, but may need to be recommenced for intolerable recurrences. Tender buccal lesions may be relieved by allowing pellets of hydrocortisone sodium succinate to dissolve slowly in the mouth, or by the use of intra-oral steroid spray. More persistent mucosal lesions may warrant intralesional or even systemic corticosteroid therapy. Surgical excision has been recommended for intractable ulceration of the mouth, and is advisable for chronic ulcerating lesions in other areas.

Severe extensive intractable lichen planus may sometimes necessitate the use of PUVA or oral retinoids, which are effective but, because of potential toxic effects, are not considered first-line treatments.

5

Vesiculobullous diseases

1. Epidermolysis bullosa
2. Pemphigus
   (a) pemphigus vulgaris
   (b) variants of pemphigus
3. Chronic benign familial pemphigus (Hailey–Hailey disease)
4. Pemphigoid
   (a) bullous pemphigoid
   (b) benign mucosal (cicatricial) pemphigoid
5. Dermatitis herpetiformis
6. Toxic epidermal necrolysis (Lyell's syndrome)

Blisters in the skin appear when layers separate and tissue fluid accumulates within the zone of cleavage. As a rough general rule, intra-epidermal blisters tend to contain clear fluid, break readily and heal without scarring, whereas subepidermal blisters are usually large, tense and stable, may contain bloodstained fluid, and heal with milia and scar formation. Classification of blistering diseases is usually based on aetiology which may be genetic, immunological or infective.

Epidermolysis bullosa

Pressure and friction of sufficient force and duration produce blisters in normal people. In some predisposed individuals, blisters can be induced by trauma which is inadequate to damage normal skin. This abnormal blistering after mechanical trauma occurs in a group of inherited diseases, collectively called epidermolysis bullosa. Sometimes the term 'mechanobullous diseases' is used because, in some varieties, blisters form beneath the epidermis rather than within it, as the name 'epidermolysis' may imply. When the bulla forms due to lysis of epidermal basal cells, there is no residual scarring—the non-dystrophic type. When the plane of cleavage is below the basement membrane, scarring and other changes follow—the dystrophic type. Blistering may also take place within the lamina lucida of the basement membrane (junctional type); this results in atrophy.

Electron microscopy of the dermo-epidermal junction, and monoclonal antibodies directed against antigens of the junctional zone, have enabled many varieties of this rare group of diseases to be better defined.

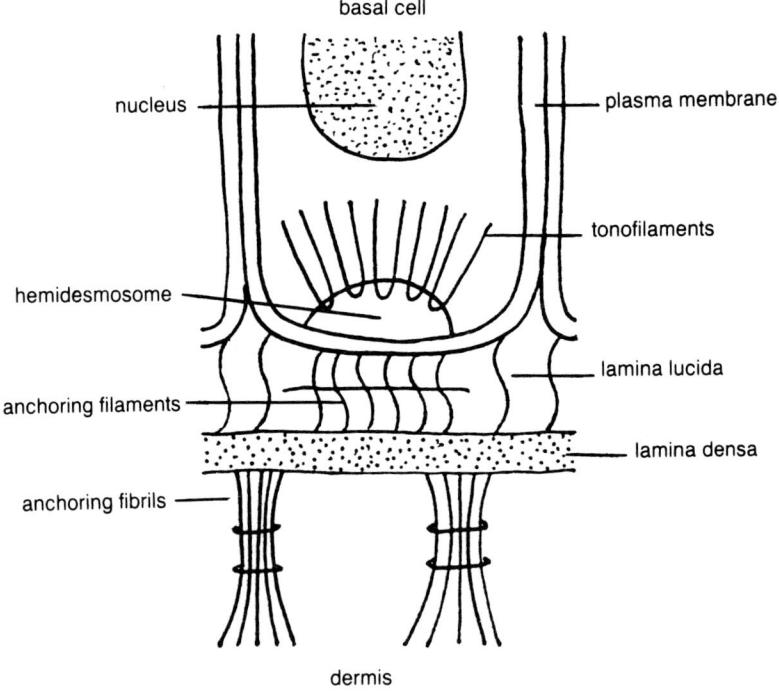

Basement membrane zone

Aetiology

The junctional forms are inherited as an autosomal recessive trait, the non-dystrophic forms are autosomal dominant, and the dystrophic varieties as both autosomal recessive and autosomal dominant. In general, the recessive forms are more severe.

The dystrophic forms have reduced or absent anchoring fibrils. In the dominant types, this abnormality is most commonly localised to the blistered areas, whereas in the recessive types anchoring fibrils are absent in both abnormal-looking and clinically unaffected skin. It is not yet known if this is a primary characteristic or secondary to other changes that occur. Patients with the recessive dystrophic forms also have fibroblasts that produce increased amounts of an altered but functional collagenase.

Most junctional forms show rudimentary hemidesmosomes which are few in number.

A rare acquired dystrophic form (epidermolysis bullosa acquisita) is well documented, with onset usually in the fifth or sixth decades of life. Immuno-electron microscopy demonstrates IgG deposits beneath the lamina densa of the basement membrane zone. The antibody is bound to type VII procollagen of anchoring fibrils. These patients give no family history of epidermolysis bullosa. There is a frequent association with serious systemic disease such as amyloidosis, lymphoma, myeloma and inflammatory bowel disease.

Histology

Light microscopy can demonstrate that the non-dystrophic forms are characterised by cleavage secondary to degeneration of cells in the lower epidermis, and that dystrophic forms are the result of subepidermal separation. However, what is revealed by special stains on light microscopy as the 'basement membrane' is in fact a part of the most superficial papillary dermis and therefore electron microscopy is required to diagnose the junctional forms.

Clinical features

■ *The non-dystrophic types* usually behave as a relatively mild disease. The commonest generalised form is usually evident at birth but may remain unsuspected until the child begins to crawl. Tense clear bullae develop at such sites of trauma as the elbows, knees, hands, and feet, or where the skin is rubbed by belt, shoes or garters. Blisters form without erythema and, after rupture, leave erosions which heal without scarring. Improvement during childhood is common, and abnormal blistering may cease entirely in adult life.

The commonest localised form is confined to the palms and soles and usually begins in childhood or early adult life. Some cases are only unmasked by unusual trauma such as that associated with prolonged marching or vigorous clapping. *(Colour plate 13)*

■ *Junctional epidermolysis bullosa* also has two main varieties. A severe type manifests at birth, with large raw areas, mainly on the trunk and within and around the mouth. Most of the affected children die from severe infection within the first two years of life.

The other form also begins at birth. Blisters are large and may contain bloodstained fluid. They are most severe in the arms and legs but also occur on the trunk. With time the affected skin becomes atrophic, hair growth becomes sparse and nails and teeth become dystrophic. However, there is no scarring or milia formation. The disease may become milder later in adult life.

■ *Dominant dystrophic forms* have their onset in early infancy. Blisters are generalised but involvement is most pronounced over knees and elbows, and hands and feet. Healing is with scarring and milia formation. In one variety scars are hypertrophic but in another type scars are atrophic and white papules appear in areas that have not blistered. Nails are dystrophic but teeth are normal. These forms are compatible with long life, although squamous cell carcinoma can occur in areas of blistering.

■ *Recessive dystrophic epidermolysis bullosa (Colour plate 14)* has as its most common type a very extensive and mutilating expression. The disease begins at birth. Blisters are large and often bloodstained. Milia are present. Healing is with extensive atrophic scars that may fuse the fingers and toes together. Mucous membranes are usually involved, producing strictures that complicate feeding. There is scarring alopecia, nail dystrophy and malformed teeth. Eye involvement is common. Squamous cell carcinoma develops in scars. Survival beyond the third decade is uncommon.

Diagnosis

The clinical setting usually allows the diagnosis of epidermolysis bullosa to be made with little difficulty. The exact variety is established on the basis of clinical signs, genetic history, and examination of biopsy material using light microscopy, electron microscopy, immunofluorescence techniques and monoclonal antibodies.

Prenatal diagnosis can be achieved using foetoscopy to obtain foetal skin. However, the procedure should be delayed until the seventeenth week because the antigens and structures looked for may not all have developed until then.

Treatment

Infants with epidermolysis bullosa should be admitted to hospital for assessment and early management. Severely affected infants need careful handling and feeding, and protection from all forms of trauma. In these patients the administration of corticosteroids may be lifesaving but large doses are needed. Diphenylhydantoin, sufficient to achieve blood levels greater than 8ug/mL, is reported to produce significant improvement in almost 70 per cent of patients with recessive dystrophic disease. The clinical response may reflect the impaired collagenase activity demonstrable in explants of human skin exposed to the drug. Eroded areas benefit from corticosteroid applications, and appropriate therapy is frequently necessary for secondary bacterial infection or for superadded moniliasis. Furniture and clothing may need to be padded as the child begins to crawl. Suitable physiotherapy and plastic surgery may be necessary to prevent and relieve contractures and deformities. All varieties of epidermolysis bullosa blister more readily at high temperatures, and patients and carers should be made aware of this. For mildly affected patients, avoidance of trauma, careful selection of clothing and footwear, and a suitable occupation may be sufficient to permit a nearly normal life.

Pemphigus

Pemphigus is a group of diseases characterised by intra-epidermal bulla formation, following dissolution and disappearance of intercellular connections (acantholysis). In all variants of the disease there are circulating antibodies with specificity for an intercellular antigen. In vivo binding of these antibodies occurs at the site of epidermal pathology, and is accompanied by complement fixation. When demonstrated by immunofluorescence, the antibodies produce a characteristic intercellular pattern.

Pemphigus vulgaris

Aetiology

It is likely that auto-antibodies are directly involved in the pathogenesis of lesions. They are present in virtually all cases, bind in vivo to the site of early histological change, and show some correlation of titre with the severity of disease. Antibodies of the IgG class taken from the serum of patients with pemphigus vulgaris induce histologically similar lesions in human skin explants, and reproduce the human disease in neonatal mice. There is a significant association of pemphigus vulgaris with myasthenia gravis, thymoma, and systemic lupus erythematosus.

An eruption which closely resembles pemphigus foliaceus or, less often, pemphigus vulgaris may complicate therapy with either penicillamine, captopril or rifampicin. These drug-induced analogues of pemphigus add support to a suggested immunological basis for the spontaneous disease.

Histology

Acantholysis is characteristic but not diagnostic of pemphigus. Individual cells of the epidermis become rounded as tonofilaments detach from desmosomes and form clumps around the nucleus. Acantholytic cells are no longer drawn together by desmosomes and become detached from one another, floating free in the accumulating fluid as individual cells or in small clusters.

In pemphigus vulgaris, acantholysis occurs in the lowest layers of the stratum spinosum, while the basal cells remain attached to the dermis at the floor of the developing bulla. A variable infiltrate of leucocytes, most commonly eosinophils, may appear within the epidermis.

Clinical features (Colour plate 15)

The patient is usually middle-aged and often Jewish. In Australia, the incidence appears greater among those of Southern European extraction.

■ *Individual lesions* begin as tense or flaccid bullae, which arise on apparently normal or sometimes erythematous skin. The blisters break easily and rarely become large. Blister fluid is usually clear at first, but may become pustular or haemorrhagic before rupture. Erosions form and extend peripherally, often with a shaggy epidermal collarette around the margins. The erosions are tender, and painful with movement, with little tendency to heal. With acute disease, bullae may not be apparent, and the epidermis just slides away from the border of expanding erosions.

■ *Distribution of lesions.* Onset may be acute, with a wide scatter of bullae and erosions, but the disease often remains localised to a single region for months before becoming generalised. In about half of the patients the initial area is the mouth, where blisters break easily and are seldom seen, the patient presenting with painful erosions and dysphagia. Crusted erosions frequently form around the nose, mouth and eyes, and the intertriginous and pressure areas are often severely affected.

Course

Pemphigus vulgaris may begin insidiously with a few persistent lesions, or may be generalised from the outset with rapid progression. Complete spontaneous remission is rare. Persistent, stable low grade mucosal disease does occur but, most commonly, untreated patients progress over months or years, with exacerbations and partial remissions, to widespread involvement and death. With adequate therapy, the mortality has now been reduced to less than 25 per cent.

Complications

- Dysphagia and general debility
- Intercurrent infection
- Severe toxaemia
- Hypo-albuminaemia
- Side effects of therapy, including septicaemia and thrombo-embolism.

Diagnosis

▶ **Suspect** pemphigus in the patient with flaccid blisters that break easily to form erosions that do not heal, especially if there are also erosions on the buccal mucosa.

▶ **Consider and exclude**

- ***Bullous erythema multiforme***, which may resemble the more acute onset of pemphigus vulgaris, is usually associated with fever, 'target' lesions and involvement of the hands and feet, which is uncommon in pemphigus.
- ***Bullous pemphigoid*** has larger tense bullae with less persistent erosions. Biopsy reveals separation at the dermo-epidermal junction without acantholysis.
- ***Cicatricial pemphigoid*** lesions heal with scarring.

▶ **Confirm** the diagnosis by histology and immunofluorescence studies.

Treatment

The course of pemphigus vulgaris is variable and guides the approach to treatment. Rapidly progressing extensive disease is a threat to life and is best managed in hospital. Initial treatment is with 120 mg of prednisolone per day. The appearance of new blisters five days later indicates an increase in dose by another 60 mg and this regimen is continued until blistering stops. If the dose of 240 mg of prednisolone per day is reached and new blisters are still appearing, pulse therapy with 1 gram of prednisolone intravenously per day for five days usually controls the disease. Oral prednisolone is maintained until the majority of erosions have healed and then the corticosteroid dose is rapidly tapered to 60 mg prednisolone per day, from which stage reduction takes place very gradually. Cytotoxic drugs have a delayed onset of action of about six to eight weeks and can be introduced at this stage if there is concern regarding possible corticosteroid toxicity. Cyclophosphamide, azathioprine and methotrexate are all effective.

Patients who present with stable, moderate extent pemphigus can be treated with intermediate dose corticosteroid (60 mg prednisolone per day) in combination with one of the cytotoxic drugs. When disease activity is suppressed, dosage can be reduced with the aim of achieving low dose immunosuppressive treatment and alternate day prednisolone. Plasmapheresis to remove the antibody, plus cyclophosphamide to minimise resynthesis of the antibody, is another treatment helpful in this group of patients.

Gold is usually limited to stable minimal extent pemphigus vulgaris because it is not potent and has a six to eight week delay until effect is noticed. In this variety of pemphigus, dapsone is occasionally helpful.

These two treatments are also sometimes used as adjuvant treatments, together with other modalities.

Spontaneous resolution of pemphigus is rare and most people require life-long supressive therapy.

Variants of pemphigus

■ *Pemphigus vegetans* may be regarded as pemphigus vulgaris in a patient with unusual resistance to the disease. Denuded areas evolve to hypertrophic lesions with vegetative granulation tissue, which is often studded with vesicles or pustules. Despite the more protracted course, most untreated patients eventually succumb to the disease.

■ *Pemphigus foliaceus* results from acantholytic cleavage at the level of the stratum granulosum. Blisters are small, fragile and not always apparent. After rupture, the blisters produce shallow erosions which are soon covered with small, fine scales, attached at one side in a peculiar, leafy fashion. Generally beginning on the face, neck and upper trunk, the disease may progress to generalised exfoliative dermatitis.

■ *Pemphigus erythematosus* is a curious disease, combining clinical and histological features of both pemphigus foliaceus and lupus erythematosus. Histologically the disease is pemphigus foliaceus but, with immunofluorescence microscopy, lesions reveal deposits of immunoglobulin at the dermoepidermal junction, as seen with lupus erythematosus, as well as the intercellular antibody pattern of pemphigus foliaceus. Some patients have significant titres of circulating antinuclear antibodies, and a few have developed frank systemic lupus erythematosus.

Benign familial chronic pemphigus
(Hailey-Hailey disease)

As in pemphigus, lesions of Hailey-Hailey disease develop from acantholytic cleavage in the lower epidermis. The diseases are otherwise unrelated.

Aetiology

There is a genetically determined epidermal fragility, transmitted as an autosomal dominant defect, as a result of which the epidermis responds abnormally to friction. The role of bacteria in precipitation of lesions is not well understood, but staphylococci can frequently be recovered from intact vesicles, and temporary improvement usually follows therapy with systemic antibiotics.

Histology

The acantholysis is more extensive but less complete than in lesions of pemphigus vulgaris. Many cells in the lower epidermis are only partially separated, which produces a characteristic 'dilapidated brick wall' appearance. In addition, there is some dyskeratosis of individual cells.

71

Clinical features

■ *Typical lesions* begin as clustered, clear, thin-walled, flaccid vesicles, sometimes on an erythematous base. The vesicles quickly become turbid and rupture, leaving a crusted patch of coalesced erosions. Patches tend to extend peripherally, usually with a well-defined, often frankly vesicular border. The central area may heal with some residual hyperpigmentation, or may persist as oozing granulation with areas of warty thickening.

■ *Typical sites* include the axillae, groins and perianal region, as well as the sides and back of the neck. Recurrences tend to involve the same areas repeatedly, so that one patient may have recurrent patches in both groins, or on the neck and trunk, while another suffers recurrences only in the axillae.

Course

The onset is usually in young adults, most often during the humid summer months. The disease may clear completely in cooler weather, only to recur with increased sweating and maceration of the flexures in summer. The disease follows a fluctuating course of exacerbations and remissions, with little tendency to clear with increasing age.

Diagnosis

▶ **Suspect** the disease in the patient with a chronic recurrent intertrigo.

▶ **Consider** the following diseases, which sometimes may only be definitely excluded by biopsy.

■ *Tinea* may be difficult to distinguish clinically. Look for the inflamed margin and examine skin scrapings microscopically.

■ *Seborrhoeic dermatitis* is less sharply demarcated, is not frankly vesicular and has a different histological appearance.

■ *Histiocytosis X* usually has a petechial component. Biopsy reveals the characteristic cells in the upper reticular dermis.

■ *Darier's disease* often has papules evident, and nail changes when present are a helpful sign. Biopsy reveals acantholytic cells only in a suprabasal location.

■ *Psoriasis* in the flexures has a glazed red appearance. Signs are often present elsewhere.

■ *Subcorneal pustular dermatosis* is a very uncommon inflammatory dermatosis, encountered most often in middle-aged women. Successive waves of flaccid pustules are replaced by superficial crusts or leafy scales. The eruption generally affects the major flexures and may resemble Hailey–Hailey disease clinically. However, the primary lesion is a pustule rather than a vesicle, there is usually an associated monoclonal gammopathy (typically IgA), and histology is that of a spongiform pustule.

▶ **Confirm** the diagnosis by biopsy and exclude true pemphigus by obtaining negative results using immunofluorescent antibody techniques.

Treatment

Systemic antibiotics provide the most effective therapy and should be prescribed according to the results of culture and sensitivity testing. Mild cases may respond to topical antibacterial agents. Therapy with systemic corticosteroids is effective, but inadvisable in the doses which are necessary to maintain suppression. For severe, intractable disease affecting limited areas, surgical excision and split-thickness grafting may provide very useful relief, although minor recurrences are common at the periphery of the graft.

Pemphigoid

Bullous pemphigoid

Bullous pemphigoid is a relatively benign chronic blistering disease, mainly of elderly people. Bullae form just below the basal layer, so that the blister roof is thick, being formed by the whole of the epidermis.

Aetiology

More than 80 per cent of patients are older than 60 years, but occasional cases occur in children. Most patients with active disease have serum antibodies which react with a transmembrane antigen within hemidesmosomes and the underlying upper portion of the lamina lucida of the basement membrane of skin. In vivo binding occurs at the dermo-epidermal junction with fixation of complement, but the antibody titre does not correlate well with the clinical course. Bullous pemphigoid has been reported as a rare complication of frusemide therapy and of PUVA treatment of psoriasis.

Histology

It is important that the biopsy be taken from an early blister, preferably a small one which can be excised intact. Regeneration is so rapid that in lesions already present for a few days the split may appear to be intra-epidermal.

Bullae develop just below the basal layer within the lamina lucida. On light microscopy, the epidermis is lifted by accumulating fluid, the basement membrane remaining attached to the dermis at the floor of the blister. Bullae contain coagulated serum and a variable number of leucocytes with a high percentage of eosinophils. Within the dermis there may be a heavy inflammatory infiltrate containing many eosinophils, or there may be no infiltrate at all.

Direct immunofluorescence demonstrates a homogenous band of antibody deposited in the basement membrane zone of normal-looking skin surrounding the blister.

Clinical features *(Colour plate 16)*

■ *Bullae* are multiple, thick-walled and tense. They are round, oval or pear-shaped, and may reach 5 cm or more in diameter. The blister fluid is usually clear and viscid, but may become haemorrhagic. The bullae arise on normal or erythematous skin, and are sometimes resorbed without breaking. When rupture occurs, the erosions, unlike those of pemphigus, heal well with little tendency to peripheral extension.

■ *Distribution of lesions* is typically over the abdomen and flexor surfaces of the limbs, but may be haphazard over the whole skin surface. Bullae may be confined to a single region for months before spreading to other areas and, occasionally, never spread beyond the initial area of involvement.

■ *Mucosal lesions* are uncommon and arise as small firm blisters, usually on the buccal mucosa. Although somewhat tender, they do not produce the severe discomfort of pemphigus involving the mouth.

Course

The onset is usually gradual, often with a nonspecific urticarial or eczematoid rash on the extremities. This early premonitory phase may persist for weeks before bullae begin to appear. The subsequent course is chronic over many months or years, but the disease is eventually self-limiting. Even without treatment the mortality is not high, except in feeble patients who are prone to bronchopneumonia or other intercurrent illness.

As association with visceral malignancy has been claimed. If the association is valid, bullous pemphigoid must be a rare presentation of internal neoplasm.

Diagnosis

▶ **Consider and exclude**

■ *Bullous erythema multiforme* occurs at a younger age, mucosal lesions are almost invariably present and systemic disturbance is marked.

■ *Dermatitis herpetiformis* also affects younger patients, is polymorphous and symmetrical, and is intensely itchy.

■ *Stasis dermatitis and urticaria* resemble the early changes in some cases of developing pemphigoid.

■ *Herpes gestationis* occurs during pregnancy.

■ *Bullous insect bites* appear in the elderly but are usually localised to the legs, and non-bullous lesions are often found elsewhere.

Treatment

Corticosteroid suppression can generally be achieved with initial doses of 40 mg to 60 mg of prednisone daily. Occasional patients are less responsive. For these, the addition of azathioprine or another immunosuppressive drug may avoid the need for very high doses of steroid. For most patients, however, prednisone is sufficient and can be reduced fairly quickly to maintenance levels of 10 mg to 15 mg daily. After three to four months of suppressive therapy, withdrawal should be attempted and will often be followed by a sustained remission.

Occasionally, when the disease has a prominent urticarial component and histology reveals an intense inflammatory infiltrate, pemphigoid will respond to oral erythromycin and high dose nicotinamide.

Benign mucosal pemphigoid (cicatricial pemphigoid) *(Colour plate 17)*

Like bullous pemphigoid, this rare chronic blistering disease predominantly affects elderly people. As in bullous pemphigoid, blisters develop beneath the basal epidermal cells but the zone of cleavage involves the lower portion of the lamina lucida and the basal lamina. Therefore blisters have a marked tendency to heal with scarring.

Although not life-threatening the disease leads to serious complications. The oral mucosa is involved in most patients, and may be the only site for many months. The conjunctivae are affected in 75 per cent and the skin in about one-third of patients. Conjunctival vesicles are small and inconspicuous, but scarring may lead to conjunctival adhesions, entropion, and to vascularisation and opacity of the cornea. At other sites, scarring may result in distortion of the pharynx, larynx, and oesophagus, and stenosis of the anogenital orifices.

Direct immunofluorescence will reveal the antibody deposited in the basement membrane zone but titres of circulating antibody are very low and testing may be interpreted as negative.

Treatment

Treatment cannot reverse the scarring. Orally administered dapsone reduces activity of the disease but there is a delay of about three months before response can be noted and from then on there is a slow and gradual improvement evident as a reduction in the amount of blistering. Dapsone is excreted by the kidneys, and as renal function is often reduced in the elderly patients who typically have this disease, the dose should begin much lower than is usual for dermatitis herpetiformis.

Dermatitis herpetiformis

Dermatitis herpetiformis is an uncommon, intensely itchy eruption of unknown cause, most often seen in young to middle-aged men. Although lesions are at least microscopically vesicular, frank blistering is not a prominent feature of the disease.

Aetiology

Most, if not all, patients with dermatitis herpetiformis have a patchy, partial or subtotal villous atrophy of the jejunal mucosa, closely resembling the changes seen with coeliac disease. Patients with dermatitis herpetiformis and those with coeliac disease share an increased frequency of histocompatibility antigens HLA-B8, DRW3 and DQW2. Dermatitis herpetiformis is accompanied by deposition of IgA and complement at the site of developing lesions, and at the dermo-epidermal junction of clinically uninvolved skin.

However, indirect immunofluorescence fails to detect a circulating antibody directed against components of skin even though there may be other antibodies present in high titre directed against gliadin, smooth muscle endomysium, reticulin, or thyroid antigens.

The enteropathy associated with dermatitis herpetiformis is usually mild, producing a biochemical steatorrhoea that is rarely apparent clinically. It responds to a gluten-free diet, but the link between the skin disease and enteropathy is not well understood. It has been suggested that the immunological reactions in the small bowel lead to the formation of immune complexes that are deposited in skin, where they induce lesions.

Histology

The characteristic lesion develops high in the dermal papillae. The tips of papillae become oedematous and infiltrated with neutrophils and a varying number of oesinophils to form small papillary abscesses. Fluid accumulates and vesicles develop from coalescence of several papillary foci. Direct immunofluorescence reveals granular deposits of IgA at the tips of the dermal papillae in the normal skin surrounding the vesicles.

Clinical features

- *Typical lesions* begin with burning itch, as clustered reddish papules or small vesicles develop on an urticarial or erythematous base. Some papules are surmounted by a tiny vesicle, but scratching soon reduces the area to an erythematous patch of crusted papules and nondescript excoriations. Bullae are rare, except in recurrences after cessation of treatment. Healing leaves temporary hyperpigmentation, but scarring is slight.

- *Distribution* is bilateral and often strikingly symmetrical. The extensor surfaces of knees, elbows and forearms, the shoulders, scapular region, buttocks, and particularly the skin around the natal cleft, are frequently involved. The scalp is commonly affected, but the face is usually spared.

Course

This is fluctuating but chronic and, without treatment, is likely to extend over many years.

Diagnosis

▶ **Consider and exclude**

- *Scabies*, which rarely affects the scalp, except in infants, but frequently involves the genital area. A careful search usually reveals a characteristic lesion between the fingers or elsewhere.

- *Papular urticaria* differs histologically and lacks the characteristic deposition of IgA in clinically uninvolved skin of patients with dermatitis herpetiformis.

- *Nummular dermatitis* tends to produce more discrete plaques. Distribution is usually more peripheral and seldom shows the typical mirror-image symmetry of dermatitis herpetiformis. Biopsy differentiates doubtful cases.

- *Linear IgA disease* is a blistering disorder in which a homogenous linear band of IgA is deposited at the dermo-epidermal junction. Although separation occurs at the dermo-epidermal junction, blisters are typically large. Occasionally small vesicles occur around the rim of polycyclic erythematous areas. In the childhood variant, blisters are usually localised to the buttocks, upper thighs and pubic region. Unlike dermatitis herpetiformis, mucosal lesions are common and there is no enteropathy. However, there is dramatic clearing with dapsone.

- *Bullous lupus erythematosus* may present as grouped vesicles on an erythematous base, produce the same histology and IgA deposition as dermatitis herpetiformis, and may even respond to dapsone. However, this disorder is seen only during active systemic lupus erythematosus and usually involves the trunk. Direct immunofluorescent testing of skin shows the additional immunoreactant deposition pattern typical of systemic lupus erythematosus.

■ *Other bullous eruptions* are rarely a source of confusion. Bullous erythema multiforme has an acute onset with systemic features, and oral lesions are almost invariably present. Bullous pemphigoid is distributed more to the flexor surfaces, with large monomorphic bullae.

Treatment

Dapsone is dramatically effective in the great majority, but the frequency of haemolytic anaemia warrants a cautious approach. Treatment should be preceded by a haemoglobin estimation, blood count, and exclusion of glucose-6-phosphate dehydrogenase deficiency. Starting with 50 mg daily, the dose is increased to the minimal level adequate for suppression. Regular haematological monitoring is necessary and, from time to time, attempts should be made to withdraw the drug gradually, in the hope of a sustained remission. Other sulphones such as sulphapyridine are also effective but they are difficult to obtain and also require haematological monitoring. Topical therapy is relatively ineffective, although with the application of corticosteroid creams, the dose of dapsone necessary for suppression may be reduced.

The importance of a gluten-free diet in the management of dermatitis herpetiformis remains controversial. There seems no doubt that the enteropathy improves with the diet. In some cases avoidance of gluten leads to control with a reduced dose of dapsone and occasionally the manifestations of dermatitis herpetiformis can resolve completely. However, those who have had the skin changes clear have been on the diet for six to twelve months before improvement was noted. As the diet is difficult to follow, most patients become discouraged and reject the diet.

Toxic epidermal necrolysis (Lyell's syndrome)

The distinctive appearance of toxic epidermal necrolysis, with large areas of tender erythema which progress to epidermal separation as if by scalding, produces a characteristic clinical picture well described as the 'scalded skin syndrome'.

Aetiology

In children, there is generally a preceding infection with *Staphylococcus aureus*, commonly of phage group 2. Organisms of this group produce an exotoxin which reproduces the disease in laboratory animals. A clinically similar syndrome occasionally complicates drug therapy, especially with sulphonamides, phenylbutazone, barbiturates and allopurinol. In some patients, viral infections have preceded the reaction, while in others no cause is apparent.

Histology

In the staphylococcal form, splitting of the epidermis develops immediately below the stratum granulosum, with little associated inflammatory change in or beneath the epidermis. In the non-staphylococcal type, the whole affected epidermis is necrotic and blister formation subepidermal.

Clinical features

- **_Prodromal phase._** The staphylococcal type is rare after the sixth year, although a few cases have been reported in adults who are immunosupressed or who are unable to excrete the toxin due to hepatic or renal insufficiency. There is often purulent conjunctivitis or a discharging ear for a day or two before the onset, and many patients have pharyngitis. As the skin begins to change, there is fever and toxaemia, but patients who are more than one year old generally appear fretful and miserable rather than seriously ill. Septicaemia can occur, but is rare. The onset in adults is more abrupt, with pain and tenderness at the site of developing lesions.

- **_The cutaneous phase_** usually commences in the large flexures or around the orifices, where large areas of skin become red and tender. Affected skin may be confined to a few patches, or may spread to involve most of the surface. The mucosae are involved in more than one-third of patients, but there is relative sparing of hair-bearing areas. Flaccid bullae may be superimposed, or the epidermis may simply become sodden and crinkled, separating in sheets without recognisable blisters. In badly affected infants, the whole skin takes on a 'boiled lobster' appearance.

Course

Healing occurs in one to two weeks without scarring, unless secondary infection has been added. Especially in children, marked desquamation follows the acute phase and may continue as a scaly exfoliation for 10 to 14 days. The prognosis is relatively good for children with the staphylococcal type, but the disease is more serious during the first year of life, especially with involvement of areas greater than half the skin surface. Patients with the non-staphylococcal form have a reported mortality of 25 per cent or more. Worrying features include widespread involvement, mucosal lesions, and extremes of age.

Diagnosis

▶ **Consider and exclude**

- **_Bullous erythema multiforme_**, which is characterised by discrete blisters which lack the shreddy epidermal separation of toxic epidermal necrolysis. Nevertheless, there is considerable overlap between these two diseases.

- **_Bullous impetigo_** may be confirmed by Gram stain of a smear from eroded areas, but staphylococcal impetigo may precede and accompany toxic epidermal necrolysis.

- **_Severe epidermolysis bullosa_** in infants may resemble toxic epidermal necrolysis, but there is no prodromal phase, no early toxaemia, and the bullae arise on clinically normal skin.

Treatment

In infants and children, the associated staphylococcal infection is treated with flucloxacillin.

Administration of systemic corticosteroids may be advisable for the drug-induced type, but would be inappropriate for children with the staphylococcal syndrome. Attention to fluid and electrolyte balance, careful nursing, and prevention of ocular complications are important whatever the cause.

6

Disorders of pigmentation

1. Localised hyperpigmentation
2. Generalised hyperpigmentation
3. Localised hypopigmentation
4. Generalised hypopigmentation
5. Poikiloderma
6. Abnormal pigmentation not due to melanin

The dominant component of normal skin colour is provided by melanin. In the epidermis melanin contributes shades of brown or black which, under Wood's light, look even darker. Dermal melanin imparts a bluish colour which does not change when examined under long wavelength ultraviolet light. Oxygenated blood adds a pink or reddish hue and, in some areas, carotene imparts a faint yellow tinge. Without melanin, however, the skin is pink or milky white.

The capacity for the synthesis of melanin is genetically determined, but is modified by endocrine and local factors. Melanocyte-stimulating hormone (MSH) and, to a lesser extent, adrenocorticocotrophic hormone (ACTH) promote melanogenesis, with darkening of skin colour. Oestrogen and progesterone also stimulate melanin production, but some areas are more susceptible, particularly the nipples, areolae, genital skin, and linea alba. Testosterone appears to be involved, pale skin and inability to tan being characteristic of the eunuch. Of the local factors which influence melanocyte function, by far the most important is exposure to ultraviolet light.

Disorders of pigmentation are mainly disorders of melanin synthesis or distribution. Those which are most frequently found are listed above.

Localised hyperpigmentation

Freckles and lentigines

The freckle is a small brown macule, coloured by abundant epidermal melanin without any increase in the number of melanocytes. Freckles occur only on light-exposed skin and tend to darken in summer and fade in winter. The brown to black colour of lentigines is also produced by epidermal melanin, but in the lentigo there is an increased number of melanocytes scattered along the basal layer.

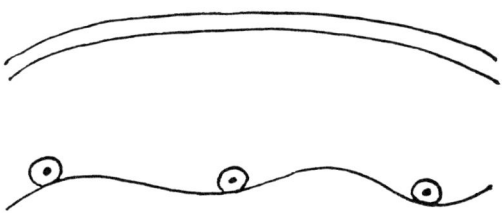

Melanocytes in normal skin and freckle

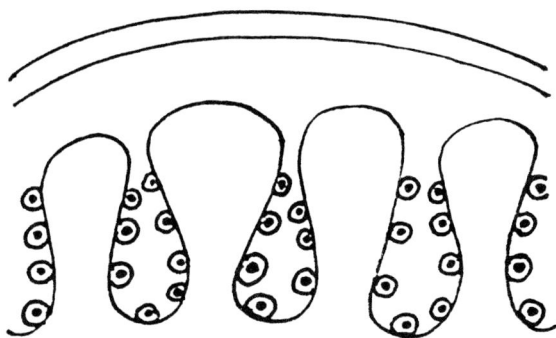

Simple lentigo

Lentigines are small, rounded, brown to black areas, which may coalesce to form macules or slightly elevated lesions, a centimetre or more across. They are very common, most white-skinned children having twenty or thirty lentigines distributed in a haphazard fashion over the surface. They usually appear in childhood, but may erupt during pregnancy or with elevated levels of ACTH. There is no seasonal variation of colour, and distribution is not confined to light-exposed areas. However, light can induce their appearance. Lentigines often appear in the sundamaged skin of the elderly, and are also a feature of long-term PUVA therapy.

Lentiginosis syndromes

In some families, multiple lentigines are inherited as an autosomal dominant characteristic. The distribution may be generalised or restricted to the centrofacial area. Various developmental defects, particularly of the central nervous system, have been described in association with either type.

■ *The 'leopard syndrome'* is one such variant of generalised lentiginosis in which the outstanding features of the syndrome are summarised in mnemonic fashion by the designation 'leopard': Lentiginosis, Electrocardiographic changes, Ocular hypertelorism, Pulmonary stenosis, Abnormalities of the genitalia, Retardation of growth, and Deafness.

■ *Peutz–Jeghers syndrome.* The Peutz–Jeghers syndrome is the association of intestinal polyposis, usually confined to the small bowel, with multiple mucocutaneous lentigines. The syndrome is inherited as an autosomal dominant trait, but there is a significant incidence of sporadic cases. In some patients only part of the syndrome is expressed, and carriers may be asymptomatic.

The lentigines are usually noticed early in life and are distributed over the fingers and toes, the lips, around the mouth, nose and ears, and on the hard palate, gums and buccal mucosa. They tend to become more prominent during childhood but may fade in adult life, with the exception of those in the mouth, which persist unchanged.

Polyps of the small intestine lead to episodes of severe colicky pain, believed to be due to transient incomplete intussusception. Management should generally be conservative, but surgical relief is sometimes necessary. Haematemesis and melaena are less frequent complications. Polypoid lesions of the stomach, duodenum and colon are occasionally present, and may undergo malignant change.

Mongolian spots

Mongolian spots are poorly defined, slate grey to brownish macules, present at birth, which generally occur over the lumbosacral region or buttocks. Up to 10 per cent of Australian infants have one or more of these macules, and the incidence exceeds 80 per cent in infants born to black or oriental parents. The naevus darkens in colour for a time after birth, but later fades and usually disappears completely before the child is 10 years old.

Histologically, the macule is composed of spindle-shaped melanocytes which lie deep in the dermis, parallel to the surface. Similar dermal deposits of melanocytes may occur, most often in oriental females, over the forehead and periorbital region on one side of the face ('naevus of Ota') and frequently involve the sclera on that side.

Hereditary syndromes with hyperpigmentation

Pigmented (*'café au lait'*) macules are a regular feature of neurofibromatosis and Albright's syndrome, and are commonly present in tuberous sclerosis. Pigmentation may be mottled or diffuse in Fanconi's syndrome, or form a reticulate pattern in Rothmund–Thomson and other rare hereditary syndromes.

Pigmentary changes are a relatively minor component of these diseases, but are the outstanding feature of another inherited disorder, incontinentia pigmenti.

Incontinentia pigmenti

This is an uncommon disorder, almost completely confined to girls. The disease develops through three overlapping phases to culminate in a spectacular pattern of pigmentation, often accompanied by other ectodermal abnormalities.

■ *Cutaneous changes* usually begin soon after birth as irregular linear erythematous bands, often with superimposed bullae. This early inflammatory eruption is gradually replaced by warty, hyperkeratotic plaques, which slowly flatten over a few months. During, or soon after, the hypertrophic phase, an irregular pattern of pigmented streaks and whorls develops. The appearance is bizarre and best described as resembling the coloured pattern in marble. The pigmentation is brown to slate-grey, and deepens over a few years before fading, usually completely, by the end of the second decade.

■ *Associated features.* The inflammatory phase often involves the scalp, leaving a residual patchy alopecia in about 25 per cent of patients. Nearly two-thirds of patients have other ectodermal defects involving the eyes, teeth or central nervous system.

Other causes of localised hyperpigmentation

Hyperpigmentation may follow any inflammatory process which involves the epidermis, particularly when the inflammation is centred about the basal layer. Post-inflammatory pigmentation is accompanied by release of melanin into the dermis, where it is engulfed by macrophages ('pigmentary incontinence'). Pigmentation is confined to the previously inflamed area and is often transitory, but may persist for months or years.

Post-inflammatory pigmentation may be a sequel to any pattern of dermatitis, but is characteristic of the phototoxic type. Continued handling of such phototoxic agents as creosote and tar may darken skin on the back of the hands and forearms. Degeneration of the basal layer is a feature of such diseases as lichen planus and cutaneous lupus erythematosus, so subsequent pigmentation is not surprising. Epidermal changes leading to hyperpigmentation may be secondary to pathological changes in the dermis, as in mastocytosis (urticaria pigmentosa) and the cutaneous lesions of porphyria, or may follow thermal, mechanical or other forms of injury by physical agents.

Endocrine and metabolic causes usually produce more generalised pigmentation, but there are two forms in which melanosis remains more or less localised—melasma and acanthosis nigricans.

Melasma (chloasma)

Melasma is a sepia to brown, blotchy melanosis, which is usually confined to symmetrical areas of the cheeks and forehead, but sometimes extends onto the upper lip, chin and neck. Although precipitated by sunlight, melasma appears to be endocrine-induced. It most frequently develops during pregnancy or in women taking the contraceptive pill, but occasionally occurs in women, and even men, without discoverable cause. Pigmentation indistinguishable from melasma is a rare complication of therapy with diphenylhydantoin.

Acanthosis nigricans

Acanthosis nigricans is a distinctive, pigmented thickening of the skin of large flexures, with a variable involvement of other areas. In most cases, acanthosis nigricans is a benign sequel to intertrigo in obese adolescents or adults, but may develop as a manifestation of pituitary or other endocrine disorders. It is occasionally inherited as an autosomal dominant characteristic, and is a rare complication of therapy with nicotinic acid, corticosteroids and diethylstilboestrol.

However, the appearance of acanthosis nigricans for the first time from middle age onwards, especially in a patient who is not obese, is a reliable pointer to malignant disease, often of the gastro-intestinal tract. The cutaneous changes usually develop in parallel with the neoplasm, but may precede its clinial onset, sometimes by years. Onset of acanthosis nigricans in adults necessitates a thorough search for visceral or lymphoreticular malignancy. When the disease appears for the first time after the fourth decade, the risk of malignant disease is so great that bronchoscopy and even laparotomy are justified when simpler investigations have been unrewarding.

■ **The benign form** is usually confined to intertriginous skin of the major flexures. There is no pruritus except that caused by intertrigo. Affected skin darkens and the skin markings are increased as a velvety thickening slowly develops. Warty or nodular swellings may be added as the colour deepens to dark brown or black.

■ **The malignant form** tends to be more severe and spreads beyond the large flexures. Pigmentation is not restricted to thickened skin and frequently involves the buccal mucosa. Pruritus is common, and pigmentation is progressive.

Generalised hyperpigmentation

Endocrine

Addison's disease is the prototype of the diffuse melanoses. Elevated levels of MSH and ACTH, unrestrained by adrenal feedback, lead to a generalised increase of melanogenesis. The increase is more apparent in areas where melanin synthesis is normally greater, as in light-exposed skin and areas of friction. The areolae, genital and flexural skin, palmar creases and developing scars all tend to be more deeply pigmented. Moles darken and lentigines may become more numerous. Hair colour may deepen, and the buccal mucosa is almost always spotted with black or bluish macules. The skin may darken to brown or black, but in fair-skinned patients there may be no more than a moderate tan, of a colour which is normal in healthy people of darker complexion.

Exogenous ACTH or its synthetic analogue, tetracosactrin, may cause hyperpigmentation indistinguishable from that of Addison's disease. Diffuse melanosis occurs in nearly half of those with acromegaly and in some patients with thyrotoxicosis. Addisonian pigmentation may develop in Cushing's syndrome, but more often follows therapeutic bilateral adrenalectomy. Increased pigmentation is the rule during pregnancy, particularly over the face, nipples, anogenital region and midline of the abdomen. A less pronounced pigmentation of similar pattern precedes menstruation in some women. A rare endocrine cause of generalised hyperpigmentation is phaeochromocytoma.

Metabolic and nutritional

Starvation and malabsorption may lead to patchy or diffuse hyperpigmentation, and melanosis complicates the jaundice of biliary cirrhosis. The pigmentation of haemochromatosis, renal and hepatic failure is at least partly due to increased melanin synthesis.

Connective tissue diseases

Lupus erythematosus, scleroderma and dermatomyositis may all be accompanied by hyperpigmentation, often diffuse and sometimes Addisonian in distribution.

Drugs

Pigmentation may be a non-specific sequel to drug eruptions, or may develop without a preceding rash. Cytotoxic agents, especially busulphan and, less often, cyclophosphamide, bleomycin and procarbazine may cause diffuse melanosis. Amiodorone and high doses of chlorpromazine may slowly produce a diffuse bluish-grey colour, more marked on light-exposed areas. Similar pigmentation may complicate therapy with chloroquine and hydroxychloroquine, often with pigmentation of the buccal mucosa and nail beds. The prolonged use of minocycline for the suppression of acne has occasionally been associated with a generalised muddy discolouration, but is more frequently reported as causing a bluish-black, macular pigmentation of acne scars and sites of inflammation of the face, chest and limbs.

Chronic intoxication with inorganic arsenic may cause diffuse pigmentation, sometimes dotted with small pale macules producing a characteristic 'raindrop' pattern. Silver salts are now a very rare cause, but large cumulative doses of gold salts lead to diffuse melanosis, more marked on light-exposed areas, with relative sparing of the flexures.

Lymphoma and carcinoma

Lymphoma and carcinoma may be accompanied by generalised darkening of the skin, usually in the late stages of the disease.

Localised hypopigmentation

In the scarred atrophic lesions of cutaneous lupus erythematosus and lichen sclerosus et atrophicus, melanocytes are destroyed and leucoderma is permanent. Similar depigmentation may develop in plaques of lupus vulgaris and after thermal or chemical burns; hypopigmentaion is a common feature of tuberculoid leprosy and may occur in healed lesions of secondary syphilis. The pallor of pityriasis alba and pityriasis versicolor is reversible and probably secondary to reduced melanin synthesis.

Chemical agents may reduce pigmentation by scarring or as a sequel to severe inflammation, but certain chemicals induce leucoderma in some individuals at the site of contact, without preceding inflammation. These chemicals, usually phenolic compounds, appear to exert a direct toxic effect on melanocytes. Monobenzyl ether of hydroquinone may cause a vitiligo-like leucoderma, not only at sites of direct contact but in apparently unexposed skin as well. Depigmentation in affected areas is total and frequently irreversible.

Some regressing melanocytic naevi develop a halo of leucoderma ('halo naevi'), which may persist after complete resolution of the naevi. Discrete macules of hypopigmentation may occur as congenital malformations, either alone or as part of such complex hereditary syndromes as tuberous sclerosis. A more common inherited cause of localised hypopigmentation is piebaldism, in which a white forelock is accompanied by circumscribed areas of leucoderma on the trunk and limbs.

Idiopathic guttate hypomelanosis

Idiopathic guttate hypomelanosis is a common pigmentary disorder in which small, white, circumscribed macules appear in areas of light-exposed skin, particularly the front of the legs.

From the outset, these white spots are about 0.5 cm to 1 cm across, and persist indefinitely without further change. They occur in both sexes from adolescence onwards, but with greater frequency in older people. Idiopathic guttate hypomelanosis is probably no more than one form of 'ageing' produced by the cumulative effect of ultraviolet irradiation from sunlight.

Vitiligo

Vitiligo is a common disease which affects more than 1 per cent of the population. About one-third of patients have a relative who also suffers from the disease, and it is likely that predisposition to vitiligo is inherited as an autosomal dominant characteristic. There is a significant association with pernicious anaemia, Addison's disease, thyroid dysfunction, uveitis and halo naevi, which suggests the possibility of an auto-immune mechanism.

Histology

Melanin and melanocytes are absent in mature lesions, but at the hyperpigmented borders melanin is increased and the melanocytes unduly large. As the melanocytes disappear, they are replaced by Langerhans cells. In early lesions there may be a dermal infiltrate of lymphocytes and histiocytes.

Clinical features

■ *Lesions* are round, oval or irregular white macules with a well-defined, often scalloped border. Extending lesions are usually surrounded by a band of hyperpigmentation, but the macules are themselves a uniform opaque white. Hairs in affected areas are usually white, but in early lesions pigment may persist in and around hairs, producing a spotty appearance.

■ *Distribution* is usually bilateral and roughly symmetrical, but may be unilateral and occasionally follows an approximately dermatomal pattern. Vitiligo may appear at any site, but has a predilection for skin over bony prominences, about the body orifices, the flexures and light-exposed areas.

Course

Onset may be at any age, but begins before the age of 20 in 50 per cent of patients. Lesions may slowly expand, coalesce to form large patches, and occasionally may involve most of the skin surface. In many, however, the macules soon reach a maximum size, with little change thereafter. Limited spontaneous regression is not uncommon, pigmentation spreading out from uninvolved follicles. Complete spontaneous repigmentation is very rare.

Complications

■ *Sunburn of the macules*, unprotected by melanin, is common and may be severe.

■ *Disfigurement* of normally dark-complexioned patients may be marked.

Diagnosis

▶ **Consider and exclude**

■ *Pityriasis alba* and *pityriasis versicolor*, which are distinguished by the light surface scale and incomplete depigmentation.

■ *Lichen sclerosus et atrophicus* and *morphoea* are palpable plaques, rather than macules as in vitiligo.

■ *Hypopigmented lesions of tuberculoid leprosy* are always anaesthetic.

■ *Post-inflammatory depigmentation* can be differentiated by history.

Treatment

When lesions are small and cosmetically insignificant, vitiligo is better left untreated. For ugly lesions on the face or hands, effective masking preparations are available. When all but a few small areas are involved, it is often more practical to achieve depigmentation of unaffected areas, using monobenzyl ether of hydroquinone, rather than to attempt repigmentation of the vitiligo.

Psoralens may be used with ultraviolet light to attempt repigmentation. Oral administration is better than topical preparations, and trimethylpsoralen (trisoralen) is more effective than the 8-methoxy compound. Activating wavelengths are in the UV-A range, so natural sunlight is quite suitable. The initial adult dose is 30 mg of trioxsalen followed after two hours by exposure to sunlight, beginning with ten minutes of exposure and gradually increasing to half an hour. The 'effective dose' is a product of drug dosage and duration of exposure to utraviolet radiation, so the patient should be protected from exposure to sunlight except during the treatment time. Because of a theoretical risk of cataract formation, the eyes need to be shielded by suitable sunglasses designed to incorporate side protection from UV-A. In experimental systems, psoralens are mutagenic and may be carcinogenic. Although there is no unequivocal evidence to relate these experimental findings to the clinical situation in humans, unnecessary exposure should be avoided, and this treatment should not be offered to those with past exposure to other carcinogens such as arsenic or X-ray therapy.

In countries with insufficient sunlight for adequate exposure, artificial sources of UV-A are used. Response to treatment begins as pigmented dots that are perifollicular. These dots then enlarge and coalesce.

Repigmentation is slow and unpredictable, and treatment may need to be continued for many months. A disadvantage of psoralen therapy is the increased pigmentation of normal skin during treatment, which accentuates the contrast with affected areas. Satisfactory repigmentation occurs in less than 25 per cent of light-skinned patients.

Generalised hypopigmentation

Some inherited disorders of amino acid metabolism are associated with diminished pigmentation of skin and hair, and poor ability to tan. In phenylketonuria there is a general dilution of colour, while pale skin and fair hair are characteristic of homocystinuria.

Albinism

Albinism is a heterogeneous cluster of disorders linked by an impaired capacity for melanin synthesis. Patients can be grouped on the basis of genetic transmission as:
1. X-linked recessive
    (a) ocular albinism
2. Autosomal recessive
    (b) oculocutaneous albinism
        (i)   tyrosinase-positive
        (ii) tyrosinase-negative
        (iii) variants
3. Autosomal dominant
    (c) oculocutaneous hypomelanism.

Ocular albinism

The skin and hair are pigmented normally, but affected males have translucency of the iris, defective pigmentation of the retina, nystagmus and photophobia. Female heterozygotes are less severely affected.

Oculocutaneous albinism

Individuals with oculocutaneous albinism demonstrate a generalised dilution of pigmentation in the skin, hair and eyes, despite normal numbers of melanocytes. Tyrosinase is absent in some patients and demonstrable in others, but the more severely affected are tyrosinase-negative. In the tyrosinase-positive form there is a tendency for pigmentation to increase with age, but in both types there is a partial or total absence of melanin in melanosomes. Inheritance is autosomal recessive and in heterozygotes the disease may be incompletely expressed.

Clinical features

■ *Hypopigmentation* is uniform and severe. In the very rare complete form, the skin completely lacks melanin. The hair is white, the skin pale pink or white, and the iris is pink. More commonly, albinism is incomplete, with yellowish hair, a pink or pale blue iris, and an abnormally pale skin. In black races, the incomplete form may produce colouring comparable to that of a normal Caucasian.

■ *Low tolerance to sunlight* is a feature, and the skin is easily sunburned. Wrinkling and 'senile' atrophy develop at an early age and, in tropical or subtropical regions, skin cancers may appear in the first decade.

■ *Associated features*. There is photophobia, with a squinting expression in bright light; refractive errors and nystagmus are common. Mental retardation, deafness and skeletal abnormalities are less frequent associations.

Variants

One rare variant of albinism presents changes indistinguishable from the tyrosinase-negative form at birth, but the hair gradually develops a reddish colour, the blue colour of the iris deepens a little, and patients have some limited capacity to tan with light exposure. There is a variant which includes pseudohaemophilia, another with deafness but normal eye colour, and a rare form associated with cataracts and serious defects of the central nervous system.

Management

There is no treatment available for albinism. Management is directed to protection of the vulnerable skin from the effects of sunlight, and to early detection and treatment of malignant and premalignant changes.

Oculocutaneous hypomelanism

In some families, relative hypomelanosis is transmitted as an autosomal dominant gene. The iris is pale blue, and the skin lighter in colour than that of unaffected siblings, but without the marked pallor of albinism.

Poikiloderma

Poikiloderma is a descriptive term applied to lesions in which there are atrophy, telangiectasia, and a blotchy or reticulate pattern of hyperpigmentation and hypopigmentation.

Congenital causes

Poikiloderma is a prominent feature of a few rare congenital diseases, particularly the Rothmund–Thomson syndrome.

Acquired causes

■ *Radiation*. In Australia, poikiloderma is a common expression of chronic solar damage, occurring mostly on the sides and front of the neck, particularly in women from middle age onwards. The affected skin is rather loose and atrophic, with reddish brown reticulate pigmentation and a variable degree of telangiectasia. Striking poikiloderma is a common feature of severe atrophy following X-ray therapy.

■ *Collagen diseases*. Poikiloderma may develop in cutaneous lesions of lupus erythematosus, and is characteristic of dermatomyositis.

■ *Prelymphomatous* mycosis fungoides and, less often, other reticuloses may be preceded by areas of poikiloderma, sometimes for years before the lymphoma becomes recognisable. The characteristic changes of poikiloderma may develop in association with parapsoriasis en plaques, or may arise as large patches without apparent cause over the buttocks, breast, trunk or large flexures. Lesions may extend slowly or remain unchanged, but increasing pruritus and areas of infiltration herald the transition to lymphoma.

Abnormal pigmentation not due to melanin

The yellow or yellowish green colour of jaundice is to some extent mimicked by the yellow skin of hypercarotenaemia. However, the bronze or greenish tint of jaundice is never produced by carotene, and the sclerae are not discoloured. The discoloration of hypercarotenaemia is most marked over the face, palms and soles, and usually follows ingestion of enormous quanitites of such carotene-rich foods as carrots, squash, spinach and oranges. Occasionally the cause is hyperlipoproteinaemia, as in uncontrolled diabetes mellitus or hypothyroidism. Skin may also be discoloured yellow by the ingestion of mepacrine or picric acid, but jaundice is excluded by the relative sparing of conjunctival and other mucous membranes.

The rusty brown staining of haemosiderin complicates stasis dermatitis and some forms of capillaritis, but the pigmentation of haemochromatosis, although associated with iron deposition, is due to melanin. A melanin-like pigment is deposited in the connective tissue and cartilage of patients with alkaptonuria (ochronosis) and may be visible over the ears, extensor tendons of the hands, forehead, eyelids and sclerae.

Tattoo

The tattoo is formed by the introduction of insoluble pigment into the dermis. Accidental tattooing of wounds may occur in road accidents, and occupational tattoos may develop, for example, on the knees of coal miners. However, the majority of tattoos are produced as a 'decorative' procedure, sought on impulse and soon regretted. When removal is requested, small, easily excised tattoos should be removed surgically. Dermatitis or granulomatous reactions caused by sensitivity to a pigment can only be cured by excision.

Larger lesions can often be removed by salabrasion—the superficial abrasion of skin by ordinary salt, rubbed over the area with a damp square of gauze. Tattoos can also be removed by dermabrasion using a high-speed rotary drill, or by the heat generated by a carbon dioxide laser. However, with both these modalities severe scarring may complicate inexpert techniques.

7

Acne vulgaris and rosacea

1. Acne vulgaris
2. Variants of acne
3. Rosacea
4. Perioral dermatitis

Acne vulgaris

Acne is a very common inflammatory disease of pilosebaceous follicles, largely confined to the face, neck, shoulders and upper trunk of adolescents and young adults.

Aetiology

The precise cause of acne is unknown, but post-pubertal levels of androgenic hormone are necessary for the disease to develop. The hypertrophy of sebaceous glands, which normally occurs as an early expression of puberty, sets the stage for subsequent change and appears to depend on the tissue androgen, dihydrotestosterone. Without androgen there is little if any sebum, and without sebum there is no acne.

Infants may develop acne following stimulation of sebaceous enlargement by maternal androgens, but the disease does not otherwise affect normal prepubertal children; nor does it occur in untreated eunuchs. Acne is aggravated by the administration of testosterone and reduced by large doses of oestrogen. As a group, patients with acne produce more sebum than normal controls, and lesions are more densely distributed to areas of greater sebum production.

Acne, however, is more than just a complication of androgen-dependent sebaceous hypertrophy. Genetic factors are clearly important, and bacteria influence the development of inflammatory lesions. The relevance of dietary and psychological factors is unproven.

Pathogenesis

The primary lesion of acne is the comedo—a cellular cast of the dilated vestibule of a pilosebaceous duct. It is formed by retention hyperkeratosis and binds within its interstices hair fragments, lipid, micro-organisms and extraneous matter. It is a firm, brownish, seed-like body with a grey or black tip. The comedo at first communicates with the surface only through a tiny opening (closed comedo) and, although it may bulge

91

the surface as a 'whitehead', it is not itself visible. With increasing size, a closed comedo may dilate the pilosebaceous pore, becoming visible as a 'blackhead' (open comedo).

The more inflammatory lesions form in association with closed comedones, and the inflammation is paralleled by increasing amounts of free fatty acids in sebum. These free fatty acids probably result from triglyceride breakdown by bacterial lipases in the pilosebaceous canal, and are very irritating to the skin. Inflammatory rupture of the pilosebaceous canal may extrude keratin, bacteria and hair fragments into the dermis, which adds to the inflammation.

Clinical features

■ *The eruption* is a polymorphic mixture of whiteheads, blackheads, pustules and inflamed papules. With more severe inflammation, there may be red or purplish nodules and purulent cysts. In a particular patient, one type of lesion may predominate, but the mixture of lesions is characteristic. The severity of the eruption varies a great deal. There may be no more than a few whiteheads on the forehead or a light sprinkling of pustules and blackheads on the chin or cheeks, but the badly affected patient may have much of the face, chest and back transformed into a boggy mass of nodules and cysts, with abscesses and draining sinuses. Most patients suffer little discomfort, but nodular and cystic lesions are tender and somewhat painful.

■ *Distribution of lesions* is bilateral and roughly symmetrical. The forehead, cheeks and chin are usually involved, but the scalp and eyelids are always spared. The shoulders, back and central chest are also common sites and, in severe cases, there may be extension onto the arms, buttocks and even the upper abdomen.

Course

Onset is a little earlier in girls, but in either sex is very uncommon before the tenth year. A few lesions may begin to appear a year or two before this, but the development of overt acne in younger children indicates the need for endocrine investigation. The duration of acne is as variable as the severity. Individual comedones may remain for months, but inflammatory lesions usually resolve within three or four weeks. Nodules and cysts may persist for long periods before healing slowly with scar formation.

The course is chronic but fluctuating, with a tendency to improve in summer. However, in hot humid weather and in tropical regions marked aggravation is common. In mild cases, spontaneous resolution occurs within a few months, but typical acne normally lasts for a year or two. In some patients, the disease continues for years and, particularly in women, persistence into the fifth decade is not rare.

Complications

■ *Scarring* is a common sequel to severe acne and occasionally follows relatively mild disease. Scars develop as small pits or broader depressed areas and, in the nodulocystic type, there may be elevated bands and nodules. Cheloidal scarring is a rare but mutilating complication.

■ *Psychological*. Acne causes some embarrassment to most patients, and is an occasional trigger of serious emotional disturbance.

■ *Systemic features* are very uncommon, but may accompany acute exacerbations of the cutaneous disease. There may be arthralgia, myalgia and, less often, fever and leucocytosis. Weight loss and anaemia may be added if the severe inflammatory phase persists.

Diagnosis

Diagnosis is made on the basis of:
■ Distribution within the acne region of the face chest and back
■ Polymorphic nature of the rash—comedones, papules and pustules
■ Age of the patient

▶ **Consider and exclude**

■ *Rosacea*, which may resemble acne, but comedones are not a feature.

■ *Drug eruptions* may be acneiform, but the distribution is more widespread and lesions are monomorphic—usually papules.

■ *Oil acne* caused by contact with paraffins, insoluble cutting oils, and chlorinated hydrocarbons, all of which may produce acneiform lesions. The distribution, however, is to sites of contact, so that the arms and thighs are usually involved, with relative sparing of the face.

■ *Perioral dermatitis* may complicate topical therapy with corticosteroids and be misinterpreted as persistence or worsening of the acne itself.

Treatment

Acne occurs at an age when the adolescent is adjusting, sometimes with difficulty, to a major physical and emotional transition. The teenager is often self-conscious and unduly embarrassed by even minor grades of the disease. To dismiss acne as unimportant demonstates a considerable lack of understanding, particularly as the disease can be satisfactorily suppressed in the great majority of patients, and scarring prevented or minimised.

No single treatment is effective for all patients with acne. Therapy should be tailored to the individual patient and will need to be modified during the course of the disease.

▶ **Topical therapy**

■ *Tretinoin* (retinoic acid) is the most useful topical agent available for preventing the formation of comedones. It provides an effective treatment for comedones already present, by altering the keratin within the plug causing it to discharge to the surface rather than rupturing into the dermis where it would produce nodules and pustules which are the so-called inflammatory lesions of acne. However, quite severe irritation and peeling can complicate tretinoin therapy, and the drug should be introduced carefully, beginning with the 0.01 per cent gel or the 0.05 per cent cream. Patients should be aware that exposure of treated areas to wind or strong sunlight is apt to exaggerate the irritant effect of retinoic acid.

■ *Benzoyl peroxide* may be prescribed as a lotion or gel, and is marketed in concentrations of 2.5 per cent, 5 per cent and 10 per cent. It effectively penetrates the pilosebaceous follicle, where it reduces formation of the irritating free fatty acids, presumably by its bacteriostatic effect on the lipase-producing anaerobes which colonise the pilosebaceous canal.

It has a tendency to cause dryness accompanied by a mild desquamation, and can be rather irritating to sensitive skin. It should be introduced gradually, commencing with the less irritating 5 per cent lotion. Application should be slowly increased in both quantity and duration until tolerance has been established. If necessary, the 5 per cent preparation can be gradually replaced by the 10 per cent gel. Benzoyl peroxide must be kept away from the eyes, and patients should be warned that it bleaches clothing.

■ *Topical antibiotics* are now widely and successfully prescribed for the inflammatory component of acne. Erythromycin 2 per cent and clindamycin 1 to 2 per cent in hydro-alcoholic solution appear to be safe and effective. Contact sensitisation is very uncommon and the solutions cause little irritation. With clindamycin there is the potential problem of drug-associated colitis following percutaneous absorption, but the risk appears to be minimal. These agents appear to be particularly effective because of inhibitory effects on polymorph migration.

■ *A corticosteroid application* is occasionally helpful when other measures have failed, but corticosteroids (other than hydrocortisone acetate) carry a real risk of erythema and telangiectasia if continued for more than short periods and long-term use can actually induce acne. Intralesional injection of triamcinolone into nodular or cystic swellings relieves inflammation and can flatten hypertrophic scars.

▶ Systemic therapy

■ *Antibiotics.* Tetracycline therapy has transformed the prognosis for patients with moderate to severe acne. As little as 250 mg daily is often sufficient for good suppression, but initial doses of 0.5 to 1.0 g daily may be necessary.

The value and safety of tetracylines in doses up to 0.5 g daily, even for long periods, is now well established. Tetracycline therapy is, however, ineffective in clearing comedones and, because of effects on developing teeth, should not be prescribed for pregnant women or for children less than twelve years old. It should be remembered that antibiotics, including tetracycline, have been reported as reducing the effectiveness of oral contraceptives.

The mode of action of tetracyclines in acne is uncertain, but is probably related to their effect on micro-organisms responsible for lipolysis of triglycerides.

The bacteria that cause most of the changes that result in acne are a normal comensal anaerobic Gram-positive bacillus called *Propionobacterium acnes.* As a group, people with untreated acne have similar numbers of *P. acnes* as people without acne and the numbers after acne has resolved are still the same. Although the organism is sensitive to penicillin in vitro, the pencillins are not effective in treating acne because they are not lipid-soluble and cannot reach the region required.

However, erythromycin and minocycline are effective, as is trimethoprim-sulphamethoxasole. Lincomycin and clindamycin are also effective but, in view of their potential for serious side effects, are better avoided.

■ *Hormone therapy*. Oestrogens in sufficient dosage suppress acne but produce unacceptable side effects in boys. For girls, especially those with premenstrual exacerbation, adequate doses of ethinyl oestradiol (0.1 mg daily) or its derivative, mestranol, can be used to decrease sebum production. When oestrogen is combined with a progestagen and administered in cycles of 21 days, menstruation occurs regularly although ovulation is suppressed.

Improvement is slow and must be balanced against the risk of side effects. The anti-androgen, cyproterone acetate, has been found effective in the treatment of women with acne as has spironolactone used for its anti-androgen effect. Both of these drugs should be avoided during pregnancy because they induce feminisation of the male foetus. Spironolactone is not as potent as cyproterone acetate and is taken in a dose of 1 to 2 g per day. Sodium and potassium levels need to be monitored and occasionally menstrual irregularities may occur. Cyproterone acetate has marked effects on the menstrual cycle and therefore to maintain normal menstrual periodicity is given in a reverse sequential regimen from day 5 to day 15 of the menstrual cycle, together with ethinyl oestradiol, which is given for the usual 21 days.

■ *Oral retinoids*. Isotretinoin, which is the 13-cis derivative of retinoic acid, has a dramatic and beneficial effect in acne. While being taken, it changes sebum excretion to the prepubertal chemical composition and acne improves. Although sebum excretion slowly returns to normal when treatment is ceased, for reasons that are not understood, approximately 80 per cent of patients remain free of acne thereafter. The drug is usually given for four months, then ceased. Because of many toxic effects, including elevation of cholesterol and triglyceride, and embryotoxicity and teratogenicity, its use is restricted by law in Australia only to approved practitioners who use it for severe cystic acne unresponsive to other treatment.

■ *Dietary manipulation* has never been shown to be effective in clinical trials, despite many patients believing certain foods make their acne worse. This would suggest that if foods play any part it is merely as exacerbating agents rather than the cause; that the proportion of patients where foods are important is small; that not all patients react to the same foods; and that if there is any benefit from dietary restriction, the effects are too small to justify rigid diets that are difficult to adhere to.

▶ Physical therapy

Manipulation of lesions should be discouraged because this will cause contents to rupture into the surrounding dermis and produce more inflammation. Gentle drainage through a tiny incision is sometimes necessary for cystic lesions and may be combined with intralesional injection of corticosteroid. The use of comedo-extractors is limited to patients with superficial comedones and little inflammation.

Although most patients improve substantially after a holiday at the beach, and the beneficial effect of sunlight would seem undoubted, the use of artificially produced ultraviolet light is of minimal benefit. Because of recent advances in the management of acne, the indications for superficial X-ray therapy have been considerably reduced.

Frequent washing and cleansing of the skin is of no benefit.

Scarring due to acne improves with time and in most patients is better left untreated. Hypertrophic scars can be flattened with the intralesional injection of steroid. Depressed scars are sometimes treated with chemosurgery or dermabrasion but the scars that respond best to these treatments are broad shallow scars, which are the types that tend to improve greatly with time. This type of scar can also be improved with the injection of collagen under the depression but the effects last only a few months.

Variants of acne

Acne conglobata

This is a rare but severe variant, usually occurring in men. There are many nodules and multiple abscesses which burst onto the surface or burrow into adjoining nodules to form interconnecting sinuses. Response to treatment is much less satisfactory than with other forms of acne and severe scarring is the rule.

Infantile acne

In the first few months of life, mainly in boys, comedones may develop on the face, particularly the cheeks. There may be a few papules and pustules, but more severe manifestations are rare. The course is mild, and significant scarring very unusual.

Less frequently, infantile acne does not appear until three to four months of age, or even later. The disease then tends to follow a more severe course and to be more persistent.

Drug-induced acne

Acneiform lesions may develop in patients treated with systemic corticosteroids. Comedones may be recognisable, but the papules are more uniform and the eruption less polymorphic than in spontaneous acne. Pre-existing acne may be aggravated by systemic corticosteroid therapy, as well as by androgens, diphenylhydantoin, and trimethadione.

Acneiform drug eruptions lack comedones, and are not true variants of acne. Drugs noted to cause acneiform eruptions include iodides, bromides, isoniazid, lithium carbonate, quinine, chloral hydrate, thiourea and cyclosporin.

Acne cosmetica

Patients are mainly women between 30 and 50 years of age. In many cases the disease appears to be precipitated by the prolonged use of

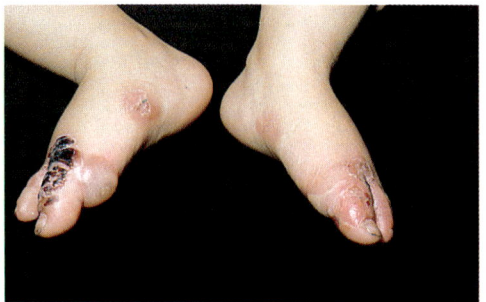

13. Epidermolysis bullosa—non-dystrophic

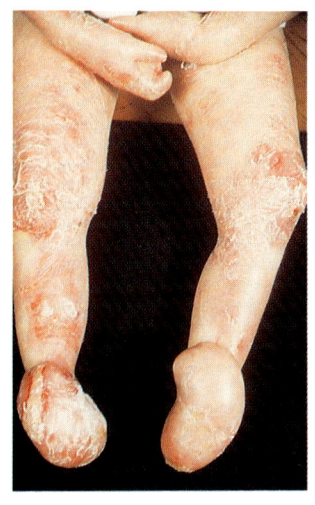

14. Epidermolysis bullosa—recessive dystrophic

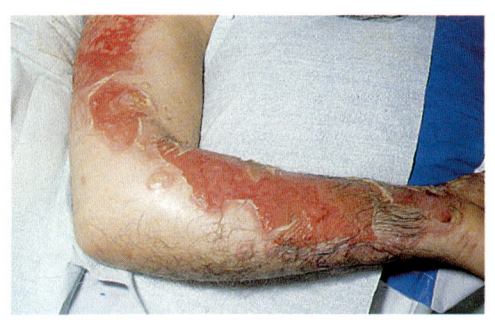

15. Pemphigus vulgaris

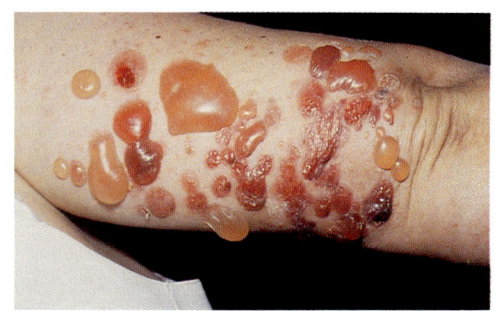

16. Bullous pemphigoid

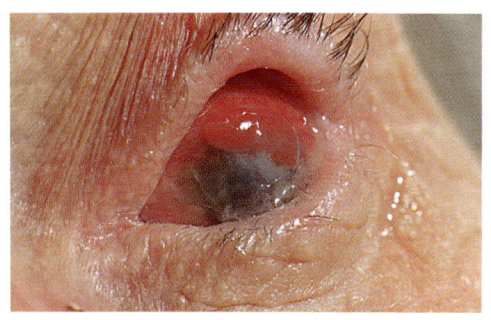

17. Cicatricial pemphigoid

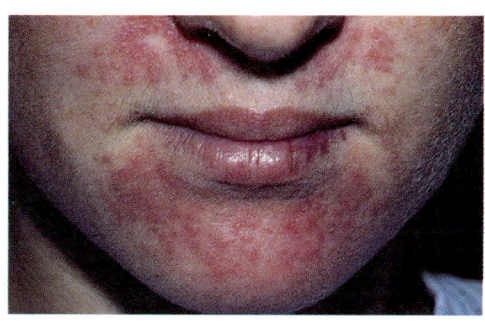

18. Peri-oral dermatitis

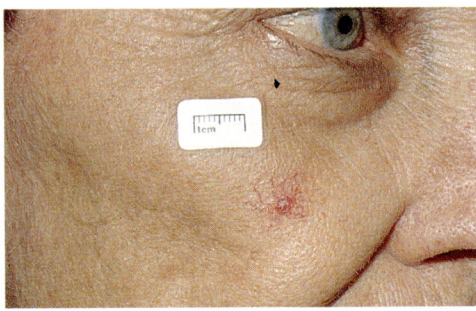

19. Spider naevus

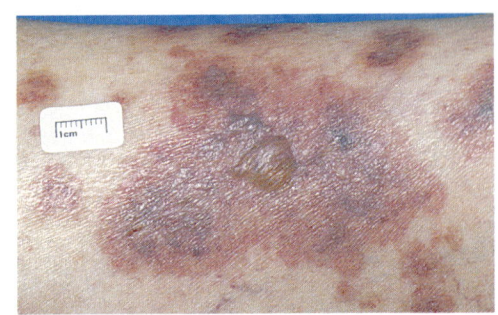

20. Leucocytoclastic vasculitis

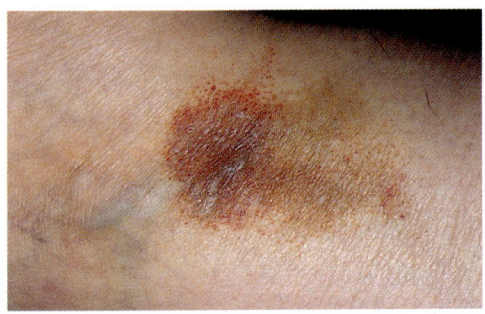

21. Pigmented purpuric dermatosis

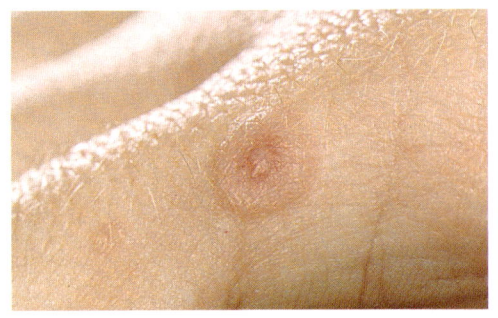

22. Target lesion—erythema multiforme

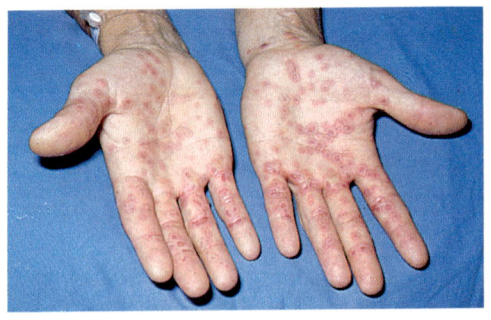

23. Erythema multiforme

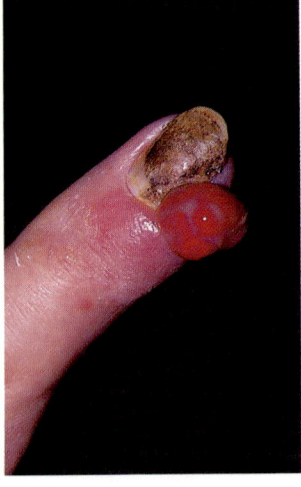

24. Granuloma telangiectaticum

cosmetics, especially those containing lanolin or petrolatum. There is usually no past history of severe acne, and the distribution is mostly over the lower part of the face. Comedones are present, but lesions are less inflammatory than in teenage acne. The disorder responds well to tetracyclines, provided that the relevant cosmetics are discontinued.

Acne excorié

Some minor trauma to acne lesions is very common among patients of all ages, but acne excorié is a distinct variant largely confined to young women. A mild degree of acne is present, but it is altered out of all proportion by incessant picking and scratching at even the most minor blemish. Significant scarring is common. Whatever acne is present should be treated, but management is directed more to controlling the obsessional squeezing and picking responsible for most of the changes seen. Some of these women are seriously disturbed and are in need of psychiatric help.

Rosacea

Rosacea is a common disorder affecting facial skin and characterised by both vascular and inflammatory components.

Aetiology

The cause of rosacea is unknown. It may develop at any age in either sex, but more often begins in women between 30 and 50 years of age. In men, rosacea tends to begin earlier and to be more severe. Factors which cause flushing in normal people may aggravate rosacea and render it more apparent, but there is no evidence that these factors are involved in the basic aetiology of the disease.

Clinical features

The eruption is a composite of vascular and inflammatory components. The vascular changes are erythema and telangiectasia, and the inflammatory lesions develop as papules or pustules—but any of these may predominate. The earliest change is usually a recurring or persisting erythema of the nose and cheeks. The erythema gradually becomes constant, varying only in intensity. The skin is usually oily, and may become somewhat thickened. Papules and pustules appear over the areas of erythema and, with time, telangiectasia may be added. In some patients, telangiectasia dominates the appearance from the outset, while in others erythema may be the dominant feature, with only occasional pustules developing.

Severely affected patients may develop nodular thickening of the nose, cheeks and chin. The nose becomes grossly swollen with irregular knobbly thickening, sometimes with little change on the rest of the face (rhinophyma); this disfiguring variant, 'potato nose', is almost completely restricted to men.

Distribution usually involves the 'flush areas' of the nose and cheeks. Less often the chin, glabellar region, forehead and ears are affected and, occasionally, the front of the chin.

Course

This varies from a few recurrences followed by permanent remission to a steadily progressive, disfiguring disease. Typically, the disease is chronic and persistent, with fluctuations of severity and occasional brief remission.

Complications

■ *Blepharitis and conjunctivitis* are common. Patients often feel a grittiness between the conjunctiva and eyelids.

■ *Keratitis, corneal ulcer and iritis* are less frequent but serious complications.

Diagnosis

▶ **Suspect** rosacea when there is:

■ *episodic flushing* papules and pustules

■ *exacerbation* with heat, alcohol, emotional upset

■ *associated eye symptoms*

▶ **Consider and exclude**

■ *Acne vulgaris*, which typically begins at a younger age, is more wide-spread and invariably has comedones present.

■ *Lupus erythematosus*, which may resemble telangiectatic and erythematous rosacea. However, pustules are not a feature of lupus erythematosus and the marked episodic fluctuation seen with rosacea does not occur.

■ *Perioral dermatitis* may be a variant of rosacea and a precise separation is not always possible.

▶ **Confirmatory tests** are usually not required as the diagnosis is made on clinical grounds.

Treatment

Agents which promote facial flushing, such as alcohol, excessive exposure to sunlight, and highly seasoned food and drink produce at least a temporary aggravation of the erythema and are probably better restricted. Tetracyclines given orally are very effective in suppressing the skin changes, often with improvement of the ocular features as well. It takes about four to six weeks to appreciate the beginnings of improvement and about three to six months to achieve clearing. However, as treatment is suppressive rather than curative, once clearing is achieved treatment is gradually reduced over a period of weeks to months to find the minimum able to maintain clearing. The oral antibiotics erythromycin and trimethoprim-sulphamethexazole are also effective.

Topical treatments are sometimes used to suppress minor rosacea and to minimise reliance on oral treatment.

Effective agents include low concentration sulphur, hydrocortisone cream and topical metronidazole, which seems to be the most effective topical agent. The potent topical steroids may actually induce rosacea and may exacerbate pre-existing rosacea.

In the rare instances where oral antibiotics and topical treatments are not helpful, oral isotretinoin is usually of benefit but, in distinction from its use in acne, does not result in lasting remission from rosacea when treatment is ceased. Concerns regarding long-term use of oral retinoids therefore restrict their use in rosacea.

Cosmetic surgery may be required when rhinophyma causes significant disfigurement.

Perioral dermatitis *(Colour plate 18)*

This distinctive eruption generally begins on the lower part of the face, most often in young women. Small delicate papules and papulo-pastules appear on a pink background and typically there is usually a zone of normal skin sparing a few millimetres around the vermilion of the lips.

In most patients the rash follows the repeated application of a potent fluorinated topical steroid to the face for some minor disorder such as mild seborrhoeic dermatitis of the nasolabial folds. On ceasing the application there is a rebound flare which is likely to be retreated with the same or similar preparation with further progression which culminates in a severe rosacea-like dermatitis involving much of the face. Although in some females there is no history of topical steroid use, fluorinated steroid application is almost invariably associated with a periorbital variant (seen more commonly in males) in which telangiectasia is an additional feature.

The disease responds to oral tetracycline 250 mg twice daily for six to eight weeks and withdrawal of the fluorinated steroid application. Patients should be specifically warned against reusing these applications during the rebound phase. The use of hydrocortisone cream may provide some relief during this uncomfortable period.

8

Diseases involving peripheral vessels

1. Telangiectasia and livedo reticularis
2. Vasculitis and related hypersensitivity syndromes
3. Urticaria and angioedema
4. Leg ulcers
5. Lymphoedema

Vascular changes are a feature of many congenital, inflammatory and neoplastic diseases included in other chapters. The ensuing discussion is restricted to the listed diseases.

Telangiectasia and livedo reticularis

Telangiectases may develop in skin which appears to be otherwise normal, but more often occur as a complication or accompaniment of other changes. Prolonged exposure to cold or to repeated applications of corticosteroids may so reduce capillary blood flow that deeper and larger vessels become permanently dilated. Telangiectases may complicate rosacea and other diseases characterised by prolonged vasodilatation. They are a common feature of scleroderma, lupus erythematosus, dermatomyositis and polycythaemia vera, and are a frequent sequel to any process leading to cutaneous atrophy—as on the exposed, sun-damaged skin of the elderly or in areas of post-irradiation atrophy.

Hereditary haemorrhagic telangiectasia

Hereditary haemorrhagic telangiectasia is a familial disease of autosomal dominant inheritance, characterised by vascular malformations of skin, mucous membranes and viscera. Defective haemostatic mechanisms and exaggerated fibrinolysis within lesions may contribute to the pronounced tendency to haemorrhage which may occur at any affected site.

Cutaneous lesions are composed of dilated, tortuous vessels below a thinned epidermis. They generally begin to appear in late childhood or early adult life as small, ruby-red macules or papules. They are discrete, non-pulsatile and blanch with pressure. They are most often found on the lips, face, palms, nail beds and upper trunk. Similar lesions are almost always visible on the nasal and oral mucosae.

The most common presenting symptom is haemorrhage, usually from the nose. Recurrent epistaxis may begin in childhood, becoming more frequent and more severe in adult life. Haematemesis, melaena and haematuria are less common. Visceral complications may result from pulmonary arteriovenous fistulae, and from vascular malformations in the liver or brain.

Generalised essential telangiectasia

Generalised essential telangiectasia is predominantly a disease of females and often begins around adolescence. Individual lesions may resemble those of the haemorrhagic type, but there is no familial clustering of cases, and bleeding is not a feature. Telangiectases usually develop as broad asymmetrical sheets, most often on the lower limbs, but frequently progress to an extensive, bilateral distribution.

Spider telangiectasis (spider naevus)

Vascular spiders are very common, and occur in at least 10 per cent of normal adults, and more frequently in children. They are present in most pregnant women, and may develop in large numbers in patients with hepatocellular disease.

Histology

From deep in the dermis, a central arteriole coils towards the surface, becoming progressively thinner until it reaches the papillary dermis where it expands into a thin-walled ampulla. From this arteriolar expansion, fine branches pass out in radial fashion towards a peripheral venous network.

Clinical features

■ *Individual lesions* vary from a few millimetres to two centimetres in diameter, with a central pulsating vessel revealed by light diascopy. Small surrounding vessels are barely visible to the naked eye as they radiate outwards and may appear as a circular blush surrounding the central punctum. *(Colour plate 19)*

■ *Distribution* is to the upper part of the body, lesions rarely forming below the umbilicus. Mucosal surfaces may be involved, but bleeding is seldom a problem.

■ *During pregnancy* spider naevi tend to erupt in the early months and usually resolve spontaneously a month or two after parturition.

Treatment

When removal is requested for cosmetic reasons, a very satisfactory result can be achieved by careful electrodesiccation of the feeder arteriole.

Livedo reticularis

When normal skin is cooled, a mottled web of purplish discolouration may develop, especially over the legs. This web-like pattern of bluish colour is evidence of sluggish blood flow in the affected ares, but the reasons for the reticulate pattern are obscure. When a normal limb is rewarmed, the pattern disappears. In livedo reticularis the discolouration is more or less permanent, showing only limited variation with temperature changes. In severe cases, ulceration may develop at the darker areas of diminished flow.

In infants and chubby children, the livedo pattern is physiological. In older patients, particularly when the distribution is in discontinuous patches, an organic cause should be sought. Arteriosclerosis, vasculitis or connective tissue diseases may be responsible. Intravascular causes include polycythaemia vera, cryoglobulinaemia, and arterial embolism. Livedo reticularis should be distinguished from a similar pattern of pigmentation in those who habitually warm their legs close to fires and radiators.

Vasculitis and related hypersensitivity syndromes

Cutaneous changes resulting from vasculitis are largely determined by the size and site of affected vessels, and by the severity of necrosis and inflammatory reaction. The varying combinations of size, site, and severity result in a wide range of clinical manifestations, which are in no way specific for cutaneous vasculitis. Diagnosis rests more on histological than clinical criteria and is suggested by:

■ necrosis of vessel wall and surrounding tissue;
■ a perivascular deposition of fibrinoid material;
■ marked leucocytic infiltration, mainly of neutrophils, in and around the vessel wall;
■ a characteristic disintegration of the nuclei of neutrophils in and around vessel walls ('nuclear dust');
■ endothelial swelling and proliferation, which leads to a narrowed lumen and often to thrombosis.

There is a group of disorders which lack the histological criteria for vasculitis, but are characterised by altered function of cutaneous vessels. There is no true vasculitis, but vascular permeability is increased. The altered permeability may result in a leakage of fluid only, as in urticaria, or the fluid may be accompanied by an exudate of cells, as in erythema multiforme or erythema nodosum.

    1. Necrotising vasculitis
       (a) leucocytoclastic vasculitis of small vessels
       (b) granulomatous vasculitis
       (c) polyarteritis nodosa
    2. Related syndromes
       (a) pityriasis lichenoides
       (b) pigmented purpuric dermatosis
       (c) pustular vascular reactions
       (d) erythema nodosum
       (e) erythema multiforme
       (f) erythema perstans

Leucocytoclastic vasculitis of small vessels ('allergic vasculitis')

Leucocytoclastic vasculitis of small vessels is a necrotising vasculitis, which involves arterioles, venules and capillaries of the skin and viscera.

Aetiology

A history of recent streptococcal infection is fairly common, and some patients achieve a sustained remission after treatment of associated chronic infection, such as pyelonephritis. Drugs have frequently been held responsible, although in many cases the same drugs have been administered later without recurrence. Occasionally, leucocytoclastic vasculitis is the presenting feature of patients with lupus erythematosus, rheumatoid arthritis, and cryoglobulinaemia.

An immunological basis is suggested by the histological resemblance to the experimental Arthus reaction and is supported by the demonstration within a newly developed lesion of immunoglobulin and complement at the site of vessel necrosis. Circulating immune complexes are probably involved and may be filtered off in a non-specific way at sites of relative stasis or increased permeability. It is likely that the size and solubility of circulating complexes are more important than the specificity of antibodies.

Clinical features (Colour plate 20)

■ **The cutaneous lesion** begins with exudation and inflammation, so that small areas of erythema and oedema are common early signs. These erythematous and oedematous papules may be the only cutaneous expression of small vessel vasculitis, but a purpuric component is frequently added. In contrast to the macular petechiae of thrombocytopaenia, purpuric lesions of vasculitis are palpable because of the dense inflammatory infiltrate and oedema which, as in any tissue, are part of the infarction process. The purpuric papule ('palpable purpura') is a common and distinctive feature of vasculitis.

Exudation may be more marked, with the formation of vesicles, sometimes haemorrhagic. Thrombosis of superficial vessels is usually insufficient to produce epidermal necrosis, but ulceration may follow thrombosis of deeper vessels. With less acute changes in deeper vessels of the dermis and subcutis, tender reddish nodules may form. Cutaneous changes therefore range from erythema to papules, nodules, purpuric lesions, blisters and ulcers which are frequently small, painful and punched-out.

■ **Distribution** involves the legs in the great majority of patients. Other areas are affected with variable frequency.

■ **Systemic features.** There may be fever, headache, malaise, weight loss and arthralgia. Gastro-intestinal lesions are not infrequent, and there is at least microscopic haematuria as evidence of renal involvement in more than one-third of patients. Myocardial, pulmonary and other visceral features are less common.

Course

This is unpredictable. There may be only a single crop of lesions, which resolve over two or three weeks, leaving no residual evidence of the attack. Other patients suffer repeated recurrences, with varying visceral involvement, over months or years, even if the cause is removed.

Variants

■ *Henoch-Schoenlein purpura* is a distinctive clinical presentation of leucocytoclastic vasculitis which occurs mainly in children. Cutaneous lesions are polymorphic, and generally include urticarial and purpuric elements. Characteriscally, the distribution in addition to the lower legs also includes the extensor aspects of upper arms, the buttocks, and the anterior thighs. Unlike other varieties of small vessel leucocytoclastic vasculitis in which direct immunofluorescence of skin biopsy reveals vascular deposition of immunoreactants of mixed immunoglobulin class, biopsy of Henoch-Schoenlein purpura reveals predominantly IgA.

■ *Other variants* have been assigned syndrome status on the basis of one or more predominant features. These syndromes are no more than variations of severity, duration and organ of maximal involvement.

Investigations

■ *A biopsy* should be taken from an early lesion to confirm the diagnosis. The specimen should extend down to subcutaneous fat and, as the changes are frequently patchy, more than a single biopsy may be required.

■ *Special tests* are necessary to assess involvement of other organs, particularly the heart and kidneys.

■ An attempt should be made to *uncover underlying disease*, the treatment of which may prevent recurrences.

Granulomatous vasculitis

Particularly when subcutaneous tissue is involved, histiocytes and giant cells may be added to the inflammatory infiltrate to form granulomas in or around the walls of damaged vessels.

Wegener's granulomatosis

This is a rare form of granulomatous vasculitis in which necrotising granulomas of the respiratory tract and focal necrotising glomerulitis form part of a generalised vasculitis involving, particularly, small arteries and veins. Antineutrophilic cytoplasmic antibodies (ANCA), which block proteinase inhibitors, characterise this disease. It has been suggested that, as a consequence, uncontrolled effects of proteinases produce the respiratory tract pathology. Oral cyclophosphamide has dramatically improved the prognosis in patients with this disease, by comparison with the past treatment using oral steroids, which merely provided supression of disease activity.

Allergic granulomatosis

This begins as chronic respiratory disease characterised by asthma and hypereosinophilia. After a variable period granulomatous vasculitis becomes evident as the deep nodules and haemorrhagic lesions of cutaneous and subcutaneous involvement and the accompanying serious visceral disease.

Giant cell arteritis

An uncommon variety of granulomatous vasculitis, giant cell arterilis involves medium to large muscular arteries, particularly those of the carotid system.

The disease is predominantly one of old age, rarely affecting patients younger than 55. Unilateral or bilateral headache, pain with mastication, and pain or stiffness of the proximal limb muscles are common early complaints. Ocular manifestations are frequent and may lead to blindness. Involved arteries are tender and may be palpably thickened, with oedema and redness of the overlying skin. Thrombosis of affected arteries may produce blisters, ulcers or gangrenous areas on the scalp. The ESR is elevated, often to very high levels, and biopsy of affected vessels is diagnostic. The disease responds dramatically to large doses of corticosteroids.

Polyarteritis nodosa

Polyarteritis nodosa is a multisystem disorder caused by necrotising vasculitis of small to medium-sized muscular arteries. The disease is three times as common in men and is believed to result from a hyper-sensitivity reaction. Onset has been associated with drug therapy in many patients and with streptococcal infection in others.

Histology

Cutaneous lesions are largely the result of subcutaneous vasculitis, although small arteries deep in the dermis may be involved. There is a panarteritis, which begins with foci of necrosis in the media or adventitia, but soon spreads to the intima. Infiltration by neutrophils, with some eosinophils and lymphocytes, follows. The necrotic areas are invaded by granulation tissue, which leads to fibrosis which, with intimal proliferation, may narrow or obliterate the arterial lumen.

Clinical features

■ *Cutaneous lesions* are usually non-specific. There may be a livedo pattern of erythema or purplish discolouration, purpuric lesions, ulcers caused by small infarcts, or digital gangrene. Distinctive subcutaneous nodules may develop along the course of an artery, but are uncommon.

■ *Other organs.* Fever, weight loss, tachycardia and polymorphonuclear leucocytosis are common early features. Renal involvement, hypertension, cardiac failure, abdominal pain and polyneuritis are frequent manifestations.

Diagnosis

Polyarteritis nodosa should be suspected in a patient who has multisystem disease, with fever, leucocytosis, elevated ESR, and hypertension or urinary abnormalities. However, the diagnosis is histological, and cutaneous or subcutaneous lesions provide accessible sites for biopsy.

Treatment

The disease is modified by treatment with corticosteroids and other immunosuppressive drugs, but remains a serious threat to life.

Pityriasis lichenoides

Pityriasis lichenoides is an inflammatory disorder of unknown aetiology involving small vessels of the dermis. The disease ranges in severity from a very acute ulcerative process accompanied by fever and considerable systemic disturbance to a chronic papular eruption devoid of extracutaneous features.

Histology

Lymphocytes surround dermal capillaries and, in acute lesions, permeate capillary walls, with an extravasation of erythrocytes into the dermis. The lymphocytic infiltrate extends to the dermo-epidermal junction and may penetrate the epidermis. A variable degree of epidermal spongiosis follows and, in the acute form, foci of epidermal necrosis and erosion develop.

Clinical features

■ *The acute form* most often presents as a generalised eruption of reddish brown papules which may involve much of the body, although the face and scalp are generally spared. The papules usually evolve quickly into vesicular and then crusted lesions, which may become haemorrhagic or necrotic. Individual lesions heal over two or three weeks, often with scarring, but new crops continue to evolve, producing a polymorphous appearance. Pruritus is unusual.

■ *The chronic form* is more common in young men and is characterised by a monomorphous eruption, mainly on the trunk, of reddish papules surmounted by an adherent scale. Individual lesions resolve without scarring over a few weeks, but new papules may continue to erupt for months or years.

Treatment

Topical corticosteroids are sometimes helpful, and the more acute scarring disease can often be suppressed with prednisone in doses of 15 mg to 20 mg daily for an adult. However, recurrences usually follow withdrawal of the steroid, which does not appear to alter the duration of the disease. Tetracycline (1 g daily) has been reported effective in some patients, as has erythromycin in children. Exposure to natural sunlight is usually of great help in the chronic form, as is treatment with UV-B and PUVA. Mild, chronic cases (which are sometimes asymptomatic) may be better left untreated.

Pigmented purpuric dermatosis

Pigmented purpuric dermatosis is a distinctive clinical pattern of benign capillaritis, most frequently encountered on the legs of men. Although the cause remains undiscovered in most patients, very similar changes may develop as a drug eruption, particularly from carbromal or the chemically related meprobamate, or as a reaction to colouring agents and preservatives in food.

Histology

Capillaries of the upper dermis are altered and surrounded by a lymphocytic infiltrate. Haemosiderin deposits result from the destruction of red cells escaping into the dermis.

Clinical features

Irregular rusty brown patches are formed from closely aggregated pinpoints of haemosiderin. The patches expand slowly and may become confluent. Lesions may develop at any site, but are often restricted to the lower limbs. Pruritus is seldom a feature, the disease persisting in most cases as a minor disfigurement with slow extension for many years. *(Colour plate 21)*

Pustular vascular reactions

This group of conditions have in common a histology in which vascular change, ranging from true vasculitis to mild endothelial swelling, is associated with a very intense and heavy neutrophilic infiltration of the dermis. Diagnosis is based on the clinical setting and exclusion of other diseases because there are, as yet, no diagnostic tests for these conditions.

Acute febrile neutrophilic dermatosis (Sweet's Syndrome)

Aetiology

The exact mechanism is unknown but it is thought to be a reactive process in predisposed individuals, with the precipitating factor often being either a preceeding infection, an underlying myeloproliferative disease or an auto-immune disorder.

Histology

The upper mid-dermis contains a massive neutrophilic infiltrate with leucocytoclasis and vascular endothelial swelling but no necrosis of vessels or fibrin deposition.

Clinical features

Typically, an acute onset of fever is accompanied by a peripheral neutrophilia and boggy red tender plaques which are characteristically located on the head and neck region and upper limbs. Middle-aged females are particularly prone to this disorder. Arthralgia and glomerular involvement may be present. Despite the name, the disorder may be chronic or recurrent, and fever or neutrophilia may be absent, but the skin neutrophilia is constant. The skin changes may preceed the systemic features by up to ten days.

Treatment with prednisolone 40 mg per day usually produces a dramatic rapid clearing. Other treatments used have included dapsone, indomethacin, colchicine and oral potassium iodide. Untreated, the condition often resolves spontaneously over a period of one to two months.

Behcet's disease

This is a rare multisystem disease in which cutaneous features include ulcers and pustules. Systemic features are produced as a result of vascular involvement.

Aetiology

A genetic predisposition and immunological factors, as yet undefined, seem to be involved. The disorder is most common in those from Japan and Middle Eastern countries. There appears to be a linkage with HLA-B51 genotype. Immunological abnormalities reported have included circulating immune complexes, reduced killer cell activity, lymphocytotoxicity to oral epithelial cells, and enhanced neutrophil migration but, as yet, no test is consistently abnormal.

Histology

Microscopic examination of early ulcers and skin lesions reveal changes that range from a neutrophilic infiltrate around almost normal looking vessels, to frank leucocytoclastic vasculitis. However, in old lesions the perivascular neutrophils are replaced by lymphocytes.

Clinical features

Behcet's disease usually begins with recurrent crops of oral or genital ulcers. The mouth ulcers may be superficial and indistinguishable from aphthous ulcers, or deeper and more persistent. Genital ulcers are similar and occur on the scrotum or labia majora. Pustules are common on the trunk and limbs, particularly at the sites of minor injury such as venepuncture wounds. Superficial thrombophlebitis occurs in up to 50 per cent of patients and may precede thrombosis of the superior and inferior vena cava.

Ocular involvement occurs in 80 per cent of patients and generally begins with episodes of conjunctivitis and photophobia, which may progress to iritis or uveitis and ultimate blindness. Other features include arthritis, vasculitis, aneurysms and arterial or venous occlusions, gastrointestinal ulceration and pericarditis. Focal or diffuse involvement of the central nervous system has a grave significance, with a 50 per cent mortality within a year.

Treatment

Mild mucosal lesions can be successfully treated with topical or intralesional injection of corticosteroids. Pustular or vasculitic lesions may be helped by oral colchicine or dapsone. Systemic corticosteroids, used alone or in combination with cytotoxic drugs such as azathioprine, chlorambucil or methotrexate, are used to contol systemic vasculitis, neurologic disease and severe ocular involvement. Cyclosporine has been helpful in some patients resistant to other treatments.

Bowel bypass syndrome

First observed following small intestinal bypass surgery for obesity, bowel bypass syndrome has now been seen in other situations with functionally blind loops that occur following peptic ulcer surgery or are produced by inflammatory bowel disease.

Aetiology

Evidence suggests that overgrowth of bowel flora within a blind loop generates circulating immune complexes that contain bacterial peptidoglycans as the antigen, and it is these complexes that mediate the changes producing clinical disease.

Histology

Appearances are identical to those seen in Sweet's syndrome. Frequently there is marked oedema of the papillary dermis with subepidermal pustule formation.

Clinical features

Crops of papules appear on the trunk and arms. Lesions evolve within days to pustules on a purpuric base then resolve over a week or two. Arthralgia of wrists and small joints of the hands is a common accompanying feature. Other associations include fever, myalgia and flu-like illness.

Treatment

Reversal of the blind loop is the definitive treatment. Systemic treatment with antibiotics such as tetracycline, erythromycin and metronidazole is also effective.

Pyoderma gangrenosum

A characteristic pattern of cutaneous ulceration occurs.

Aetiology

Although often associated with ulcerative colitis, granulomatous colitis, and seropositive rheumatoid arthritis, pyoderma gangrenosum may complicate leukaemia, myeloma and virtually any severely debilitating disease. However, in almost 50 per cent of cases, there is no detectable associated disease. The mechanisms involved in the pathogenesis of lesions are unknown, but are likely to be immunological.

Histology

There is no universally accepted diagnostic biopsy appearance. Although many reports indicate that early lesions have a neutrophilic infiltrate, others describe a lymphocytic invasion of the dermis. However, there is unanimity that the bullous variant is characterised by a heavy neutrophilic infiltrate similar to Sweet's syndrome. Vascular change can range from nil to severe necrosis with fibrin deposition. Established lesions of pyoderma gangrenosum may also show marked tissue necrosis with an inflammatory infiltrate that includes giant cells.

Clinical features *(Colour plate 58)*

The early lesion begins as an inflamed papule or nodule, which rapidly becomes pustular, enlarges and develops a central area of necrosis. The ulcer that follows has a characteristic appearance, with a dusky, oedematous, overhanging border, surrounded by an erythematous band up to a centimetre wide. The ulcer may slowly expand to cover a large area, or quickly reach a stable maximum. The ulcer may be solitary but, when associated with ulcerative colitis, lesions are frequently multiple. When treatment is successful, healing produces a cribriform atrophic-looking but strong scar.

Diagnosis

Biopsy is required for exclusion of squamous cell carcinoma, granulomatous vasculitis, and deep fungal infections; culture to exclude bacterial, fungal, protozoal and mycobacterial infections; biochemical analysis to test for halogenoderma as a cause; and psychiatric evaluation to ensure the lesion has not been artefactually induced.

Treatment

Topical therapy alone is rarely successful, although claims have been made for injections of triamcinolone into the active borders of the ulcer. Systemic therapy with sulphapyridine is often effective, but blood levels of the drug need to be monitored and the doses required are poorly tolerated by many patients. Systemic corticosteroids are generally effective in initial doses of 80 mg to 100 mg of prednisone or its equivalent daily. The dose is reduced stepwise as healing occurs, but months of therapy are usually necessary and the incidence of side-effects has been high. Dapsone, minocycline, and clofazimine are possible alternatives for difficult cases. Cyclosporin is often effective but renal toxicity and extreme expense prevent this from being a first-line treatment.

Erythema nodosum

Erythema nodosum is a distinctive, self-limited eruption of subcutaneous nodules, usually confined to the front of the legs. Incidence is greatest in schoolchildren and young adults, with a predominance of females.

Aetiology

Erythema nodosum is believed to be a pattern of allergic hypersensitivity triggered by various agents in predisposed individuals. The reaction may be provoked by drugs or by fungal, viral and bacterial infections, especially streptococcal and tuberculous ones. Non-infectious associations include sarcoidosis, enteropathies, and malignant tumours.

Histology

Changes are restricted to the subcutis and adjoining dermis, where an infiltrate of neutrophils and lymphocytes surrounds vessels and invades the septa between fat lobules. Lymphocytes soon predominate, with a variable admixture of histiocytes, giant cells and erythrocytes. Vessel walls are thickened, but necrosis is not a feature.

Clinical features

The eruption appears abruptly, as slightly raised, bright red, painful nodules over the shins or sides of the legs. There may be only three or four, or dozens may erupt over the legs and thighs. The arms are occasionally involved, but other sites are rare. The nodules are poorly demarcated at the edges and range from 2 cm to 6 cm in size.

The colour slowly deepens to purplish red, and may fade to yellowish green as the lesions resolve over three to six weeks. A little surface scaling is common as the nodules heal.

Fever is common at the outset, but constitutional disturbance is generally mild. Arthralgia, usually involving the knees and ankles, is present in more than half of the patients.

Diagnosis

▶ **Suspect** the diagnosis when a patient presents with red nodules on the anterior lower legs.

▶ **Consider and exclude**

■ *Vasculitis*, which tends to involve also the backs of the legs, but may produce nodules distinguishable only after biopsy.

■ *Thrombophlebitis* is suggested by tender, palpable veins.

■ *Insect bites* are itchy rather than painful, and often have a recognisable central punctum.

■ *Bruises* may be very similar. When the history and morphology are insufficient for diagnosis, biopsy should be undertaken.

■ *Necrobiosis lipoidica*, although often beginning as nodules, evolves to atrophic yellowish plaques.

▶ **Confirmation** of diagnosis is often not necessary when the setting is typical. If there is doubt a deep incisional biopsy is required. Tissue removed by a punch biopsy will not provide enough fat to enable the diagnostic features to be seen.

Treatment

The important treatment is that of the underlying cause, which should be sought in every case even though a cause is not evident in 30 per cent of cases. Bed rest and salicylates relieve discomfort. Systemic corticosteroids should not be prescribed unless indicated for the primary disease. Spontaneous resolution takes place over three to six weeks.

Erythema multiforme

Erythema multiforme resembles erythema nodosum in being a characteristic pattern of hypersensitivity which develops as a reaction to many primary causes.

Aetiology

In 50 per cent of patients the provocative agent is never discovered. The most frequently recognised trigger is herpes simplex, which typically appears seven to 14 days before the rash, but a wide range of infections and vaccinations may precede the eruption. Erythema multiforme may also complicate rheumatoid arthritis, lupus erythematosus, lymphoma, leukaemia and visceral carcinoma. Drug causes include sulphonamides, penicillin, salicylates and phenylbutazone.

Histology

There is a variable mixture of epidermal and dermal changes, and either may predominate. Epidermal changes can range from no more than scattered necrotic cells in the stratum spinosum to more severe damage with liquefaction degeneration of the basal layer. The dermal component may sometimes be barely evident but commonly shows vasodilatation, dermal oedema and a perivascular cellular infiltrate, mostly lymphocytic. In bullous lesions, the plane of separation is subepidermal.

Clinical features *(Colour plates 22, 23)*

- *The primary lesion* is a small reddish macule or oedematous papule, which increases in size for a day or two, reaching a centimetre or more in diameter. The centre darkens and is sometimes purpuric, while a distinct ring tends to develop at the periphery, producing a target-like appearance (iris lesion). This pattern is produced by varying degrees of ischaemia in the cone of skin supplied by the vessels involved in this disorder. With more severe ischaemia, central blistering can be seen.

- *Distribution* is bilateral and centrifugal, with relative sparing of the face and trunk. Palms, soles, the back of the hands and extensor surfaces of the limbs are the common sites.

- *Mucosal involvement* is variable. Vesicles and bullae develop from macules of erythema and quickly rupture to form painful, shallow erosions, covered with a greyish-white pseudomembrane. There may be no mucosal lesions at all, or the mucous membranes may be severely affected, with only a few scattered lesions on the skin.

- *Toxaemic variant (Stevens–Johnson syndrome)* is a less common, more severe illness, dominated by severe constitutional disturbance and painful mucosal erosions. Cutaneous lesions of erythema multiforme are present, but with a pronounced tendency to bulla formation.

There is fever, headache and tachycardia. The mouth is eroded and painful, and the lips crusted. Severe conjunctivitis may progress to corneal ulceration and anterior uveitis. Pneumonia, urinary retention, and cardiovascular complications may be added. The mortality among untreated patients approaches 10 per cent.

Course

Onset is sudden and the evolution of lesions rapid. Individual lesions fade in seven to ten days, but new crops may continue to appear for two or three weeks.

Treatment

An attempt is made to discover the primary cause of the eruption and, in older patients, particular attention is directed to the possibility of occult malignant disease.

The minor form resolves spontaneously without incident and requires no treatment. Recurrent erythema multiforme is usually due to herpes simplex and can be prevented by the prompt treatment of that infection with oral acyclovir.

Patients with the severe bullous form should be admitted to hospital and are probably better treated with systemic corticosteroids to improve the toxaemia.

An initial dose of 40 mg to 60 mg of prednisone daily is reduced slowly over two weeks. Antibiotics may be necessary for secondary infection, and the fluid–electrolyte balance should be monitored. With ocular involvement, ophthalmological consultation is essential.

Erythema perstans ('the annular erythemas')

This group of related diseases is characterised by slowly spreading rings or bands of erythema. No cause is found in most patients, although there is good evidence that some cases are manifestations of hypersensitivity much as is the case in erythema multiforme and erythema nodosum.

Lesions begin as oedematous reddish papules or plaques which enlarge peripherally with central clearing. The spread may be eccentric and lesions may coalesce, forming polycyclic, arcuate, and horseshoe patterns. New lesions may form within old ones, producing concentric rings of erythema—a pattern sometimes sufficiently marked to simulate a woodgrain appearance. This striking variant has a well-documented association with internal malignant disease.

Urticaria and angioedema

Urticaria ('hives')

Urticaria is a very common pattern of vascular reaction which is manifested by transient, well-circumscribed areas of dermal oedema. When the reaction is more marked, the subcutaneous tissue and mucosal surfaces may be involved as well. The condition is then called angioedema. Urticaria and angioedema often occur in the same patient at the same time, or there may be urticaria at one time and angioedema at another. The difference is only one of degree.

Aetiology

The cardinal feature of urticaria, the weal, is produced by an extravasation of fluid from capillaries and venules altered by increased permeability. This temporarily enhanced permeability implies the intervention of vasoactive mediators and, in many patients with acute urticaria, histamine is probably the mediator of importance. In others, kinins, prostaglandins and products of complement activation have been implicated.

Many cases of episodic urticaria (acute urticaria) are a manifestation of the type I allergic reaction, but urticaria can also be a feature of the type III response. However, some substances can have a direct histamine-releasing effect on mast cells and thereby produce urticaria without involving any immunological mechanisms at all. Substances with this property include drugs like aspirin, quinine, dextran, codeine and morphine; and foodstuffs such as azo dyes, preservatives, some shellfish, and some fruits—particularly strawberries.

It is customary to speak of allergic and non-allergic urticaria but in practice the distinction is seldom possible to establish and it is of more relevance to speak of acute urticaria or chronic urticaria.

■ *Acute urticaria* is a suddenly appearing episode which settles within six weeks. Drugs are a frequent cause. Commonly incriminated are aspirin, penicillins, sulphonamides, iodinated X-ray contrast media, and vaccines. Foods often responsible for acute attacks of urticaria are eggs, nuts, chocolate, cheese and fish. Acute urticaria is an uncommon and rare presentation of systemic disease such as viral hepatitis, infectious mononucleosis, hydatid disease, infestation with intestinal parasites, and the connective tissue diseases.

■ *Chronic urticaria*, which is urticaria lasting longer than six weeks, is sometimes seen as a response to chronic sinusitis or readily visible dental sepsis. Emotional factors are often suggested, but their role if any, is controversial. Even after careful investigation, no cause is found for most cases of chronic urticaria.

Multiple causes may be contributing to urticaria in any one patient, and some agents are important as secondary elements rather than as primary causes. Approximately half of those with chronic urticaria are made worse by aspirin. Tartrazine and other food dyes are frequent aggravants, as are the benzoates and hydroxybenzoates used as preservatives. The relevance of small quantities of salicylate and penicillin in food is suspected but unproven.

Clinical features

■ *Lesions* are generally raised and almost always itchy. They are white or pink in colour, often with an erythematous halo around the well-defined border. Size varies from barely visible papules to large plaques many centimetres across. The shape is usually round or oval, but may be quite bizarre. Linear weals may form along scratch lines and there may be broad bands at sites of pressure from clothing. Occasionally, mainly in children, lesions are vesicular or even bullous.

■ *Distribution* is haphazard and may involve any site.

Course

Individual weals are transient. Resolution within a few hours is the rule, and persistence for more than a day is rare. In an acute attack, lesions continue to erupt for several days, and sometimes for two or three weeks after withdrawal of the cause. Unless the aetiological factors are found, chronic urticaria may persist in episodic or continuous fashion for many years, although spontaneous resolution within two years occurs in the majority of cases, even when the cause is not removed.

Hazards of acute urticaria

Particular attention should be directed to the patient with a swollen tongue, or one who complains of tightness in the throat. The onset of hoarseness warns of laryngeal oedema, and is a serious sign in patients with urticaria. A feeling of tightness in the chest may be accompanied by bronchospasm and progress with increasing respiratory distress to asphyxiation. Other badly affected patients have no respiratory discomfort, and complain only of feeling light-headed before collapsing from hypotension.

Diagnosis

▶ Consider and exclude

■ *Mastocytosis*, which is characterised by urtication after light rubbing. However, the persistence and colour of lesions differ from urticaria.

- *Insect bites* are suggested by distribution, history and often by a visible central punctum.

- *Bullous pemphigoid* may present as an urticarial component, but tense blisters eventually appear as well.

Establishing the cause

The weals of urticaria are not hard to identify; detection of the cause is a far more difficult problem. A careful history provides the most helpful information and all patients should be questioned about drugs, particularly salicylates. A 'food diary' may be used to list all ingested food and drink, noting the time of onset of new lesions, in an effort to pinpoint the agents responsible. A diet which eliminates salicylate, dyes and other food additives may be usefully followed after two weeks by oral challenge tests with these agents, provided that the urticaria is no longer evident. Physical examination and relevant investigations occasionally reveal a systemic cause. Immunological testing with prick tests is usually only of benefit in patients where acute episodes occur many months apart with no obvious cause.

Treatment

- *Systemic antihistamines.* Unless the cause can be identified and removed, treatment is symptomatic. H_1 antihistamines provide relief for the majority of patients, provided that the dose is adequate. An average adult will need 16 mg to 32 mg daily of cyproheptadine to achieve initial supression. In some patients, these doses may prove unacceptably sedating and where that is the case, antihistamines that do not cross the blood-brain barrier may be helpful. These include astemizole and terfenadine. Although H_2 antihistamines are not of additional benefit, some patients respond better to one pharmacological group of antihistamines than to another, and, if adequate relief is not obtained with one group, another should be tried. Hydroxyzine is a particularly useful alternative. It usually takes many days until oral antihistamines produce clinical improvement.

- *Systemic corticosteroids* are seldom indicated. In severe acute episodes, steroid therapy may be necessary to relieve intolerable pruritus which remains uncontrolled by adequate doses of antihistamines, or for the patient with involvement of the respiratory tract. However, in an emergency, an intramuscular injection of adrenaline acts more quickly, and should be combined with intravenous administration of hydrocortisone. An airway and tracheostomy tray should be nearby. Systemic steroids should not be prescribed for chronic urticaria.

Variants of urticaria

Pressure urticaria

If you firmly stroke the skin of normal people, more than 5 per cent of them will develop an exaggerated weal along the line of pressure (dermographism). This response should not be confused with pressure urticaria, which develops in predisposed people at sites of moderate rubbing or pressure. Swelling is slow in onset, commencing three or four hours after provocation, and lasting eight to twenty-four hours.

Common sites are the buttocks after sitting, the soles, and beneath the waistband of clothing.

Pressure urticaria is neither prevented nor noticeably modified by antihistamines.

Cold urticaria

This is an uncommon variant, which develops in predisposed individuals after cooling of the skin. Although usually idiopathic, cold urticaria may be an association of cryoglobulinaemia and, rarely, of cold haemolysins. Provocation by application of cold is accompanied by histamine release, but other vasoactive peptides are also involved.

Typically, there is swelling—for example, of the palm after handling a cold object, or of the lips, and sometimes of the oral and pharyngeal mucosa after a cool drink. Large areas may be involved when attacks are precipitated by a cold wind or by swimming, and may be accompanied by tachycardia, hypotension and syncope. The systemic effects of histamine release are particularly dangerous when induced by swimming.

Antihistamines provide only partial relief for most patients. Tolerance to cold can often be substantially increased by gradually increasing exposure to cold water at 15°C over two or three weeks, but the method has been generally unsatisfactory for long-term management.

Cholinergic urticaria

This is a common disorder characterised by the eruption of small urticarial papules with sweating. It occurs mostly in young adults and may be precipitated by heat, exercise or emotion. The papules are surrounded by areas of erythema, which may dominate the appearance. Attacks last up to two hours and itching is often severe. Of all the antihistamines, hydroxyzine pamoate is the most consistently effective for this variety of urticaria.

Contact urticaria

Urticarial weals are a rare expression of contact sensitivity and most frequently follow contact with certain plants and caterpillars. Occasionally, however, urticaria may develop as a true contact allergy to foods and to relatively simple compounds that are harmless to most individuals. The hands are the most commonly affected site and it is likely that contact urticaria is a significant aetiological factor in the persistence of some cases of chronic hand dermatitis.

Hereditary angioedema

This is a rare disease which is caused by defective inhibition of C_1 esterase, and is transmitted as an autosomal dominant defect. Patients develop large areas of circumscribed subcutaneous oedema, spontaneously or after minor trauma, especially dental procedures. There may be colicky abdominal pain, but pruritus is not a feature. Laryngeal oedema is common during attacks, and is a frequent cause of death. Maintenance therapy with tranexamic acid has prevented recurrences in some patients. Danazol is also effective, but is unsuitable for use by pregnant women.

Urticarial vasculitis

Leucocytoclastic vasculitis may occasionally produce urticaria with no other skin signs of vasculitis. In contrast to all other varieties of urticaria, where typically individual weals fade within a few hours, the characteristic feature of urticarial vasculitis is that individual welts of urticaria persist fixed and unchanged for 48 hours or more. Joint pain is reasonably common and renal involvement may occur. However, this pattern of vasculitis is seldom associated with vasculitis of other internal structures, even though the list of causes is the same as for other varieties of leucocytoclastic vasculitis. Urticaria seen during an acute phase of lupus erythematosus is always urticarial vasculitis. Oral antihistamines are not usually of benefit.

Leg ulcers

The cutaneous circulation of the lower leg normally has less reserve than other areas. The relative stasis below the knee is reflected in the frequency with which lesions of cutaneous vasculitis occurs on the legs alone. The poorer nutrition of skin over the lower leg explains the intractable ulceration which may follow doses of X-ray therapy that are well tolerated at other sites. The poor reserve is further reduced with increasing age, and by the effects of diabetes, hypertension and arteriosclerosis.

When the efficiency of the muscle-vein pump is destroyed by deep vein thrombosis and the stasis syndrome is added, very minor trauma or infection may be sufficient to precipitate ulceration.

Stasis ulcer

The stasis ulcer usually develops on the inner side of the lower leg, overlying an incompetent perforating vein. The edge is sharp with little undermining, the border is curved and somewhat irregular. The base is oedematous, red and granulating, often with a cover of exudate. The surrounding skin is frequently inflamed by a low-grade cellulitis, and some staining by haemosiderin is almost invariable. Much of the lower leg may show the pigmentation and fibrosis of prolonged stasis.

The ulcer may be a centimetre or two across, or it may replace most of the skin of the lower third of the leg, erode the subcutis and cause periostitis. Recurrent infection may lead to chronic ill health, and immobility may lead to fibrous ankylosis of the ankle. Squamous cell carcinoma is a very rare, late complication.

Ischaemic ulcer

The ischaemic ulcer usually begins at the tip or base of the toes, or around a fissure on the heel, but may develop on the lower leg, particularly in the diabetic. The edges are well-defined, and the ulcer is painful, especially when the limb is warmed. The toes may be pale, bluish or dull red, and feel cool to the touch. The skin tends to be dry and flaky, but may be moist. The nails are dystrophic and hair is lost from the dorsum of the toes. The fat pads under the toes and heel are often atrophic.

Hypertensive ulcer

Ischaemic ulcers in hypertensive patients are frequently multiple, painful, punched-out and, at first, covered by a dark scab. They may occur anywhere on the leg, but commonly develop around the ankles.

Diabetic ulcer

Patients with diabetes have many potential reasons for developing ulcers. Neuropathy may render the foot insensitive to pain so that an ulcer develops at a site of pressure on the toes or at a weight-bearing region on the sole, where the ulcer may extend deeply, sometimes to bone. The ischaemic leg ulcer is more common in diabetics than in other patients with arteriosclerosis, because of associated diabetic microvascular disease. Also, areas of necrobiosis lipoidica are very prone to ulceration.

Other causes of leg ulcers

Patients with vasculitis, lupus erythematosus and scleroderma may present because of leg ulcers, and the leg is a common site for pyoderma gangrenosum. Bowen's disease on the leg may become crusted and ulcerate, particularly with progression to frank carcinoma. The leg ulcer may be a manifestation of lymphoma, leukaemia, and tertiary syphilis, and is a rare presentation of basal cell carcinoma. A bizarre ulcer which resists adequate therapy should raise the possibility of artefact, but this is a diagnosis to be made with caution.

Management

The patient with a leg ulcer should be carefully assessed, in regard both to local factors and to general health. Arteriosclerosis, diabetes, renal disease, and cardiac failure may all contribute to the pathogenesis of a 'typical stasis ulcer'. The chronic ulcer may itself cause ill health, with anaemia, depression, and apathy. The ischaemic limb requires evaluation by a vascular surgeon. The use of tobacco is discouraged, and the patient warned of the dangers of local heat and inexpert paring of corns and calluses.

The patient should understand the vulnerability of the leg ulcer to chemical and mechanical trauma. Applications should be bland, non-irritating, and have a low potential for contact sensitisation. Apart from such simple measures as those described in relation to stasis dermatitis with ulceration, topical therapy seldom provides more than marginal benefit. The important treatment is that of the cause.

Lymphoedema

Lymphoedema may follow surgical removal or malignant invasion of lymph glands, or their destruction by radiotherapy. The lymphatic drainage of a region may also be compromised by recurrent streptococcal infection, or by tuberculosis or parasitic infestation of the draining nodes.

Primary lymphoedema may be transmitted as an autosomal dominant defect, but most patients give no family history of the disease. Whether hereditary factors are present or not, varicose or hypoplastic lymphatic vessels are demonstrable in the majority of cases.

Clinical features

Primary lymphoedema may be present at birth, but generally appears in the second decade or later. The legs are the common site, but the arms, face and genitalia may be affected.

Soft, pitting oedema develops in one ankle, disappearing at first with elevation of the limb. The oedema becomes more persistent, progresses proximally and may involve the other leg. The swelling becomes firm and non-pitting, while the skin thickens, ultimately forming an irregular, verrucoid surface. The course is punctuated by episodes of cellulitis, which further compromise lymphatic drainage.

Treatment

Progression is retarded by firm bandaging and the use of diuretics. Infection should be promptly treated, and regular prophylactic doses of an antibiotic may be necessary to prevent recurrences. Surgical attempts have been made to improve lymphatic drainage, but the main value of surgery in primary lymphoedema is to reduce deformity in badly affected limbs.

Yellow nail syndrome

This very uncommon disorder of adults is characterised by lymphoedema, usually of the ankles, a yellowish or greenish discolouration of all 20 nails, and recurrent pleural effusion. Episodes of paronychial inflammation with shedding of individual nails are common.

9

Tumours of the skin

1. Epidermal tumours
2. Cutaneous cysts
3. Appendageal tumours
4. Mesodermal tumours
5. Neural tumours

Tumours of the skin, like those of other organs, are classified as benign or malignant usually on the basis of predicted future behaviour, and the division is sometimes arbitrary. Solar keratoses have some histological features of malignancy, yet it is likely that only a small proportion would ever become truly malignant. Kerato-acanthomas show many mitoses, disorganised arrangement of cells, and send proliferating columns of cells down into the dermis, but are benign in behaviour. Despite many microscopic features of malignancy, Bowen's disease may persist for many years before invasive carcinoma supervenes. Basal cell carcinoma is locally destructive and may destroy life by invasion of vital structures, but almost never metastasises.

Cutaneous tumours are described according to the tissues they resemble, but this does not imply origin from such tissue. The resemblance of cells of basal cell carcinoma to epidermal basal cells does not signify that the tumour has arisen from the basal layer. Apocrine tumours are not confined to areas where apocrine glands are normally found and apocrine differentiation does not indicate aprocrine origin. Epithelial cells of the skin and its appendages are pluripotential and may differentiate in various directions.

Many tumours of the skin are more accurately described as hamartomas. The term 'naevus' is used by dermatologists to describe almost any developmental abnormality of the skin, and many naevi are hamartomas. The nomenclature and classification of cutaneous tumours contain many inconsistencies. The ensuing discussion is designed to present the important features of tumours of the skin and, to achieve this, clarity will take precedence over academic niceties.

Epidermal tumours

1. Benign
   (a) seborrhoeic keratosis
   (b) kerato-acanthoma

2. Premalignant
   (a) solar keratosis
   (b) cutaneous horn
   (c) Bowen's disease
   (d) arsenical keratosis
   (e) erythroplasia of Queyrat
   (f) leukoplakia
   (g) post-irradiation keratosis
3. Malignant
   (a) squamous cell carcinoma
   (b) basal cell carcinoma

Benign epidermal tumours

Seborrhoeic keratosis (seborrhoeic wart)

This very common benign tumour occurs predominantly in middle-aged and elderly people.

Aetiology

In some families seborrhoeic keratoses occur as if by autosomal dominant inheritance. However, the disease is extremely common and familial distribution may be coincidental. The sudden eruption of numerous, itchy seborrhoeic keratoses is a well-documented, but very rare manifestation of internal malignancy.

Histology

Typically, the lesion sits up above the skin, with the dermo-epidermal junction more or less level with the stratum corneum of surrounding skin. The surface is irregular, with marked thickening of the stratum corneum. The whole epidermis is thick and uneven, and sections may give the impression of small cysts of stratum corneum within the stratum spinosum. Cells of the stratum spinosum are small and immature, but lack the disorganisation and mitoses of malignancy. Dermal papillae are elongated and irregular, and melanocytes are usually more numerous in the basal layer.

Clinical features

Seborrhoeic keratoses are most common on the face and trunk, but may occur anywhere on the skin, except the palms, soles and mucocutaneous junctions. The typical lesion begins as a round or oval, honey-coloured or brownish thickening, from a few millimetres to two centimetres or more in diameter. Early lesions may be scraped off with a fingernail, but recur. As the keratoses thicken, they darken to deep brown or brownish black, and may project half a centimetre or more above the surrounding skin. *(Colour plate 25)*

The surface is usually irregular and, with a hand lens, is seen to be pitted with small depressions, many of which are plugged with keratin. Occasional lesions are smooth and black, but remain sharply demarcated. The surface often has a greasy appearance, but is dry and rough to the touch. The sharp borders and elevation give the impression of a lesion which is stuck onto the surface of the skin, rather than being part of it.

Seborrhoeic keratoses may be solitary, but are usually multiple. Some elderly people have hundreds of these on the trunk at various stages of evolution. In heavily pigmented races, adults often have many small dark papular seborrhoeic keratoses on the malar regions of the face. Itch is uncommon, most lesions remaining asymptomatic. They may cause annoyance by catching in clothing and occasionally become inflamed, either from trauma or by irritation from the contents of plugged cysts. There may be crusting and bleeding, which can make differentiation from melanoma more difficult.

Diagnosis

▶ **Consider and exclude**

■ *Lentigo maligna*, which is not elevated, occurs only on sun-damaged skin, and lacks the pitted surface and sharp borders of the seborrhoeic wart.

■ *Pigmented basal cell carcinoma* usually has a gelatinous appearance and a thickened border which is more apparent when the skin is stretched.

■ *Melanomas* lack the rough pitted surface of a seborrhoeic keratosis, but occasional lesions need to be excised or biopsied to exclude melanoma with certainty.

■ *Solar keratosis* may be difficult to distinguish from early lesions, but is suggested by superficial scaling.

Treatment

The vast majority of seborrhoeic keratoses need no treatment. When disfiguring lesions occur on the face, removal can be accomplished, with little or no scarring, by light cautery, which softens the keratosis so that it can then be wiped off with a gauze square. Thicker lesions may require curettage. Bleeding is not troublesome and can be controlled with firm pressure. Freezing with carbon dioxide and acetone slush, or liquid nitrogen, is effective for very thin lesions.

Kerato-acanthoma

A tumour-like nodule of characteristic architecture, which grows rapidly to a maximum size before undergoing spontaneous resolution.

Aetiology

As a rule, kerato-acanthoma (KA) occurs in the same group of predominantly fair-skinned people who are predisposed to the development of squamous cell carcinoma (SCC). The site, on light-exposed skin, corresponds to the distribution of most SCCs, and the incidence bears a fairly constant ratio of one KA to three SCCs. Like SCCs, KAs are more frequent among workers who handle tar and mineral oils but, unlike SCCs, KAs generally arise in apparently normal skin showing no evidence of precancerous change.

There is a rare group of patients in whom multiple KAs continue to erupt over many years, without the usual association with SCC. Distribution is not confined to light-exposed areas and even mucosal surfaces may be involved. The first tumours begin to appear in the second decade and the scars from numerous healed lesions eventually become most disfiguring. Kerato-acanthomas are more numerous and appear to grow more rapidly in immunosuppressed patients.

Histology

Differentiation of KA from SCC on the basis of cellular characteristics alone is often difficult and sometimes impossible. The overall architecture of the lesion is then of great importance in diagnosis. If only part of the nodule is excised, the biopsy must therefore traverse the lesion completely from side to side, and extend downwards to the full depth of the nodule.

In the early stages, epidermal cells proliferate downwards as poorly demarcated strands, with atypical cells and many mitoses. A keratinous invagination of the epidermis produces a thick, chalice-shaped shell of proliferating epidermis which encloses a central keratinous core. The core progressively expands to form a large keratin-filled crater surrounded by proliferating epidermis which bulges over the crater as an overhanging lip. There is a dense inflammatory infiltrate in the dermis below the epidermal downgrowth.

Clinical features *(Colour plate 26)*

More than two-thirds of KAs occur on the face, with most of the remainder on the dorsum of hands and forearms. The lesion begins as a firm, pink or reddish papule, which is tender and rapidly growing. With increasing size, the nodule becomes smooth and dome-shaped, and has a well-demarcated edge. Palpation reveals extension of the nodule well below the surface, but laterally there is no surrounding infiltration.

Within a few weeks, the nodule reaches a centimetre or two in size, and rare lesions grow to many centimetres. Usually within four or five weeks, the centre of the dome either forms a hard keratinous plug or develops a crater which is packed with friable material. As the KA matures, the sides of the crater shrink, with expulsion of the central plug. Slow spontaneous resolution occurs over two to six months, but the healing margins pucker and may leave an ugly stellate scar.

Diagnosis

The history and appearance are generally distinctive. However, a rapidly growing SCC may mimic an early KA, and a KA occasionally grows slowly enough to resemble SCC. In most cases, an adequate biopsy will allow the pathologist to make a confident diagnosis, but in a few patients is not possible even after biopsy. Such doubtful lesions should be treated as SCC.

Treatment

Although KAs resolve spontaneously, the complications produced by uncontrolled scarring makes active treatment advisable. Small lesions are readily excised and examined histologically. Larger lesions may be removed by curettage and cautery of the margins, after preliminary biopsy. Radiotherapy is curative and gives satisfactory cosmetic results, but should not be used for the early-onset group with multiple lesions. For this rare group, cytotoxic agents and oral retinoids have been successfully substituted for more destructive measures, but their use in this context must still be regarded as experimental.

Premalignant epidermal tumours

The great majority of basal cell carcinomas form without any preceding lesion. Squamous cell carcinomas too may arise on apparently normal skin, but are more often preceded by lesions of borderline status. Some of these premalignant lesions have a relatively benign histology. Others show histological features of carcinoma, but remain on the epidermal side of the basement membrane. Transition from pre-cancer or cancer in situ to squamous cell carcinoma is accompanied by disappearance of the basement membrane.

Solar keratosis

An adherent scaly thickening which occurs on light-exposed areas, and has a definite potential for malignant change.

Aetiology

The term 'senile keratosis' is sometimes applied, but is inappropriate. Although the incidence of solar keratoses increases with age, it is not uncommon in Australia to see typical lesions in the third decade.

There are two major factors involved in the development of solar keratoses—the cumulative amount of solar radiation which reaches the skin surface, and the ability of the skin to protect itself from solar damage. The amount of solar energy which reaches the skin is affected by the geographical region, habits of recreation and dress, occupation, and measures taken to protect the skin from ultraviolet light. The ability of the skin to protect itself from actinic damage is largely influenced by genetic factors, particularly the ability to produce melanin.

Histology

There is a sharply-demarcated area of altered stratum spinosum, with variable thickening of the overlying stratum corneum. The cells of the stratum spinosum are disorderly in arrangement, and some atypical cells have large hyperchromatic nuclei. The epidermis is usually thickened, but may be atrophic. There is epidermal down-growth, but the basement membrane remains intact. The underlying dermis shows chronic solar degeneration and, usually, a chronic inflammatory infiltrate.

Clinical features (Colour plate 27)

The vast majority of solar keratoses occur on the face, ears and scalp of those with little hair, and on the forearms, back of the hands and, less often, the legs and dorsum of the feet. The patient first notices a small rough patch of skin; the colour may match surrounding skin, but is often yellowish-brown or red. He or she may be aware of mild stinging of the lesion with sweating, or minor discomfort when using a towel. The early keratosis is often picked or scratched off, but usually reappears. The scale is adherent and when pulled off leaves an oozing surface, sometimes with a little bleeding. The scale may separate spontaneously only to reappear later.

Natural history

The early keratosis is usually only a few millimetres across, but may be more extensive. Slow thickening follows and a horny protuberance may develop. Most solar keratoses then persist at this stage relatively unchanged. A small percentage may actually resolve.

Malignant transformation to squamous cell carcinoma is rare, with less than one per cent undergoing this change unless the person is chronically ingesting immunosuppressive agents, in which case the likelihood of this happening approaches almost thirty per cent. Induration of the base is the earliest sign to look for in determining whether the lesion being examined is a solar keratosis or a squamous cell carcinoma.

As metastasis of squamous cell carcinoma arising in sun-damaged skin is rare, and very few solar keratoses evolve to squamous cell carcinoma, metastasis of a squamous cell carcinoma arising in a solar keratosis must be an extremely rare event in the normal patient who is not immunosuppressed.

Diagnosis

▶ **Consider and exclude**

■ *Early seborrhoeic keratoses*, which may be difficult to distinguish from solar keratoses. Unlike a solar keratosis, these have a greasy rather than a gritty feel. Also, a pitted surface is usually visible, and extreme magnification will reveal the pseudo-horn cysts.

■ *Small areas of lupus erythematosus* may be similar, but the scale is more easily peeled off and shows tiny prolongations on the undersurface.

■ *Xeroderma* is common in elderly people and is frequently accompanied by small, scaly areas which may resemble multiple solar keratoses. However, senile xeroderma is not confined to light-exposed areas and responds to simple emollients.

■ *Stucco keratoses* are harmless keratinous papules, usually occurring on the back of the legs, dorsum of the feet and, sometimes, on the thighs and upper limbs. They are greyish white and easily scratched off, leaving a small depression free of bleeding and oozing.

Treatment

Cryotherapy is simple, safe and effective for superficial keratoses. Liquid nitrogen gives good results, but should be used with caution around the eyes or where a peripheral nerve lies close to the skin. A swab stick may be moistened with liquid nitrogen for application to the keratosis, or a fine jet of evaporating nitrogen can be directed under pressure onto the lesion. Carbon dioxide is also quite satisfactory. Solidified carbon dioxide is mixed with acetone to form a firm slush which is lightly applied with a swab stick for five or six seconds. More prolonged application will produce blistering, especially over the back of the hand, and is not necessary.

Within a half an hour, the frozen area of skin becomes oedematous and reddened. Over a few days, a surface crust forms and separates within a week. Scarring does not occur, but the skin is at first redder and later paler than normal. Repigmentation usually occurs over several months.

Blistered lesions are less likely to repigment. In some patients a temporary post-inflammatory pigmentation occurs and may be quite disfiguring for a time.

■ Thicker lesions may be excised, but cautery is effective and, if carefully used, leaves a cosmetically acceptable scar. With any suspicion of malignancy, keratoses should be biopsied or excised for microscopic examination. The risk of persistent ulceration warrants caution in the use of cautery, and even cryotherapy, on lesions below the knee.

■ *Topical 5-fluorouracil (5-FU)* can be used to treat solar keratoses. Lesions on the face and scalp respond well. However, clearing may not be as complete when this treatment is used in other regions. As a 5 per cent cream or 1 per cent lotion, 5-FU is applied to the keratoses once or twice daily for three to four weeks. The skin, especially where keratoses are present, becomes inflamed and, ultimately, eroded. Treatment is ceased, a bland ointment applied to relieve discomfort and the erosions then heal within a week or two without scarring. If it is thought that a satisfactory end point has been reached but erosions have not appeared, treatment can be ceased. If the inflammatory reaction is too severe, treatment can be interrupted and then recommenced. The concurrent use of a topical steroid lessens the likelihood of a severe painful response to 5-FU, but does not reduce efficacy. When 5-FU is used, follow-up examinations are essential. If basal cell carcinoma is knowingly or inadvertently treated with 5-FU, the surface may heal while the deeper component persists. Where there is the slightest suspicion of carcinoma, 5-FU should not be used. A practical difficulty is the frequency with which patients pass on their cream to friends, who then treat their self-diagnosed 'sun spots'.

■ For the elderly patient with a mixture of xeroderma and keratoses, 2 to 4 per cent salicylic acid in an emollient base applied daily for a week or two will allow recognition of keratoses in need of cryotherapy. When large areas are treated in this way, it should be realised that percutaneous absorption of salicylic acid may be significant and is additive to salicylate taken orally.

Cutaneous horn

A variant of solar keratosis in which keratinised cells remain adherent, to form a slowly growing horn-like tumour.

Clinical features

The horn forms on skin which shows other evidence of chronic solar degeneration and, usually, typical solar keratoses. The lesion is hard, brownish and often arises from a reddened, somewhat infiltrated base, sharply demarcated from surrounding skin. Neglected cutaneous horns may reach a considerable size. Frank carcinoma may develop and is suggested by a firm thickening beneath and around the base of the horn. *(Colour plate 28)*

Diagnosis

The hard 'horny' texture is rarely duplicated by other protruding lesions.

▶ **Consider and exclude**
- seborrhoeic keratoses
- viral warts
- ruptured keratinising cysts

Treatment

When the base is reddened and indurated, the lesion is better excised and examined histologically. For obviously benign lesions, cautery and curettage of the base is safe and effective.

Bowen's disease

A reddish, circumscribed, scaling or crusted plaque, with the potential for transformation to squamous cell carcinoma.

Aetiology

Chronic sun damage is responsible for most cases and even when it occurs in non-exposed areas, the patients are middle-aged or elderly.

Prolonged ingestion of inorganic arsenical compounds predisposes to the development of the disease. Eight per cent of people treated in the past with potassium arsenite (Fowler's solution) developed Bowen's disease after latent periods of up to 20 years. Ingestion of arsenic is also associated with an increased incidence of basal and squamous cell carcinomas of the skin, and with carcinoma of other organs.

Sometimes, when Bowen's disease is found extensively in non-sun-exposed areas, there is no history of past arsenic exposure. Several surveys of these patients indicate an increased incidence of visceral neoplasia. However, because patients have had to recall events that occurred up to 20 years earlier, it is not clear how much of this increased incidence can be ascribed to visceral carcinogenesis induced by arsenic.

Histology

The epidermis is irregularly thickened, with deep rete ridges reaching down between the dermal papillae. The stratum corneum is thicker but less compact than normal. The cells of the stratum spinosum are atypical, many with deeply staining nuclei and mitoses. Cell maturation is disturbed, with keratinisation of individual cells and vacuolisation of others. A few giant cells may be present. The whole appearance is of an evolving, well-differentiated squamous cell carcinoma, but atypical cells are confined to the epidermis and there is no dissolution of the basement membrane.

Clinical features

The typical lesion begins as a slowly enlarging, sharply demarcated, slightly thickened red plaque. At first the surface is lightly scaling, but may later become yellowish-brown, irregularly thickened and sometimes crusted. The plaque may persist more or less unchanged for years, with only slow, gradual extension. The development of nodular thickening or ulceration often reflects carcinomatous change.

Plaques of Bowen's disease are few or solitary, and no site is exempt. Multiple lesions suggest an arsenical cause. In the large flexures, lesions may be itchy, pigmented, macerated and nondescript in appearance. When the nail bed is involved, the disease may resemble warts, carcinoma or melanoma.

Diagnosis

▶ **Consider and exclude**

■ *Plaques of psoriasis*, which are usually multiple, with a suggestive distribution.

■ *Superficial basal cell carcinoma* has a raised border, a gelatinous appearance and may be distinguished with certainty by biopsy.

■ *Bowenoid papulosis* presents clinically as reddish-brown to purplish papules on the genital skin of either sex, or in the perianal region. The lesions closely resemble Bowen's disease histologically. Even though wart virus DNA can be recovered from the lesions, a true potential for biological malignancy remains doubtful, and spontaneous resolution may occur.

■ *Fixed drug eruption* is darker in colour, is often vesicular, and has a fluctuating course.

■ *Lichen simplex chronicus* is less defined at the edges, is itchy, and has thick adherent scale.

Treatment

Small lesions should be excised. Larger plaques, which would require grafting after excision, can be satisfactorily treated by cautery and curettage in two or three stages. This piecemeal removal gives a very satisfactory result, but should be avoided on the lower leg where healing is slow and a persistent ulcer may result.

Radiotherapy is curative, but presents difficulties with large lesions and may not be used below the knee. Cryotherapy is followed by a high recurrence rate because the abnormal cells involve hair follicle epithelium and may therefore be beyond the depth of the freeze.

Arsenical keratosis

A premalignant, horny papule or nodule which results from chronic absorption of inorganic arsenic.

Clinical features

After a latent period of years, keratinous thickenings rather like corns develop on the palms, soles, dorsum of the hands and feet, and on the sides of the digits. They are yellowish in colour and range in size from a millimetre or two to half a centimetre or more in diameter. Initially discrete, the keratoses may coalesce as they increase in size and number. They may remain more or less unchanged for long periods, but some eventually progress to squamous cell carcinoma—a change marked by infiltration, surrounding erythema and ulceration.

Arsenical keratoses are usually accompanied by multiple plaques of Bowen's disease in other areas, particularly the trunk. Superficial basal cell carcinomas may also be present. Carcinogenesis induced by arsenic is not confined to the skin. The cutaneous lesions are associated with a high incidence of pulmonary, genito-urinary and other visceral carcinomas.

In the past, arsenic mixtures were ingested for the treatment of psoriasis and eczema, peptic ulcer and asthma. It can be absorbed through the skin and is found in sheep dip, some antifungal fruit sprays, 'treated' pine and varieties of pottery glaze.

Diagnosis

▶ Consider and exclude

■ *Corns*, which are less numerous, are confined to areas of friction and are not accompanied by multiple plaques of Bowen's disease.

■ *Focal hyperkeratosis* of the palms and soles does not involve the dorsum of the hands and feet and is not associated with Bowen's disease.

Treatment

The number of keratoses precludes their routine removal, but regular examinations are essential so that suspicious lesions can be excised. At each examination, the whole skin surface should be searched for areas of Bowen's disease and other tumours. Regular chest X-ray examinations should be arranged.

Erythroplasia of Queyrat

A premalignant lesion of distinctive appearance which occurs at mucocutaneous junctions or on mucosal surfaces.

Histology

The histology is that of Bowen's disease.

Clinical features

Erythroplasia is predominantly a disease of uncircumcised men, in whom it usually occurs on the glans, coronal sulcus, or adjoining prepuce. The vulva, oral mucosa and conjunctivae are rare sites.

The characteristic lesion is a solitary, slightly thickened, bright red velvety plaque with a well-defined border. Areas of thickening or ulceration suggest carcinomatous transformation.

Treatment

Preliminary biopsy is essential for accurate diagnosis. Surgical excision of the plaque with a margin of normal tissue is curative, but is not readily accepted by many patients. Cautery, cryotherapy, and local excision may not eradicate areas of involvement too small to be recognised clinically, and radiotherapy has proved unsatisfactory. Excision by the Mohs' technique, as used for carcinoma, gives better results.

The use of 5-fluorouracil under plastic occlusion is reported to be effective and may provide an acceptable alternative. The absence of hair follicles renders the site less likely to recurrences from involved follicular epithelium than with Bowen's disease in other areas. However, treatment extends over several weeks, is very uncomfortable and requires careful and prolonged follow-up. Transition to carcinoma necessitates partial amputation of the penis.

Leukoplakia

Leukoplakia is defined as an abnormal hyperplastic reaction of a mucosal or mucocutaneous surface, which microscopically shows epithelial atypia suggestive of carcinoma in situ.

Aetiology

Much confusion has resulted from imprecise criteria for the diagnosis of leukoplakia. Too often leukoplakia has been interpreted as any persistent white patch on a mucosal surface or mucocutaneous junction. There are many causes of such lesions, some of which have no malignant potential.

On the lower lip, long exposure to sunshine is an important pre-disposing cause. On the buccal mucosa, continued irritation from dentures or tobacco may be important, while on the vulva, mucosal atrophy has been reported as a predisposing factor.

Histology

On the lip, there is hyperkeratosis and irregular thickening of the stratum spinosum with a disorderly arrangement of atypical cells. Buccal and vulval lesions are similar, but hyperkeratosis is inconstant and the epithelium may be atrophic. A dense subepithelial infiltrate of inflammatory cells is a regular feature.

Clinical features (Colour plate 29)

The common presentation is of a symptomless, slightly thickened, well-defined white area on any part of the lower lip. The patch may be more obviously thickened, in a regular or irregular fashion.

The appearance on the buccal mucosa is similar and, as on the lip, nodules of thickening or ulceration should suggest the possibility of carcinoma.

Vulval leukoplakia may involve the clitoris, labia minora or mucosal surfaces of the labia majora. Lesions are solitary or multiple, and consist of well-demarcated, white or greyish, thickened plaques. Unlike labial or buccal leukoplakia, the vulval lesions may cause considerable pruritus.

Diagnosis

When a patient presents with a suspicious area of leukokeratosis, it is reasonable to remove causes of mechanical and chemical trauma and, in the case of vulval lesions, to prescribe a corticosteroid cream to relieve itch and minimise scratching. If, however, the plaque persists, biopsy is essential.

▶ **Consider and exclude**

■ *In the mouth and on the lip*, causes of leukokeratosis include lichen planus, lupus erythematosus, cheek-biting, submucous fibrosis and trauma from badly-fitting dentures.

■ *On the vulva*, lichen sclerosus et atrophicus, vulval atrophy, lichen planus, and Bowen's disease may all be confused with leukoplakia.

Treatment

Small patches should be removed either by cautery or excision. Larger areas on the vulva may necessitate vulvectomy. Any doubtful area of thickening or ulceration requires biopsy to exclude carcinoma, and more than one biopsy may be needed. Carcinoma which arises in an area of leukoplakia, like that arising in Bowen's disease, has a greater potential for metastasis than carcinoma which evolves from a solar keratosis.

Post-irradiation keratoses

Skin which has been exposed to large doses of X-rays becomes atrophic, with telangiectasia and altered pigmentation. Light scaling is common, and lesions which resemble solar keratoses may develop. These post-irradiation keratoses frequently become carcinomatous, and should be excised or destroyed with the cautery.

Malignant epidermal tumours

Squamous cell carcinoma

Squamous cell carcinoma is a common malignant tumour of the epidermis, with a variable capacity for maturation of cells towards keratinisation.

Aetiology

Squamous cell carcinoma (SCC) may arise as a consequence of prolonged exposure to chemical carcinogens. The carcinogen may be topical, as with soot, tar, lubricating oils and creosote, or it may be systemic, as with inorganic arsenicals. SCC may form at the site of old injuries, as in burn or vaccination scars, in relation to longstanding ulcers or sinuses, or in an area of radiation atrophy. An aetiological role has been postulated also for a particular strain of wart virus which can be regularly demonstrated in association with certain rare forms of cutaneous SCC. However, such cases are exceptional. The vast majority of SCCs are due to the cumulative effect of actinic damage in genetically predisposed people, and occur on light-exposed areas.

■ The incidence is high in outdoor workers, especially those with fair or freckled complexions who tan poorly. While not uncommon on the lower lip, SCC is rare on the shaded upper lip. In most studies, 70 per cent of lip cancers have occurred in elderly, fair-skinned white men who worked out of doors. Compared to whites the incidence is low in black races and there is no predilection for exposed skin. When the protective melanin is absent, as in albinism, the incidence rises and the distribution then corresponds to that in caucasoids.

Most patients with SCC have many solar keratoses. Occasionally, histology may confirm SCC arising within a solar keratosis. More commonly sun damage is evident under the microscope only as elastotic change within the dermis. SCC which develops in sun-damaged skin differs in behaviour from SCC at other sites. The tumour is more differentiated, less aggressive and metastasises less often. When metastases do appear, they usually originate from lesions on the lip or ear.

■ Although factors are of critical importance for most patients, systemic factors may also have a significant role. In general, malignant tumours are increasingly common with advancing age, and immunological factors appear to be relevant to this. The incidence of SCC, as of other tumours, is greater in immunosuppressed patients. Among recipients of cadaveric renal transplants, the frequency of cutaneous SCC is increased twentyfold, and the mortality tenfold.

Histology

There is an irregular downward proliferation of epidermal cells, with invasion of the dermis and disruption of the dermo-epidermal junction. There are varying proportions of undifferentiated and differentiated keratinising squamous cells, and the proportion varies in different parts of the same tumour.

In well-differentiated tumours, desmosomes are well formed and there are small areas where concentric layers of squamous cells show increasing keratinisation towards the centre (horn pearls). More anaplastic areas show variation of cellular size and shape, and hyperchromatic nuclei. In such areas, the intercellular attachments are loosened, and cells are keratinised individually rather than in a concentric pattern. Mitoses are frequent and atypical. Attempts have been made to grade SCC on the basis of the degree of differentiation. In a broad sense, lack of differentiation is an index of aggressiveness, but depth of invasion is just as important as maturation of cells in assessment of the tumour.

Clinical features *(Colour plate 30)*

The early lesion is noticed as a firm thickening of the skin, usually on a background of chronic solar damage and in association with a premalignant lesion. On the lower lip, the preceding lesion may be a patch of leukoplakia, often with dryness and scaling of the remainder of the vermilion border. The carcinoma may begin as a persistent fissure which becomes firm and ulcerated, or as a warty lesion or fleshy red nodule.

On other areas of the face and on the hand or forearm, SCC usually begins as a firm thickening at the base of a keratosis, with surrounding erythema. Less often, the early lesion is a warty nodule or plaque, or a firm ulcer with rolled, solid borders of a dull reddish colour. At first, the ulcer crater has a keratinous surface which, unlike the central crust of a basal cell carcinoma, is difficult to remove. Later the keratinous centre separates, or is knocked out, leaving a reddish crater which develops a yellowish exudate.

When carcinoma arises in an area of Bowen's disease, there may be a localising thickening, an exuberant red nodule, or a firm ulcer. Squamous cell carcinoma occasionally arises on apparently normal skin. The early lesion is then usually a quickly growing red nodule, rather like granulation tissue. The nodule is firm, but lacks the hardness of more differentiated carcinomas, and soon ulcerates. These lesions are more anaplastic, with a greater incidence of metastasis to regional nodes.

Haematogenous dissemination is very uncommon with cutaneous SCC. Lymph node involvement occurs in less than 0.5 per cent of patients when the cancer arises in sun-damaged skin; when the carcinoma complicates leukoplakia or Bowen's disease, or arises on the lower lip, or on normal skin, lymph node involvement is much more frequent. Palpable draining lymph nodes found on examination of a patient with SCC are often due to secondary infection. Carcinomatous glands are hard, and soon become fixed to surrounding tissue. *(Colour plate 31)*

Diagnosis

▶ **Suspect** SCC when dealing with any keratotic indurated lesions or persistent non-healing ulcer.

▶ **Consider and exclude**

■ *Kerato-acanthoma*, which has a history of initial rapid growth, a central keratotic plug, and seems to emerge abruptly from the surrounding skin.

■ *Solar keratosis*, which does not have an indurated base.

■ *Amelanotic melanoma*, which may resemble anaplastic carcinoma—emphasising the importance of routine histology for all tumours removed from the skin.

■ *Chondrodermatitis nodularis helicis*, a small painful keratotic nodule most commonly found on the superior pole of the helix of the ear in men past middle age. Asymptomatic during the day, pain is produced at night when lying down with the affected side in contact with the pillow. The lesion is produced by chronic exposure to sunlight and cold, but trauma may also play a part. The central keratotic plug fills a small depression which is centrally placed within an area of inflamed dermis overlying a zone of perichondritis. When there is no doubt regarding the diagnosis, intralesional steroid injection may cause resolution. However, most commonly the treatment is for the lesion to be excised with some underlying cartilage, and for the diagnosis to be confirmed by histology.

■ *Basal cell carcinoma* that is ulcerated may look similar but a pearly edge can usually be demonstrated by stretching the skin.

■ *Other inflammatory ulcers* may pose difficulty when biopsied during a healing phase and histology reveals pseudo-epitheliomatous hyperplasia.

■ *Pseudo-epitheliomatous hyperplasia* is a descriptive histological term for a proliferating thickened epidermis with many mitoses and an exaggerated rete ridge pattern. The cells, however, remain essentially normal without atypical features or bizarre mitoses. This change appears at the edge of a chronic ulcer, over fungal or other dermal granulomas, or even overlying true tumours. The clinical appearance depends upon the underlying pathology. Over granulomas, the skin may be irregularly thickened and rough while, in association with a chronic ulcer, there may be red granulation-like thickening indistinguishable from underlying carcinoma.

▶ **Confirm** the diagnosis by histology whenever SCC is considered a possibility.

Treatment

As the lesion is visible, most patients with skin cancer present early, and cure rates better than 95 per cent should now be the rule. The method of treatment will vary to some extent with the site of the lesion, and the experience of the physician. Whatever form of treatment is used, therapy must be preceded by palpation of draining lymph nodes. When the tumour is too large for simple excision, treatment should be preceded by an adequate biopsy, not only for confirmation of the diagnosis, but also to assess the malignant potential of the carcinoma.

1. Office procedures
2. Radiotherapy
3. Surgery
4. Microscopically controlled excision

■ *Office procedures.* Tumours up to 1 cm in diameter, except on such special sites as the eyelids, nose and ear, are simply excised with a few millimetres of surrounding skin and examined microscopically. On the hand and forearms, it is permissible to destroy small, well-differentiated SCC with the cautery; the cosmetic result is satisfactory and in experienced hands the cure rate for these small tumours approaches 99 per cent. The cautery should be used with great caution around the eyes, where scarring may lead to ectropion and other problems. On the scalp, clinically unrecognised outgrowths more often extend beyond the visible and palpable margins of the tumour and may be inadequately treated. Below the knee, where healing is less reliable, careless use of the cautery may produce persistent ulceration. There is no place for the use of topical cytotoxic agents in this or any other form of skin cancer.

■ *Radiotherapy.* Radiotherapy is especially suitable for cancer of the head and neck in elderly patients. Properly fractionated radiotherapy gives an excellent cure rate and over the nose, ear, and eyelids the cosmetic result is often superior to that achieved by surgical excision. In the nasolabial folds and pre- and post-auricular regions, carcinoma often extends deeply and is not well suited to X-ray treatment. Radiotherapy is contra-indicated for previously irradiated areas and for lesions below the knee.

■ *Surgery.* Surgical excision may be used for any skin cancer, and lymph node involvement makes surgical consultation obligatory. Carcinomas of the anogenital region, and those which are invading bone or cartilage, are better treated surgically, but large lesions which necessitate grafts, especially on the face of an elderly patient, are frequently managed better with radiotherapy. At the labial commissure, surgical excision gives best cosmetic results; at other sites on the lip, X-ray therapy produces an equal cure rate, and frequently a superior cosmetic and functional result.

■ *Microscopically controlled excision (Mohs' technique).* The original method involved sequential excision and microscopic examination of chemically cauterised tissue. Repeated excisions proceeded in stepwise fashion until microscopic examination showed removal beyond all margins of the tumour. The method is painful and has been largely replaced by a 'fresh tissue' technique. The microscopic control of surgical excision combines maximal conservation of uninvolved tissue with an

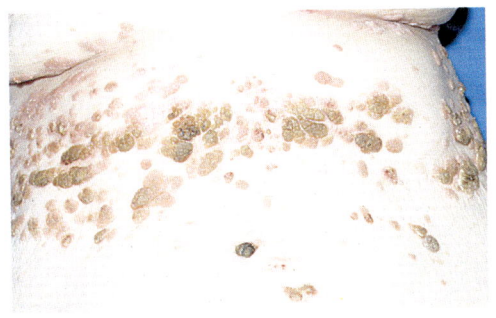

25. Seborrhoeic keratoses

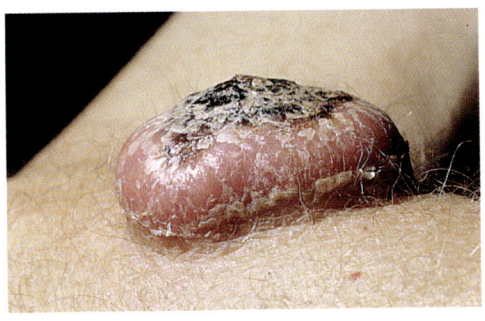

26. Kerato-acanthoma

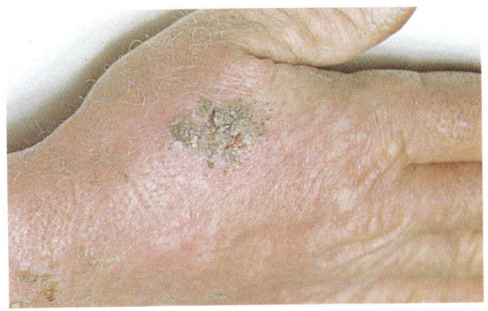

27. Typical solar keratosis

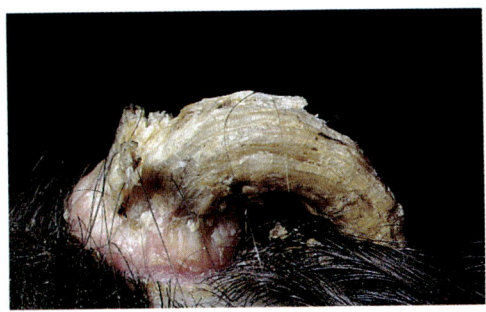

28. Squamous cell carcinoma at the base of a cutaneous horn. The scalp is a very unusual site, except in those with little hair.

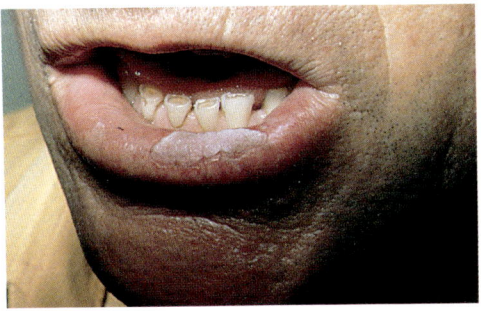

29. Leukoplakia of lip

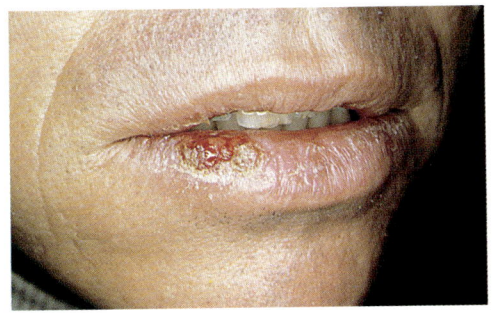

30. Squamous cell carcinoma

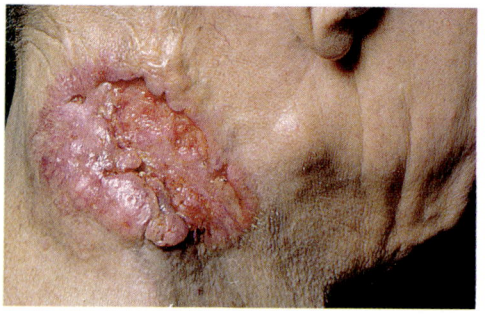

31. Squamous cell carcinoma with metastasis to lymph nodes

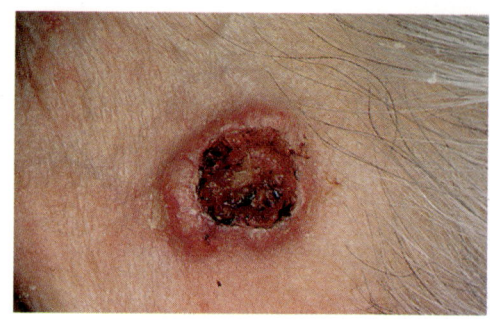

32. Ulcerated basal cell carcinoma

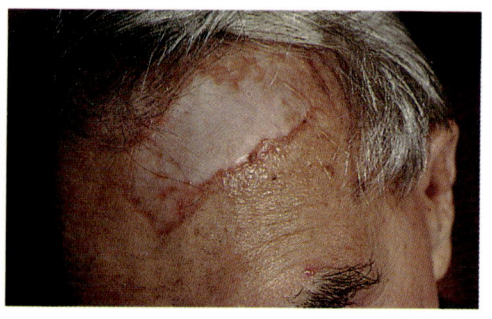

33. Morphoeic basal cell carcinoma

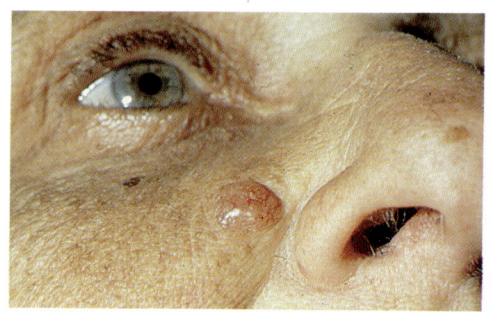

34. Basal cell carcinoma with typical telangiectatic vessels

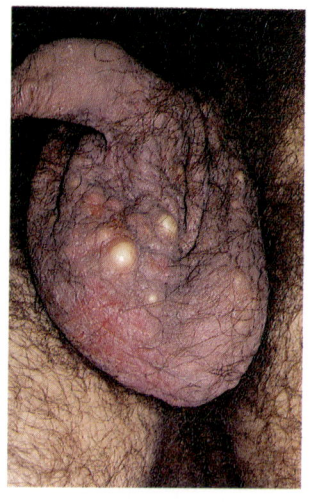

35. Pilar cysts

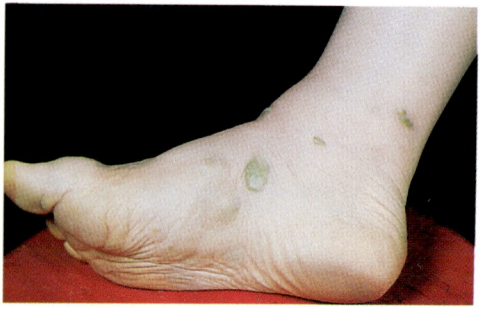

36. Kaposi's sarcoma

excellent cure rate, but is laborious and time-consuming. It is most suitable for residual or recurrent carcinoma, or for carcinoma invading bone or cartilage.

Basal cell carcinoma

Basal cell carcinoma is a common, locally invasive epidermal tumour, composed of cells resembling those of the epidermal basal layer.

Aetiology

Unlike most SCCs, basal cell carcinoma (BCC) is not preceded by a protracted premalignant phase. Rarely, the tumour arises in scars from vaccination or burns, and in areas of radiation atrophy. Certain hamartomas, such as naevus sebaceus, are occasionally complicated by BCC, but the overwhelming majority occur without any recognisable precursor lesion.

Prolonged exposure to sunlight is undoubtedly an important factor, but there is not the clear association seen with SCC. BCC is rare in deeply pigmented races but common in light-skinned individuals living in sunny climates. Most BCCs occur on the head and neck, but one-third of them are found at sites which are relatively protected from solar radiation. The eyelid is a common site for BCC, but an uncommon site for SCC. Obviously, factors other than sunlight and pigmentation are involved. The distribution of BCC closely follows the distribution of pilosebaceous follicles. BCC almost never occurs on the vermilion border of the lip nor on the palms and soles, and is never found in areas of stratified squamous epithelium other than skin.

Genetic factors are implicated, and not only in the sense of melanin production. Patients with xeroderma pigmentosum develop multiple BCCs, as well as SCC and other tumours. Multiple BCCs are also an outstanding feature of the rare, inherited naevoid BCC syndrome.

Histology

The cells of BCC are of characteristic and almost uniform appearance. They resemble cells of the epidermal basal layer or of the hair matrix. The nucleus is large, deeply staining, and oval or elongated. Cytoplasm is scanty and cell margins are difficult to define. Desmosomes are present, but the cells lack the suggestion of intercellular bridges which are normally seen with the light microscope.

The whole appearance is of uniformity, but not of anaplasia. Mitoses are infrequent and bizarre cells rare. The cell masses are often bordered by a palisade of cells whose nuclei lie parallel, whereas nuclei within the masses are haphazard in arrangement.

There is a prominent connective tissue stroma arranged in parallel bundles around the tumour masses, with young fibroblasts close to the islands of cells. The cells usually lie in large groups, but occasionally the stroma dominates the picture, with small islands or strands of cells surrounded by stroma, rather like the appearance of scirrhous carcinoma of the breast. There may be differentiation towards keratinous structures, sometimes reminiscent of cutaneous appendages.

Clinical features *(Colour plates 32, 33, 34)*

A typical BCC may be recognised as a gelatinous or waxy papule, while still as small as two or three millimetres in diameter. The tumour is well demarcated at the edges and even as a small papule usually displays tiny vessels just under the surface. The papule enlarges slowly over months or years to a pale, smooth and shiny nodule, often with a central depression. The centre eventually becomes eroded, either spontaneously or after minor trauma. The erosion may heal and recur, but ultimately persists as a frank ulcer with central crusting. The crust can usually be lifted off easily and without pain, leaving a fleshy red crater depressed below the level of surrounding skin. The border is raised, firm and waxy ('pearly'), with small vessels coursing beneath the epidermis. The rate of progression is very variable, but sooner or later the ulcer invades underlying structures, including cartilage, bone and even meninges— the 'rodent ulcer'.

Variants of BCC

■ *Pigmented BCC.* A few scattered flecks of pigment are not uncommon and haemorrhage may produce irregular darkening. Occasionally, the whole tumour has a brown or black colour and may resemble melanoma.

■ *Morphoeic BCC.* The bulk of the tumour is formed by fibrous stroma. The typical elevated border is less pronounced and the extent of the tumour may be very difficult to define. The tumour plaque is usually a little depressed below the surface and ulceration is rare. Morphoeic BCC typically occurs on the face.

■ *Superficial BCC.* Extension is mostly close to the surface, with little deeper penetration. Typical presentation is of a small slightly indurated faintly erythematous plaque. Small areas of erosion and crusting are common, and there may be nodules of localised thickening. The raised border is fine, thread-like, and easily missed unless the skin is stretched. Superficial BCCs usually occur on the trunk. When BCCs develop as a complication of arsenical intoxication, they are generally of the superficial type.

■ *Naevoid BCC syndrome.* Tumours are multiple, skin-coloured or brownish papules or nodules, which occur mainly on the face, neck and trunk. Ulceration is a late feature.

■ *BCC of the nasolabial fold.* At this site the appearance is less characteristic. The elevated border may be difficult to recognise and there is a special tendency to deep extension and ulceration.

The majority of BCCs occur on the head and neck. Although metastases are extremely rare, the tumour is destructive, and may be life-threatening. Particular attention should be directed to any doubtful lesion on the nose, around the eyes, or near the nasolabial and retro-auricular folds.

Diagnosis

After a careful examination most BCCs can be diagnosed with confidence, but mistakes easily follow cursory examination in poor light. A definite raised border is visible in most cases when the skin is stretched; even in the superficial sclerosing type, small areas of gelatinous thickening are usually present. Although it may be permissible to observe small doubtful lesions for a time, excision biopsy is generally preferable. With larger lesions, biopsy is a routine part of management. In Australia, BCC is so common that the physician should have a high index of suspicion. Early diagnosis and treatment avoid much unnecessary mutilation.

Small lesions are most frequently confused with intradermal melanocytic naevi, or the large hypertrophied sebaceous glands which are on the face of the elderly. Pigmented lesions may be mistaken for melanoma, especially of the superficial spreading type. Ulcerated BCC may mimic SCC, and Bowen's disease may be misdiagnosed for the superficial and morphoeic forms.

Treatment

1. Curettage
2. Radiotherapy
3. Surgery
4. Microscopically controlled excision

■ *Curettage*. The friability and gelatinous texture of BCC allows the removal of small, well-defined lesions by curettage. The method involves scooping out the tumour with a skin curette, and then destroying a few millimetres of surrounding and underlying tissue with the cautery or by electrodesiccation. The charred tissue is then removed with the curette, and the wound allowed to heal by granulation. The issue removed should be forwarded to the pathologist.

Curettage gives an excellent cure rate, provided that the operator is experienced in the technique and the tumour is not much larger than 0.5 cm in diameter. The cosmetic results are good, but the method is unsuitable for BCC that invades fat because in that situation there is loss of the difference in sensation imparted to the probing curette by the gelatinous BCC and surrounding fibrous stroma of the dermis. Fat involvement is likely to occur around the eye where the dermis is thin, and also where the tumour invades down embryonal fusion lines such as the nasolabial and retroauricular folds. Similarly, morphoeic BCC cannot be treated by curettage.

■ *Radiotherapy*. Radiotherapy is now being used less frequently overseas in the treatment of BCC. However, X-ray therapy remains the most suitable modality for many patients in this country. Radiotherapy is painless and does not disturb the patient, who is often elderly and apprehensive. The cure rate is at least as high as with surgery, and hospital admission is not required. Over the nose particularly, cosmetic results are often better than those achieved by excision and grafting.

Drawbacks include the necessity for fractionation into a number of treatments, and late radiation atrophy. The doses which are necessary for eradication of tumours inevitably produce marked atrophy over ten or twenty years and are better avoided in young patients.

■ *Surgery*. Small BCC can often be excised on an outpatient basis but the tissue removed should, when possible, extend at least 3 mm beyond the apparent margins of the tumour. Delineation of the tumour edge is not generally difficult with nodular lesions; with morphoeic and superficial BCC, and with tumours at such special sites as the inner canthus or nasolabial fold, particularly careful assessment is necessary.

Surgical excision has the advantage that it allows histological confirmation that removal is adequate. BCC showing microscopic involvement within one high-power field of surgical margins should be re-excised. If this is impractical, the patient should be followed carefully.

■ *Microscopically controlled excision (Mohs).* While a very effective method of treatment for 'difficult' or recurrent BCC, the technique is too time-consuming for routine use. The Mohs' technique is sometimes called 'chemosurgery', but should not be confused with the application of cytotoxic chemicals as a treatment of skin cancer. The cytotoxic applications which are presently available have no place in the treatment of BCC.

Naevoid BCC syndrome

This is an inherited disease, which is transmitted as an autosomal dominant trait and characterised by the association of multiple BCC with defects of other organs, mainly skeletal.

Clinical features

■ *Cutaneous.* Tumours may begin to appear in early childhood, but are usually first noticed during the second decade. They develop as smooth, slightly elevated, skin-coloured or brownish, dome-shaped papules. At first there may be only a few, but most patients eventually develop a large number of tumours, and there may be hundreds scattered over the head, neck and trunk. Early lesions are slow growing and non-invasive, but later ulcerate and involve underlying structures. Distinctive superficial pits are frequently present on the palms, soles, and sides of the digits. The pits are punched-out in appearance, rounded or elongated, and may have a reddish base. Rarely, BCC develops at the base of a pit.

■ *Other organs.* The face is broad, with frontal bossing and prominent supra-orbital ridges. Mandibular prognathism is common and, with the prominent forehead, produces a characteristic facial appearance. Cysts may occur in the mandible or maxilla. Other features which are sometimes present include bifid ribs, kyphoscoliosis and, less often, cataracts, mental retardation, and calcification of the falx cerebri.

Diagnosis

At least in the early stages, the BCC are atypical in appearance and may be clinically indistinguishable from melanocytic naevi or neurofibromas. However, the facies and other skeletal changes are suggestive, and the histology is characteristic.

Treatment

Small tumours are suitable for removal by curettage, and larger ones are excised. Radiotherapy should not be used. The number of BCC which are likely to develop and the age of onset preclude their treatment by irradiation. In any case, the tumours are relatively insensitive to radiotherapy.

Cutaneous cysts

1. Epidermoid cyst
2. Pilar cyst
3. Steatocystoma multiplex
4. Milia

Epidermoid cyst

The unilocular epidermoid cyst arises in the dermis, is composed of laminated keratinous material, and is surrounded by a thin wall of keratinising epithelium which is similar to normal epidermis.

Epidermoid cysts are more common in people who have had severe acne, and are most often located in areas where acne normally occurs. The early lesion usually begins in young adults as a firm dermal nodule, which slowly enlarges to a dome-shaped swelling and may eventually reach 4 or 5 cm in diameter. The cysts are subject to episodes of inflammation, during which tenderness and sudden increase in size may be followed by suppuration. They remain freely mobile over deeper structures, but may become fixed to the surface by a central punctum.

Most epidermoid cysts can be removed intact by dissection from surrounding tissue. Large inflamed cysts are more difficult, but may be drained through a small incision before removal of the cyst wall by dissection or curettage. Incomplete removal of the wall is likely to be followed by recurrence.

Pilar ('sebaceous') cyst (Colour plate 35)

Pilar cysts resemble epidermoid cysts clinically, but are far less common. The cyst wall is epithelial, and its microscopic appearance suggests external root sheath of hair follicles rather than epidermis.

The cysts are generally multiple and patients frequently give a family history of similar lesions. The majority occur on the scalp, although the face, neck, trunk and scrotum are occasional sites. Pilar cysts have less tendency to inflammation than epidermoid cysts, but may become calcified, especially on the scrotum.

As a rule, pilar cysts separate well with blunt dissection, and can be removed with little difficulty.

Steatocystoma multiplex

This uncommon disorder is characterised by multiple dermal cysts which contain sebum. The cyst wall is complex, with elements of epidermal and appendageal structure. Steatocystoma multiplex is frequently familial and is then transmitted as an autosomal dominant trait.

The cysts form relatively small nodules, seldom exceeding 2 cm in diameter. They may be present from infancy, but more often appear during the second decade of life. The nodules may be very numerous and are usually scattered over the upper trunk, particularly the front of the chest. Less common sites are the scalp, face, and more proximal parts of the limbs.

Milia

Milia are small keratinous cysts which are located in the superficial dermis, and are surrounded by a wall which is indistinguishable from that of epidermoid cysts.

Milia are very common, and occur as smooth, yellowish white papules up to 3 mm in diameter, mostly on the face, especially around the eyes. They are particularly common in areas of chronic solar degeneration, but large numbers occasionally erupt in otherwise normal skin. A few milia frequently develop on the face in infancy, but are shed spontaneously within a few months. In adults, milia are easily expressed through a tiny incision.

Appendageal tumours

A number of tumours show histological differentiation towards the various cutaneous appendages. These tumours are all uncommon, and some are very rare. Diagnosis is often difficult and, even for the experienced dermatologist, may be impossible without microscopic examination. There are, however, a few suggestive patterns.

Sebaceous tumours

An orange-yellow colour of a solitary tumour on the face or scalp should suggest sebaceous elements, as in the benign adenoma or the sebaceous carcinoma. Recognition of sebaceous tumours is particularly important because of their occasional association with gastro-intestinal and other visceral carcinomas.

Syringoma

Multiple skin-coloured or brownish papules which are confined to the eyelids of women are likely to be benign syringomas, although milia may look very similar. Syringoma is a benign tumour of eccrine sweat duct origin which produces comma-shaped aggregates of cells within the dermis.

Eccrine hydrocystoma

Benign eccrine hydrocystomas form a characteristic pattern over the cheeks or eyelids of middle-aged and elderly women. The tumours are papules or small cysts which fluctuate in size, becoming larger in a warm environment.

Apocrine hydrocystoma

This is usually a solitary cystic nodule on the face, often with a bluish tinge, reminiscent of a blue naevus.

Cylindroma

A distinctive tumour of the face or scalp is the smooth, lobulated, reddish pink apocrine cylindroma. Cylindromas may be multiple, and sometimes reach enormous proportions ('turban tumour').

Tricho-epithelioma

These form another distinctive pattern, appearing at adolescence as multiple, yellowish-pink, gelatinous papules or nodules around the nasolabial folds. Multiple cylindromas and tricho-epitheliomas may occur in the same patient.

Mesodermal tumours

1. Soft fibroma (skin tag, acrochordon)
2. Dermatofibroma (histiocytoma)
3. Granuloma telangiectaticum (pyogenic granuloma)
4. Uncommon mesodermal tumours
   (a) fibroblastic
   (b) myoblastic
   (c) vascular

Soft fibroma

Also known as 'skin tag' or 'acrochordon', soft fibroma is a very common benign tumour which occurs as a soft, sessile, pedunculated appendage on the neck, upper trunk, axillae, or groins.

Histology

There is a thin shell of epidermis covering a core of delicate loose collagen making up the dermis.

Clinical features

Tags are from 1 to 3 mm in diameter and up to 5 mm long. They are soft, skin coloured to brown, and usually multiple. They are particularly common in women from the fifth decade on and in this group of patients, numerous seborrhoeic keratoses are usually also present. Apart from their appearance, skin tags are of little significance.

Treatment

When treatment is necessary for cosmetic reasons, light electrodesiccation is sufficient and, if carefully done, leaves virtually no scarring. Very small soft fibromas also respond to cryotherapy.

Dermatofibroma (histiocytoma)

This is a common tumour-like proliferation of fibroblasts, believed to develop as an abnormal response to minor trauma.

Histology

The lesion is an unencapsulated dermal nodule which contains a variable mixture of fibroblasts and histiocytes, with occasional giant cells. There is a substantial component of young collagen, and there may be considerable vascular proliferation. The overlying epidermis is thickened, and may show a budding of basal cells, which resembles basal cell carcinoma.

Clinical features

Dermatofibromas are very firm, well-circumscribed nodules, tightly tethered to the epidermis, but freely mobile over deeper structures. Most lesions occur on the limbs, particularly the legs, and are generally few or solitary. The colour is usually pink, red or brownish, but occasional nodules are creamy white. Dermatofibromas are round to oval, 0.5 cm to 1.5 cm in diameter, and may be a little raised or a little depressed in relation to surrounding skin. Diagnosis is rarely difficult, the nodule giving a characteristic button-like feel with lateral compression. When treatment is requested, simple excision is sufficient.

Granuloma telangiectaticum (pyogenic granuloma)

This is a common, tumour-like proliferation of capillary vessels, believed to be an abnormal reaction to minor trauma.

Histology

The lesion is a mass of newly formed capillaries set in a loose gelatinous or fibrous stroma and surrounded by a thin sheath of epidermis. The vascular bulk of the lesion communicates with the dermis through an epidermal defect. An inflammatory infiltrate is added if the surface becomes eroded.

Clinical features (Colour plate 24)

Granuloma telangiectaticum may occur at any site, but is more common over the fingers or at other sites exposed to minor trauma. The early lesion is a reddish papule which grows rapidly to half a centimetre or more, and evolves to a bright red, globular outgrowth with a smooth glistening surface. Around the narrowed base of the nodule, the epidermis is thickened to form a firm collarette. Bleeding and ulceration are common, and older lesions may become dark brown or black.

Treatment

Although the lesion is easily cured by snipping off the nodule and cauterising the base, histological confirmation of the diagnosis is essential. The appearance of granuloma telangiectaticum is generally distinctive, but amelanotic melanoma and anaplastic squamous cell carcinoma should be excluded microscopically.

Uncommon mesodermal tumours

Fibroblastic

■ *The desmoid tumour* is a rare tumour of parous women, which usually occurs close to the midline of the abdomen below the umbilicus. It originates in the muscle aponeurosis and is locally invasive. Metastases do not occur.

■ *Dermatofibrosarcoma protuberans* is an invasive dermal tumour which usually presents on the trunk as a red or purplish lobulated nodule, with a broader deep component. Although locally invasive, it is well-differentiated and rarely metastasises.

■ *Fibrosarcoma* is a rare malignant tumour of the dermis, which presents as a red or purplish nodule anywhere on the skin. Ulceration, local invasion and distant metastases may occur.

■ *Atypical fibroxanthoma* is an uncommon tumour, which most frequently occurs on the ears or cheeks of elderly people. The tumour develops as a reddish-brown nodule, which may ulcerate. Simple excision is generally curative, but metastases have been recorded in rare cases.

Myoblastic

■ *Leiomyoma* is a benign nodular tumour of the dermis, with differentiation towards smooth muscle. It is often tender and spontaneously painful, and may be contractile. The tumours are usually multiple, sometimes familial, and most often occur on the limbs.

■ *Leiomyosarcoma* is a metastasising tumour which, on rare occasions, arises in the dermis.

Vascular

■ *Glomus tumours* are bluish-red papules, a few millimetres in size. They may be solitary or multiple. Solitary lesions are tender and spontaneously painful, and occur mostly on the limbs, particularly in the nail bed.

■ *Angiosarcoma* is a rare endothelial tumour which occurs mainly on the face or scalp of elderly people as red or purplish nodules or plaques. Severe haemorrhage is a frequent complication and metastases are common.

■ *Kaposi's sarcoma* (Colour plate 36) is a rare malignant tumour with both fibroblastic and vascular components. The classic form of the disease occurs in elderly men of central or eastern European origin. With this variety, purple or bluish macules begin on the feet and lower legs. Nodules and plaques which are purplish or a bluish-brown then appear on the lower legs. Later the hands and forearms may be similarly involved. The classic form of the disease progresses very slowly and may even regress for periods of time. Rapid progression with systemic involvement and death is rare.

Kaposi's sarcoma may also complicate immunosuppressive therapy in patients who have received organ transplants. The pattern of disease is similar to the classic form. Cessation of these drugs or even reduction in dose, will often induce regression and disappearance of tumour.

The acquired immunodeficiency syndrome is complicated by Kaposi's sarcoma of a different clinical pattern. Homosexual males are affected much more commonly than those with AIDS acquired by other means. Small oval macules of a purplish colour are often widespread and may even involve the oral mucosa. On the trunk, lesions follow Langer's lines. Systemic involvement occurs quickly and involves many organs.

Since this entity was first decribed, AIDS associated Kaposi's sarcoma is becoming less common. The reasons are not known.

The histology in all three varieties of Kaposi's sarcoma is identical.

Neural tumours

The true neuroma is a rare, tender and painful, benign dermal tumour. Lesions loosely referred to as 'neuromas' are usually traumatic in origin.

The only common dermal tumour related to nerves is the ***neurofibroma***. Solitary neurofibromas may occur with no other association. Multiple neurofibromas are the characteristic feature of the hereditary neurofibromatosis syndrome. Malignant transformation may occur and should be suspected when a previously stable neurofibroma increases in size.

10

Melanocytic naevi and melanoma

1. Melanocytic naevi
   (a) acquired melanocytic naevi
   (b) congenital melanocytic naevi
   (c) blue naevus
   (d) variant melanocytic naevi
2. Melanoma
   (a) superficial spreading
   (b) nodular
   (c) acral lentiginous
   (d) lentigo maligna

Melanocytic naevi

Melanocytic naevi are localised areas of altered cutaneous development (hamartomas) characterised by abnormal numbers of melanocytes. The layman often refers to melanocytic naevi as 'moles'. Melanocytic naevi are extremely common in people of all races. Most young adults have thirty or more. Like other hamartomas, melanocytic naevi behave as if there were a predetermined size for each lesion, in that the naevus grows rapidly to a certain size and then enlarges minimally in diameter thereafter.

Acquired melanocytic naevi

These are the commonest variety. They begin to appear in childhood, often with a sharp increase in number during adolescence. Crops may appear during pregnancy but in general, the appearance of new lesions becomes less common with increasing age.

Aetiology

The stimuli that induce the appearance of melanocytic naevi are unknown but it would seem that hormonal influences are possibly responsible for the onset during pregnancy and adolescence. Sun exposure during childhood is also probably important and may explain the relative paucity of melanocytic naevi on the buttocks and medial aspects of the limbs.

Pathophysiology

Within the basal layer of the epidermis, melanocytes increase in number, lose their dendritic processes, become spherical and form nests that expand the base of the epidermal rete ridge. Rounded melanocytes (naevus cells) then tend to 'drop off' into the dermis where they form aggregates within the papillary dermis. The naevus cells continue to move deeper into the reticular dermis and the intra-epidermal component diminishes. During this stage, as the naevus cell aggregates increase and enlarge within the dermis, hair follicles within the area often also undergo growth and maturation. In some old melanocytic naevi where the changes are by then purely intradermal, involution of naevus cells occurs and collagen increases in amount.

Although melanocytic naevi can undergo the complete cycle of changes as described, the process of maturation can stop at any stage. Evolution may halt with aggregates of naevus cells confined to the epidermis and papillary dermis (junctional naevus), with naevus cells purely within the dermis (intradermal naevus) or with both junctional and intradermal aggregates (compound naevus). Also, maturation of pigmentary naevi does not necessarily proceed at a steady rate and it is more usual for there to be different rates within each stage.

It should therefore be appreciated that although change in a pigmented lesion should be regarded as an indicator of malignancy, benign pigmented lesions can and do undergo a series of changes that are characteristic and recognisable.

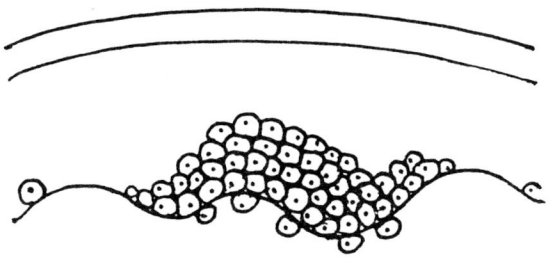

Junctional naevus

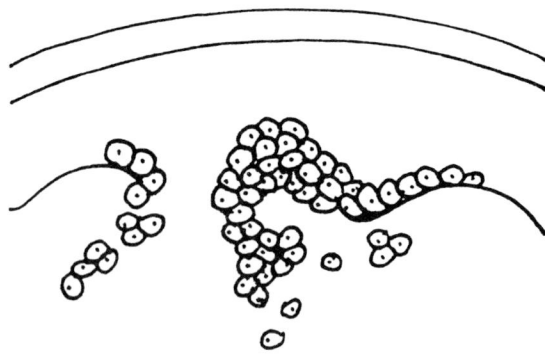

Compound naevus

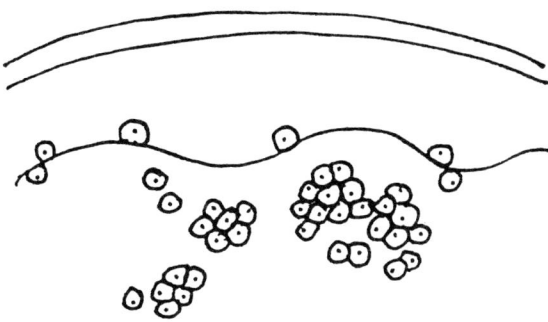

Intradermal naevus

Clinical features

Acquired melanocytic naevi can usually be diagnosed with a great degree of certainty on the basis of clinical signs which correspond to the microscopic features.

- *Junctional naevi* are usually circumscribed macules, but may be a little elevated. The colour ranges from light brown to black, often with a regular mottling or stippling rather than a uniform pigmentation. The border may be fuzzy, with a brownish halo of even, regular colour. Although vellus hair may grow through the lesion, there is not the coarse terminal hair so often associated with compound and intradermal naevi. The normal skin markings are retained and may be a little exaggerated.

- *Compound naevi* become more elevated as the dermal component increases. The lesion may be slightly raised with a somewhat corrugated surface, but is more often sessile, dome-shaped, or conical. The colour varies from light to very dark brown or black, and the surface may be smooth, rough or verrucoid. Coarse hairs may sprout from the naevus, especially after puberty.

- *Intradermal naevi* are less pigmented. They slowly evolve to firm, pink or brownish sessile nodules, or to soft pedunculated tags.

Treatment

When, as is usual, there is no doubt regarding the diagnosis, the naevus can be left untreated. However, when there is doubt regarding a certain diagnosis, the main differential diagnosis is melanoma, which is a cancer that metastasises relatively quickly yet can be cured by simple excision if removed in its early stages. Therefore, in this situation the lesion should be excised for histological examination rather than waiting for more definite clinical signs of melanoma to become apparent.

Congenital melanocytic naevi

Histology

These naevi result when melanocytes fail to complete their normal migration, which occurs during embryonal development, from neural crest to epidermis. This variety is therefore never purely junctional in type and, compared with acquired pigmentary naevi, usually has a deeper dermal component, with naevus cells often found in a perivascular location.

Clinical variants

■ *Small congenital melanocytic naevi* may look indentical to acquired compound or intradermal naevi and their true nature may only be discovered when histology has been obtained. This type, which is usually about 3 mm to 5 mm in diameter, has the same significance as acquired melanocytic naevi and therefore treatment is identical.

■ *Large congenital melanocytic naevi* (greater than 20 cm diameter) may involve any area but common sites are the head, neck and buttocks. The naevus is often bilateral, and may cover large areas (*'giant melanocytic naevus'*). The depth of pigmentation varies and the surface may be smooth, or rough and verrucoid, often with coarse hair growing through the lesion.

The incidence of melanoma in these giant naevi may be as high as 10 per cent. Prophylactic surgical removal is therefore recommended and in patients with very large lesions, removal by staged excision may be required. With scalp and nuchal lesions there is a special susceptibility to meningeal melanocytosis and hydrocephalus. Management of these child patients is an extremely difficult surgical problem.

Blue naevus

The blue naevus is a circumscribed area of slightly raised skin, with a slate grey, blue, or bluish black colour.

Histology

There is an accumulation of fusiform or elongated melanocytes in the middle and lower dermis. Melanin is present in the melanocytes, and in surrounding macrophages.

Clinical features *(Colour plate 43)*

The common blue naevus is a solitary, well-circumscribed, dome-shaped nodule, usually on the head, forearm, hand, leg, or foot. Occasionally

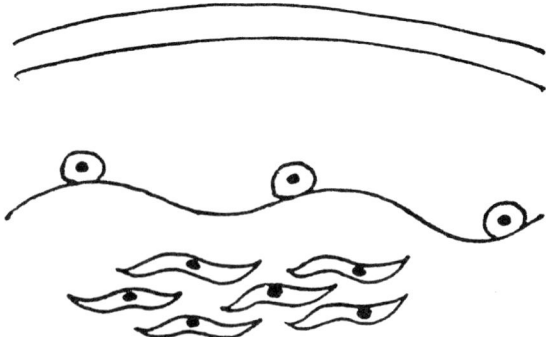

Blue naevus

the naevus presents as a larger, firm bluish plaque. As a rule, blue naevi persist unchanged throughout life. Melanoma is a rare complication, suggested by a sudden increase in size or by ulceration. When this rare event takes place, it is usually in a large blue naevus located on the scalp.

Treatment

When excised for cosmetic reasons, the depth of the naevus necessitates removal of the whole thickness of skin, with a margin of subcutaneous tissue.

Variant melanocytic naevi

Acquired melanocytic naevi can produce non-malignant disordered growth patterns or undergo benign changes which result in clinical or histological pictures so different from uncomplicated acquired melanocytic naevi that they are given a separate special name. Like ordinary melanocytic naevi, these specially named pigmentary naevi can be junctional, intradermal or compound naevi.

Dysplastic naevus

In the early 1970s it was realised that there existed families in whom members had a high risk of developing multiple primary melanomas. In these families kindred were covered with large numbers of clinically distinctive moles which showed histological abnormalities of epidermal architecture, stromal change within the dermis and cytological atypia of melanocytes. Because of this histology these clinically distinctive lesions were called dysplastic naevi even though it was realised they do not evolve to melanoma.

Clinical features

Familial dysplastic naevi are very distinctive. They are usually larger than acquired melanocytic naevi, have a cobblestoned surface, and a blurred and often poorly defined border. Pigmentation is irregularly distributed and there is usually a background erythema within the naevus that can be blanched with pressure. *(Colour plate 37)*

Histology

Dysplastic naevi are characterised by variable degrees of architectural and cytological atypia. The nests of cells are often fused horizontally and not placed regularly. The cells may vary in size and there is random slight nuclear pleomorphism. Within the papillary dermis there may be lamellar fibroplasia, telangiectasia and a mild lymphocytic infiltrate.

Significance

The clinically distinct dysplastic naevus correlates well with histological changes even when it is an isolated lesion and there is no family history. However, histological changes of dysplastic naevi may be seen in lesions that look like ordinary acquired melanocytic naevi and, in some communities, half of all melanocytic naevi examined show evidence of dysplastic change.

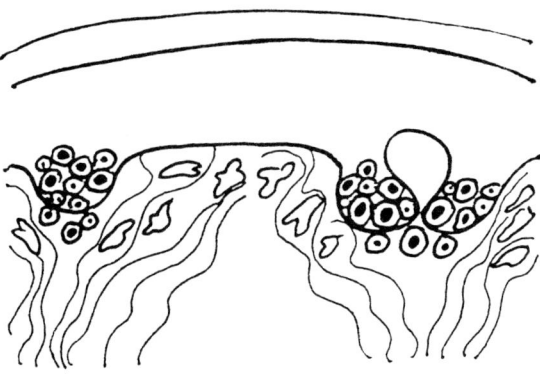

Dysplastic naevus

When a study is made of patients with dysplastic naevi, three main groups emerge. One group has a high risk of melanoma, and comprises those with a family history of dysplastic naevi and a family history of melanoma. Another group, in which the risk of melanoma is the same as that of the general community, comprises patients with only a small number of dysplastic naevi and no family history of melanoma or dysplastic naevi. A third group comprises those with a family history of multiple dysplastic naevi but no history of melanoma. This third group of patients has a risk of melanoma only slightly higher than that of the general population.

It is possible that these results may have nothing to do with dysplastic naevi and may be explained by the observations that risk of melanoma is highest in those with large numbers of acquired melanocytic naevi of any type and that families exist with a tendency to melanoma even if there are no abnormal naevi.

Treatment

Patients with small numbers of dysplastic naevi are treated as if they had ordinary acquired melanocytic naevi.

The patient with large numbers of dysplastic naevi should be managed by a dermatologist, who reviews the patient at regular intervals and uses reproducible whole body detailed photography to help identify which lesions are new or changing and therefore worth closer examination.

As with any pigmented lesion, if there is any clinical doubt the lesion is excised for histological examination to exclude melanoma.

Halo naevus

The signs in this distinctive variant of melanocytic naevus are produced by lymphokines that are released from lymphocytes that have infiltrated a compound naevus.

Clinical features *(Colour plate 38)*

The patient is generally a young adult and the lesion is usually on the trunk, particularly the back. An otherwise unremarkable mole becomes surrounded by a depigmented band 0.5cm or more wide, giving the appearance of a mole in the centre of a white, coin-shaped disc. Multiple lesions are present in 25 per cent of patients and more than 25 per cent have, or later develop, vitiligo. The mole gradually loses its colour, flattens and may completely disappear. The depigmented area may persist as a white spot, or may slowly repigment. Frequently, the patient is made aware of the lesion after exposure to sunlight, when the pale area burns and becomes tender.

Histology

Early halo naevi show an infiltration by lymphocytes. The infiltrate becomes more dense until the melanocytes are destroyed. The epidermis within the pale zone is devoid of melanocytes but is otherwise normal.

Significance

The association with vitiligo, the invasion by lymphocytes, and the presence of a circulating antibody originally thought to be specific for a melanoma antigen, all suggest the possibility of immune rejection of the naevus. It could be that the halo naevus represents the successful rejection of a naevus which is undergoing malignant change. However, melanoma does not arise from a partially regressed halo naevus.

Diagnosis

▶ **Suspect** halo naevus when the pigmented lesion is perfectly in the centre of the depigmented zone, the pigmented lesion has all the signs of a benign melanocytic naevus and the location of the lesion and the age of the patient are typical.

▶ **Consider and exclude** melanoma. Rarely, melanoma may develop a depigmented halo but the central lesion is usually eccentrically placed within the halo, the pigmented lesion is irregular in outline and colour, and the halo is an area of pallor rather than the stark white seen with a halo naevus.

▶ **Confirmation** of diagnosis by histology is usually not required because clinical features are usually very definite. However, if there are any unusual signs then the lesion should be excised for histology.

Naevus spilus ('speckled lentiginous naevus')

Naevus spilus is a relatively common lesion which may occur anywhere on the body surface. Small darkly pigmented spots are irregularly scattered over a well-circumscribed background macule of smooth, tan to sepia-coloured skin. Microscopically, the darker speckles resemble junctional naevi, and similar features have been described also in the lighter coloured background areas. *(Colour plate 39)*

Significance

The speckled naevus is a benign lesion, but the presence of melanocyte clusters in junctional zones implies the same potential for malignant change as in other junctional naevi.

Spitz naevus (juvenile melanoma)

This variety of melanocytic naevus typically appears in children although it may occur in adults. Despite the alternative name of 'juvenile melanoma', a Spitz naevus has no malignant potential and does not metastasise.

Clinical features

Typically, the lesion is a dome-shaped reddish-brown nodule on the face of a child. The nodule grows rapidly to a diameter of a centimetre or so and then remains more or less unchanged. It is a vascular nodule and bleeds easily with trauma. Crusting is common.

Histology

The tumor shows marked proliferation of naevus cells downward from the dermo-epidermal junction. Cellular pleomorphism is a feature with the naevus cells often being spindle-shaped or epithelioid rather than rounded. Mitoses and giant cells are also observed. Within the papillary dermis is telangiectasia and a chronic inflammatory infiltrate.

Significance

The inexperienced pathologist may mistakenly report these as true melanoma unless asked to consider the diagnosis of Spitz naevus by the doctor who removes a pigmented lesion from the face of a child.

Treatment

Simple excision is required to exclude melanoma.

Melanoma

Melanoma is a malignant tumour of melanocytes with great potential for metastatic dissemination.

Pathophysiology

Most melanomas which arise in the skin begin as an abnormal proliferation of melanocytes within the epidermis. In this type, which accounts for 90 per cent of melanomas, the following concepts help to understand the clinical behaviour of melanoma.

For a period, which varies considerably with the variety of melanoma, growth occurs in a lateral direction and only within the epidermis. This is known as the *radial growth phase*. Eventually the tumour becomes frankly invasive and penetrates the dermis as well. This invasive period is known as the *vertical growth phase*. Studies have repeatedly confirmed that for primary melanoma arising in the skin, prognosis relates best to how early in the vertical growth phase melanoma has been excised. For this reason pathology reports will include a measurement of depth of invasion expressed in millimeters from the top of the granular layer.

Aetiology

Many factors play a part and combine in ways that cannot yet fully explain why melanoma occurs.

■ *Sunlight* has a central role, as is demonstrated by the finding that, along the east coast of Australia, the prevalence of melanoma in the

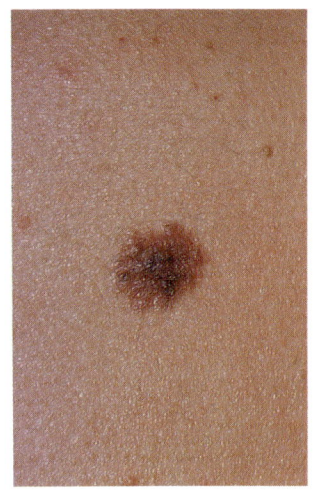

37. Dysplastic naevus

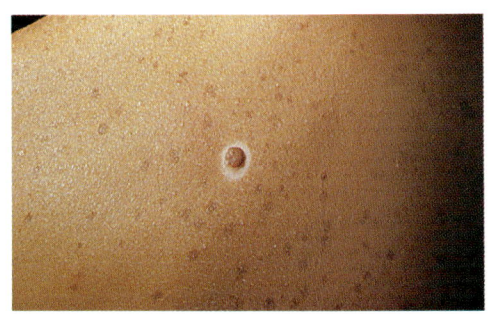

38. Halo naevus

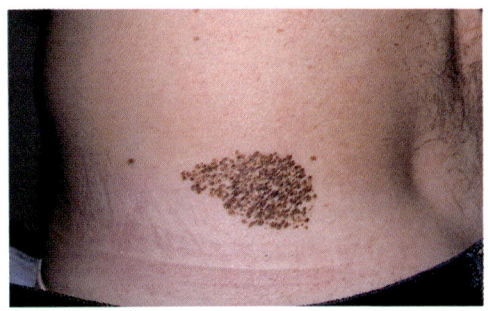

39. Naevus spilus

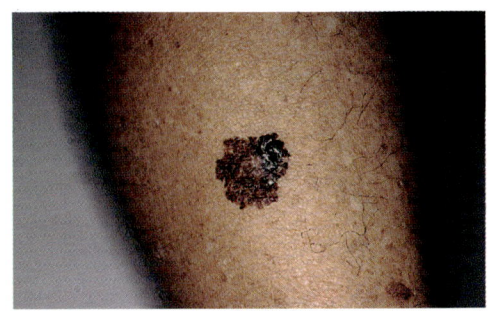

40. Superficial spreading melanoma

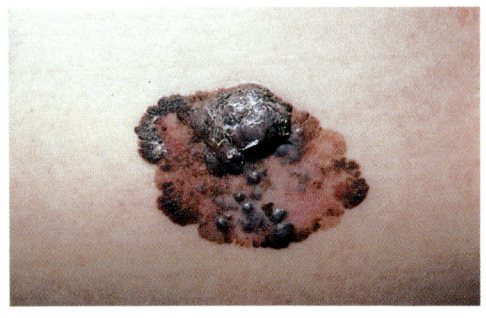

41. Nodular melanoma

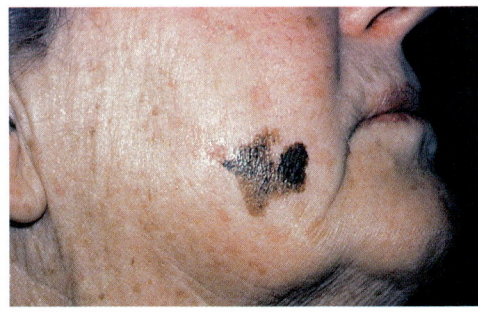

42. Lentigo maligna

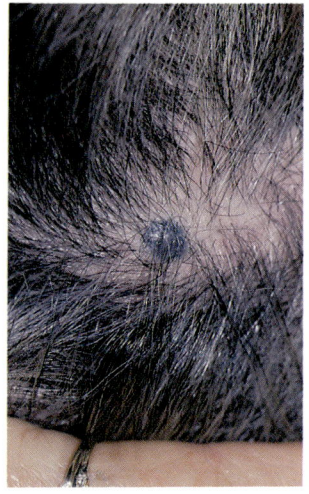

43. Blue naevus

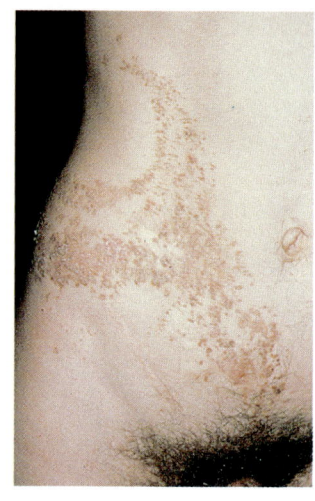

44. Extensive epidermal naevus

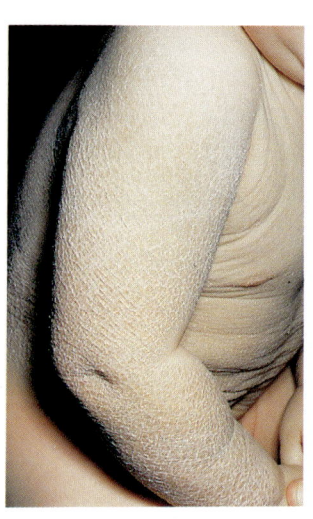

45. Ichthyosis vulgaris

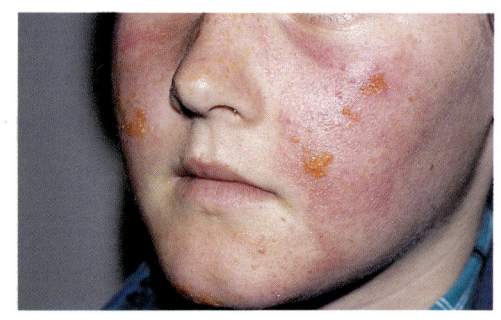

46. Impetigo

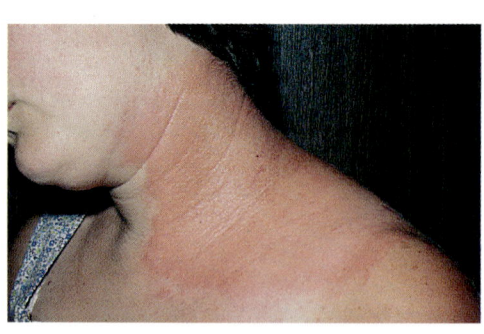

47. Erysipelas

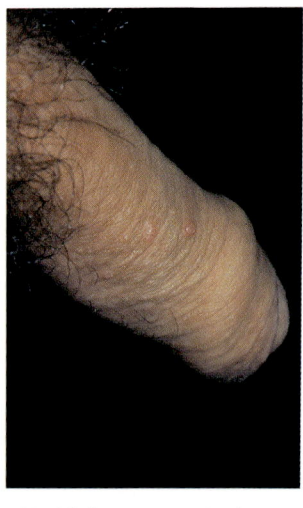

48. Molluscum contagiosum

population increases steadily in communities closer to the equator. Also people with very large numbers of acquired melanocytic naevi (which is thought to be a measure of sun exposure during childhood) are more at risk of developing melanoma even though it is not the naevi that became melanoma. Studies suggest that brief bursts of intense sun exposure, as experienced during recreational activity, are more important in producing melanoma than continuous moderate intensity exposure, which is more important in production of squamous cell carcinoma. However, although melanoma is very much less common in black-skinned races than in white, and although it is seen in patients with the disorder of defective repair of ultraviolet light damaged DNA (xeroderma pigmentosum), melanoma is not found predominantly in sun-exposed regions of skin. In fair-skinned races 30 per cent of melanomas arise on the trunk, with less than a quarter on the head and neck region.

■ *Familial tendency.* As already mentioned, xeroderma pigmentosum is a genetic disorder in which melanoma is increased. There are also families in which there are no obvious distinguishing features to explain why many members have had melanoma. However, there are also very distinctive families in which kindred develop multiple primary melanomas. These families are typified by large numbers of characteristic moles, called dysplastic naevi, which do not become melanoma but merely act as marker moles for those at-risk families.

■ *Pre-existing lesions.* Most melanomas do not arise from a pre-existing lesion and the situations when this occurs are in fact very rare.

▬ *Congenital melanocytic naevi.* Giant melanocytic naevi can evolve to melanoma in approximately 10 per cent of cases and therefore attempts are always made to excise this type of lesion.

Congenital melanocytic naevi less than one centimeter do not have an increased risk of melanoma.

▬ *Blue naevus undergoing malignant transformation* to melanoma is an extremely uncommon event. The type in which this occurs is usually very large, is on the head and neck region, and has been present many years.

▬ *Lentigo maligna (Hutchinson's melanotic freckle)* is probably best considered as a lesion which begins as a melanoma but of a variety that has a very prolonged and slowly progressing radial growth phase.

▬ *Acquired melanocytic naevi.* Approximately 30 per cent of excised melanomas have an adjacent intradermal naevus that is benign and is not obviously the origin of the melanoma. As the variety of melanoma in this situation is a superficial spreading melanoma that arises within the epidermis, any precursor naevus would have to be a junctional naevus, but this association is not seen. The role of acquired melanocytic naevi in the production of melanoma is not yet known.

Melanoma types

Superficial spreading melanoma

This type constitutes about 70 per cent of all melanomas, and is an important presentation because the lesion can be diagnosed with confidence while still superficial and amenable to removal, with a good percentage of cures.

Histology

Atypical melanocytes arise in the basal layer of the epidermis, where they form clusters and then invade higher within the epidermis, undergoing a radial growth phase that may last from months to a few years. Melanocytes do not form desmosomes and therefore the melanoma cells retract from the surrounding epidermal cells, resulting in a well outlined space around each melanocyte that falsely suggests vacuolation of the cell. This pattern of growth fancifully suggests Paget's disease and the term 'Pagetoid spread' is sometimes used by pathologists to describe this stage of intra-epidermal growth. The abnormal melanocytes then invade down through the dermis, lateral spread within the epidermis usually extending beyond the lateral margins of dermal invasion.

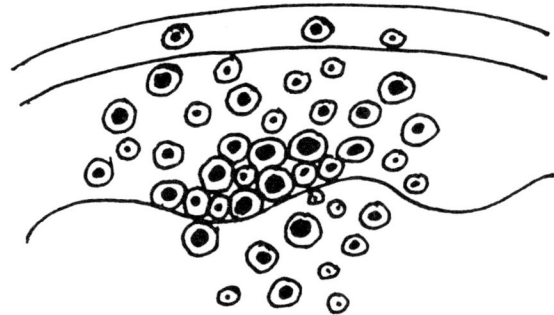

Superficial spreading melanoma

Clinical features *(Colour plate 40)*

The tumour is common on light-exposed areas, but may occur anywhere on the skin or buccal mucosa. It presents as a pigmented, slightly elevated plaque, which may extend slowly for a considerable time before invading deeply. The plaque rarely reaches more than a few centimetres in size and has a sharply demarcated border. The surface is usually dark and shiny, but there may be variation of colour within the lesion, with blue, grey or reddish-brown areas. Often the plaque is a fairly uniform brown or black. The border is irregular and notching or angular defects are common.

When the tumour becomes frankly invasive, there may be irregular thickening by nodules of paler colour than the rest of the plaque, or the nodules may be jet black. Ulceration and bleeding are inconstant, and loss of skin markings or of vellus hair in the lesion are unreliable signs, at least in the early stages. As with other forms of melanoma, examination always includes palpation of draining lymph nodes.

Nodular melanoma

This type, which accounts for 20 per cent of melanomas, has no demonstrable radial growth phase. Prognosis is usually worse with this type of melanoma only because delay in diagnosis allows for greater depth of invasion.

Histology

There is no demonstrable radial growth phase with nodular melanoma. The entire mass of abnormally proliferating epidermal melanocytes is in continuity with tumour cells in the underlying dermis, with no surrounding halo of lateral spread within the epidermis. The tumour cells are a variable mixture of cuboidal and fusiform, frequently with the addition of bizarre giant cells. Mitoses are evident, but not in great numbers. The amount of melanin varies from excessive to none visible in routinely-stained sections. There is a variable inflammatory infiltrate, which may form a dense band below the tumour or be almost completely absent.

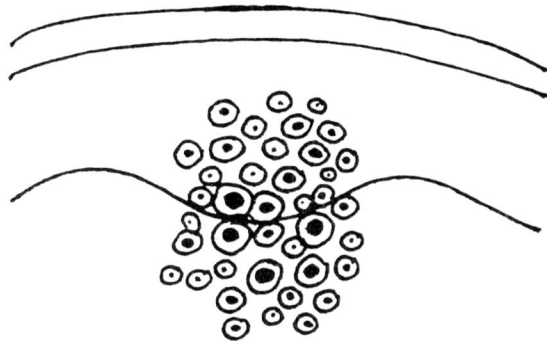

Nodular melanoma

Clinical features *(Colour plate 41)*

Nodular melanoma may occur at any site, but compared with superficial spreading melanoma, a higher proportion are seen in non sun exposed sites. The earliest change may be a small dark area noticed because of itch or some other minor discomfort, but the patient generally seeks advice after becoming aware of dark, rounded papule or nodule. The colour is usually black or bluish-grey, but may be brown or bright red with an appearance which resembles a rapidly growing squamous cell carcinoma. The nodule may show central pallor or be irregularly pigmented. Because nodular melanoma is usually more advanced than superficial spreading melanoma at time of presentation, other signs may be noted more commonly. Ulceration and bleeding reflect localised areas where melanoma cells comprise most of the epidermis. Surrounding satellite lesions, which may be nodular or linear, represent local lymphatic invasion. Enlargement of draining lymph nodes or liver may indicate distant haematogenous or lymphatic spread.

Lentigo maligna melanoma

This variety of melanoma arises in sun-damaged skin of the elderly and accounts for about 7.5 per cent of all melanomas. It is usually seen on the head and neck region, with a malar location being a very common site. This type of melanoma has a very prolonged, very slow radial growth phase; in the past, lesions presenting prior to the vertical growth phase were called a Hutchinson's melanotic freckle.

Histology

During the prolonged radial growth phase, there is proliferation of atypical melanocytes along the basal layer, with little tendency to clustering and no upward spread, although radial growth confined to the basal layer may continue down into hair follicles. The epidermis is thin and atrophic with flattening of the dermo-epidermal junction. There is considerable cellular pleomorphism and mitoses are usually evident. Excessive melanin is present in both epidermis and dermis.

With the development of the invasive vertical growth phase pigment production usually decreases, the cells within the dermis become spindle-shaped and there is sometimes a fibrous stromal reaction within the dermis.

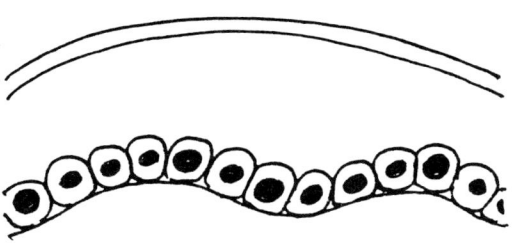

Lentigo maligna

Clinical features *(Colour plate 42)*

Lentigo maligna is a flat, pigmented macule, which almost always occurs on the sun-damaged skin of patients from middle age onwards. The usual site is the face, especially the cheek. The colour ranges from sepia to deep tan or black, and may vary in different areas of the same lesion. The border is irregular and may extend slowly in one area while regressing in another, although slow extension is the rule. After a variable time, usually many years, the change to invasive melanoma occurs. This is commonly indicated by a nodular thickening of part of the macule with either increased or decreased pigmentation, but invasion may occur without there being any obvious change. Signs of local or distant metastasis are not common because of early presentation. However, prognosis for a given depth of invasion is identical to that for other types of melanoma with the same measured depth of penetration.

Acral lentiginous melanoma

This type of melanoma occurs on the palms, soles and distal phalanges, with a much higher incidence in black-skinned people. The lesion begins as a spreading, pigmented macule, which may reach several centimetres in size before evolving to a nodule surrounded by a pigmented halo. Any age patient may be affected.

The radial growth phase is not as long as lentigo maligna melanoma but often extends over many years. During this in situ stage, there is a proliferation of melanocytes, at first as individual cells but later as irregularly shaped clusters confined to the basal layer of the epidermis within delicate club-shaped rete ridges. The histology is easily mistaken as benign hyperplasia until the tumour invades the dermis when the cells become cuboidal or spindle-shaped.

Prognosis of melanoma

Although depth of invasion at the time of excision is the single most important prognostic factor, all factors need to be considered when the individual case is discussed.

Depth of invasion

For patients with no clinically evident distant metastasis, depth of invasion is the dominant prognostic factor. A prolonged radial growth phase implies a correspondingly long period during which melanoma can be recognised before vertical growth supervenes. The very prolonged radial growth phase of lentigo maligna is associated with a lower mortality rate than with any other form of melanoma, and the superficial spreading type has a much better prognosis than nodular melanoma. For patients with the superficial spreading type, where invasion depth is less than 0.76 mm, five year survival is 95 to 100 per cent, but it is only 70 to 90 per cent for tumours 0.76 mm to 1.5 mm. Five year survival rate drops to the range of 55 to 75 per cent for tumours 1.51 mm to 4.0 mm depth, and for tumours invading greater than 4.0 mm is 30 to 50 per cent.

Tumour level is usually reported as well as an actual measurement of depth. Level I indicates tumour confined to the epidermis; level II and III, extension into the papillary dermis; level IV, involvement of the reticular dermis; and level V, invasion of the subcutaneous fat. Reporting on the level compensates for situations where the epidermis is very atrophic or, as may happen with lentigo maligna melanoma, the invasion originates from the depths of a hair follicle.

Clinical features

■ *Location.* Melanoma arising on the leg has a much better prognosis that for other locations. Although delay in observing that the tumour is present may account for the prognosis of some locations, of the common sites, melanoma of the back has the least favourable prognosis.

■ *Sex of patients.* Females have a better prognosis than males and this is further enhanced by the fact that the leg is the commonest location for melanoma in females and the back the commonest location in males.

■ *Ulceration.* Although it is an independent variable, ulceration is, as indicated previously, usually a sign that large numbers of melanocytes (which, unlike keratinocytes, cannot form desmosomes) are forming collections within the epidermis. It is therefore usually a sign of advanced invasion.

Diagnosis

▶ **Suspect** the diagnosis of melanoma with any changing pigmented lesion. Changes may be those of growth, regression, metastasis, or of host response. Features to ask about when taking the history include the following changes.

- Colour—either pallor, darkening or variation may be significant.
- Outline—changes due to growth or regression will cause asymmetry in shape.
- Size—increase in diameter is common, but increase in height occurs late.
- Surface—ulceration is particularly significant but localised areas of micro-invasion may elevate the epidermis over them, giving the impression of a papular surface.
- Inflammatory halo—is a sign of host response but is often transient and is frequently seen with irritated benign lesions.
- Satellite lesions—these represent local metastases and may be either papular or linear.
- Lymph node enlargement—it is to be hoped that patients present before this becomes evident.
- Bleeding, itching and tenderness—these symptoms are not frequent but, although more common with irritated benign melanocytic naevi, when present, indicate that those lesions require close examination.

When there is no history of change, lesions arousing suspicion of melanoma are those with

- asymmetry of either shape or colour
- irregular outline
- depigmentation and scarring suggestive of regression
- surface that is crusted, ulcerated or bleeding.

▶ **Consider and exclude** the following tumours, and bear in mind that to do so may require histology.

- *Diffuse solar keratosis* may resemble lentigo maligna, but has a scaling surface and more uniform colour.

- *Seborrhoeic keratosis,* when light-coloured and flat, may be distinguished from lentigo maligna by its rough surface, even pigmentation, and more regular border. Some degree of elevation is usually perceptible. Examination under high power magnification will usually reveal pseudo horn cysts as white dots.

- *Inflamed seborrhoeic keratoses* may mimic nodular melanoma but respond to protection from further trauma and any infection that may be present.

- *Pigmented basal cell carcinoma* retains the features of BCC, including the raised border and superficial telangiectases. Pigmented BCC never develops the peculiar bluish colour which is so suggestive of melanoma.

- *Squamous cell carcinoma and granuloma telangiectaticum* may be clinically indistinguishable from nodular melanoma, which emphasises the need for histological examination of all tumours excised from the skin.

- *Histiocytomas* may be as dark as melanomas, but are very firm and sharply demarcated. The histiocytoma can be held like a button between the fingers.

- *Small petechiae on the heel* which result from minor trauma ('talon noir') may resemble melanocytic lesions, but can be distinguished by superficial paring.

- *Other melanocytic lesions* may mimic melanoma but most are distinguished using the criteria described earlier in this chapter.

▶ **Confirm the diagnosis** of melanoma using histological examination. The sample obtained should be the whole lesion completely excised. Melanomas initially removed this way and then followed by wider excision (if necessary) do not have a worse prognosis than those initially removed with very wide margins. In contrast, melanomas initially only partially removed and then further excised have, with the exception of early lentigo maligna melanoma, a poorer prognosis. Complete removal of the lesion also removes the possibility that depth of invasion is falsely based on a small area of the melanoma that may not be representative of the whole lesion.

Treatment

Surgical excision with a margin of normal skin is the only acceptable treatment. For melanomas with depth of invasion less than 0.76 mm, margins of 1.0 cm are adequate and some studies suggest that even smaller margins are satisfactory. For lesions of high risk, with depth greater than 3.0 mm, a margin of 3.0 cm is suggested. Re-excision with a wide margin of skin reduces the risk of both local recurrence and local metastasis but the effect on long-term survival is less certain. The need for elective lymph node resection is not yet established but this extra surgery appears not to improve long-term survival in melanoma where depth of invasion is less than 0.76 mm or greater than 4.0 mm.

Most melanomas are now being diagnosed at a curable stage and the dismal statistics of past decades no longer apply. More recent studies, particularly those related to tumour thickness, indicate that the survival of patients with melanoma depends more on early diagnosis than on unnecessarily wide surgical resection.

11

Other naevi and related malformations

1. Melanocytic naevi
   (a) acquired
   (b) congenital
   (c) dermal melanocytosis
2. Epithelial naevi
   (a) epidermal
   (b) sebaceous
   (c) apocrine
   (d) Becker's pigmented hairy naevus
3. Vascular naevi
   (a) telangiectatic
   (b) haemangioma
   (c) angiokeratoma
   (d) lymphangioma
4. Connective tissue naevi
5. Cutaneous mastocytosis
   (a) solitary mastocytoma
   (b) urticaria pigmentosa
   (c) telangiectasia macularis eruptiva perstans
   (d) diffuse mastocytosis

A naevus is a localised developmental abnormality of the skin. It is composed of cells and tissues which are normally present in the skin, but the proportions are abnormal. This means that a naevus is what in other tissues would be called a hamartoma. Usually one component predominates, and the naevus is named accordingly.

Melanocytic naevi

These are the commonest hamartomas in humans, with most people having at least one and the average number in adults being about thirty. The melanocytic naevi were discussed in the preceeding chapter but are briefly reviewed again.

Acquired melanocytic naevi

Although a developmental defect, most melanocytic naevi are acquired during childhood and adolescence. All the factors responsible for their development are not known but sunlight seems to play an important part.

These begin as an increase in number of normal melanocytes in nests at the dermoepidermal function, usually at the bases of the epidermal rete ridges, to form a *junctional naevus*. Some of these cells then migrate into the papillary dermis where they lose their dendrites, become rounded and tend to aggregate in small clusters. At this stage, when there is both an epidermal and adermal component, the lesions are termed *compound naevi*. With time the clusters of naevus cells within the dermis move deeper and the epidermal component may totally disappear, which results in a lesion termed an *intradermal naevus*.

Junctional naevi are therefore mostly pigmented macules, but as the dermal component increases, the surface becomes elevated and, as the lesion becomes predominantly intradermal, the pigmentation also decreases.

Congenital melanocytic naevi

These arise during the normal migration of melanocytes from the neural crest to the basal layer of the epidermis that takes place during normal embryonal development. Becuase the abnormality disrupts migration to the epidermis, congenital melanocytic naevi can never be junctional naevi. Compared with acquired naevi, the dermal component in congenital naevi is often deeper and the naevus cells are often in a perivascular location.

Dermal melanocytosis

In contrast to the cells of the pigmentary naevi, which are rounded cells that exist in clusters within the dermis, there are also conditions in which spindle-shaped melanocytes are scattered within the dermis. These lesions have a bluish colour because, of all the colours that combine to make brown, blue wavelengths are refracted most in their passage through the dermis whereas the red wavelengths are scattered the most and therefore do not emerge to the surface.

Mongolian spot

Mongolian spots are poorly defined, slate grey to brownish macules, present at birth, which generally occur over the lumbosacral region or buttocks. Up to 10 per cent of Australian infants have one or more of these macules, and the incidence exceeds 80 per cent in infants born to black or oriental parents. The naevus darkens in colour for a time after birth, but later fades and usually disappears completely before the child is 10 years old. Histologically the macule is composed of spindle-shaped melanocytes which lie deep in the dermis parallel to the surface.

Naevus of Ota

This is a disorder of adult onset in which pigmentation similar to a mongolian spot is located on the forehead and periorbital region, with the sclera of the eye often affected. The patient is usually an oriental female. The lesion is most commonly unilateral and persists unchanged.

Histology is the same as that of a mongolian spot. No treatment is required.

Blue naevus

The blue naevus is a circumscribed area of slightly raised skin with a slate grey, blue or bluish-black colour. Lesions are dome-shaped, often with a waxy surface. *(Colour plate 43)*

The commonest locations are the distal extremities, the forehead and scalp.

Compared with a mongolian spot, the dermal melanocytes are more tightly aggregated, tend to extend deeper, are often surrounded by melanophages, may have a deeper component in which the cells are more rounded, and not infrequently are associated with an overlying compound melanocytic naevus.

Malignant transformation, which is a very rare event, may occur in large lesions in the scalp. Blue naevi in other locations can therefore be left untreated. If a blue naevus is to be removed, the depth of excision needs to extend into the fat because of the deep location of the melanocytes.

Epithelial naevi

Epidermal naevus

Clinical features

Most often located on the limbs, upper trunk or neck, the epidermal naevus is a skin-coloured or brownish plaque with well-defined borders. The surface may be finely granular, rough and warty, or irregularly papillomatous. Lesions may be solitary or multiple, and vary enormously in size. They tend to be elongated, and may form linear bands winding in zosteriform fashion along the length of a limb or obliquely across the trunk, often stopping abruptly at the midline. *(Colour plate 44)*

Histology

The major component is epidermal, but there is frequently a substantial apocrine or sebaceous contribution, particularly in those lesions which occur on the scalp, face or neck. The epidermis shows thickening, often with basiloid type cells and pseudo horn cysts similar to a seborrhoeic keratosis. At times there may be marked surface papillomatosis or at other times vacuolation of the granular layer similar to bullous ichthyosis.

Course and complications

The naevus is usually present at or soon after birth, and may extend slowly over many years, although some increase in size only in proportion to overall growth. At puberty, irregular thickening of the naevus may follow enlargement of its apocrine or sebaceous elements. Malignant change, generally to basal cell carcinoma, occasionally develops in an epidermal naevus and is suggested by localised nodular thickening or ulceration. Occasionally there are associated bone changes but this is usually only seen with the more extensive epidermal naevi.

Sebaceous naevus

Although often elongated, sebaceous naevi do not form the linear bands of the verrucous type. The typical lesion is a solitary, flat, yellowish plaque, a few centimetres long, densely covered with small elevations, and situated on the face or scalp. The naevus generally remains unchanged until puberty, when sebaceous hypertrophy produces a knobbly thickening. There is a small risk of malignant change, usually to basal cell carcinoma.

Apocrine naevus

At the usual site on the scalp, the apocrine naevus presents as a solitary pink or brownish plaque, often hairless, with an irregular surface which becomes nodular during adolescence. Less often, the lesion is a solitary nodule, sometimes umbilicated. As with sebaceous naevi, malignant change may occur.

Becker's pigmented hairy naevus

This androgen-dependent naevus that appears during the second decade of life begins as a palm-sized pigmented macule that is most commonly centred around the upper limb girdle on one side. With time, hairs within the area become coarser and darker than the unaffected side.

Histology shows elongation of the rete ridges with increase in basal layer melanin but only a mild increase in melanocytes. Although hair follicles are more numerous this may not be appreciated because hairs are widely separated.

Most cases are of no concern other than cosmetic but some may have mesodermal and tone changes similar to those seen with extensive epidermal naevi. The main significance is to avoid confusion with a giant melanocytic naevus.

Vascular naevi

Telangiectatic naevi

These are formed by persistent capillaries of the foetal circulation or a congenital malformation of mature capillaries.

The salmon patch

This very common, minor form of superficial telangiectasia is present at one or more sites in 50 per cent of neonates. Small superficial vessels are present in large numbers within the papillary dermis. There is neither alteration of texture nor elevation of affected skin. The lesion is a poorly defined, pale pink or reddish macule, most often on an upper eyelid, the forehead or the nape of the neck. The nuchal naevus may persist into adult life, but at other sites fading is almost invariable within a year. The salmon patch is an insignificant lesion, important only for the anxiety it may cause parents.

The port wine stain

The lesion consists of mature vessels that are larger than those in the salmon patch and, although also located within the papillary dermis, may involve even larger vessels within the reticular dermis or subcutaneous tissue.

Any site may be affected, but most lesions occur on the face and upper trunk. The naevus is usually solitary and unilateral, and, being composed or mature telangiectatic vessels, does not regress. Size is very variable and the colour ranges from pink to bright red or purplish. At birth, the affected area is smooth and of normal texture, but it may become uniformly or irregularly thickened during childhood and adult life.

In a variant which is known as the Sturge–Weber syndrome, a port wine stain which approximates the cutaneous distribution of one or more divisions of the trigeminal nerve is associated with vascular malformations of the leptomeninges on the same side. Sometimes other deeper locations such as the eye or oropharynx may also be involved. Epilepsy, mental retardation and ocular abnormalities are therefore common additional features.

Treatment of telangiectatic naevi

The salmon patch requires no treatment because the natural history is either that of spontaneous resolution to leave normal looking skin or of persistence confined to areas covered by hair.

The port wine stain can, with certain limitations, respond satisfactorily to the laser. Using the standard argon or copper vapour lasers, which emit wavelengths absorbed by haemoglobin, the best results are obtained by waiting until the vascular naevi change from the pale pink usually seen in childhood to a bluish-red, which usually occurs during early adult life. Recent work with flash-pumped lasers suggests that these expensive lasers can produce good results in pale pink vascular naevi and with less likelihood of residual scarring.

Haemangiomas

Superficial haemangioma ('strawberry naevus')

Histology

Early lesions are composed of numerous capillary vessels, showing considerable endothelial proliferation. In older lesions, there is gradual fibrous replacement of vascular tissue.

Clinical features

This very common naevus develops within the first three months of life and may be present at birth. The lesion evolves rather quickly to form a compressible red nodule, which is frequently lobulated. Strawberry naevi are most common on the head and neck, and are often multiple. They may be less than a centimetre in size, or they may form large tumours covering much of the face. Whatever the early size, enlargement usually continues for several months before the naevus becomes stable. In the great majority, the growing phase is followed by slow spontaneous resolution.

Regression is uncommon before six months and complete resolution is unlikely under four or five years. The first indication of regression is a deepening of colour to purplish-red, with tiny white flecks appearing at sites of sclerosing vessels. The flecks become larger and coalesce, forming pale depressed areas, generally toward the centre of the naevus. Resolution normally continues until only a pale area remains, sometimes with a slightly puckered surface.

Deep ('cavernous') haemangioma

Histology

The bulk of the naevus is formed by large irregular vascular channels, lined by a single layer of endothelium and surrounded by a wall of fibrous tissue. The cavernous vessels are located in the reticular dermis and subcutaneous tissue, and are frequently associated with an overlying superficial haemangioma.

Clinical features

The deep haemangioma varies in appearance, depending on the location of its component vessels. When the vessels are mainly subcutaneous, the colour is bluish, and the surface is smooth. When the haemangioma predominantly involves the reticular dermis, the lesion is red or purplish in colour, and the surface is irregular. When a strawberry naevus is present as well, the deeper component may be obscured and more easily felt than seen.

Most cavernous haemangiomas occur on the head, neck and trunk. They have less tendency to enlarge than strawberry naevi, and are less likely to resolve completely. When the deep haemangioma is covered by a strawberry naevus, the superficial haemangioma behaves as if there were no deeper lesion, but regression tends to be slower.

Complications of haemangiomas

■ *Unusual sites.* Feeding problems may follow involvement of the nose or mouth, and respiratory difficulty may complicate laryngeal lesions. Large naevi involving the eyelids may cause prolonged closure of the eye, with impairment of vision. Disturbance of bone growth may result from encroachment on epiphyses.

■ *Ulceration.* Rapid increase of size may precede ulceration, probably from sclerosis of vessels within the naevus. This uncommon complication does not impede resolution, but is followed by scarring which detracts from the ultimate cosmetic result. Infection of the ulcer is not a serious problem, and significant bleeding is rare.

■ *Haemorrhage.* Haemorrhage after trauma is uncommon and rarely serious. When bleeding is not controlled by firm pressure, there is usually a deep cavernous component but, even then, serious haemorrhage is very uncommon.

■ *Thrombocytopenia.* Rarely, a large rapidly growing haemangioma is complicated by thrombocytopenic purpura, associated with multiple small thromboses and sequestration of platelets within the naevus.

■ *Visceral haemangiomas.* There is an increased incidence of visceral haemangiomas in patients with angiomatous naevi, particularly when multiple. Cavernous haemangiomas may occur as compressible, blue to purplish, rubbery nodules in the skin and subcutaneous tissue, and are then frequently associated with intestinal haemangiomas. Recurrent bleeding and anaemia are common complications ('blue rubber-bleb naevus syndrome').

Treatment

■ *Superficial haemangiomas* have an excellent prognosis, most lesions resolving spontaneously with satisfactory cosmetic results. With large naevi, redundant skin may persist after resolution, and necessitate minor surgery. Cryotherapy may be used for small lesions, but there is a risk of necrosis and haemorrhage when large lesions are treated in this way. Radiotherapy accelerates resolution, but is rarely indicated. Systemic corticosteroids are effective in the suppression of large, rapidly growing lesions, and are indicated for such complications as airway obstruction, cardiac failure, and impairment of vision.

■ *Deep haemangiomas* are less likely to resolve completely than superficial and mixed lesions, but active interference is generally better avoided. The lasers used to treat superficial vascular naevi cannot penetrate beyond the upper mid dermis and are therefore not helpful for deep haemangiomas. Surgical excision is unnecessary for small lesions and difficult for large ones. Systemic corticosteroid therapy has largely replaced radiotherapy in the management of large naevi with thrombocytopenia, or the rare rapidly growing naevus which threatens the function of other organs. As with the superficial haemangioma, treatment should generally be restricted to the surgical improvement of baggy skin which persists after spontaneous resolution.

Angiokeratoma

Angiokeratomas are bright red, purplish or black papules composed of telangiectatic dermal vessels, with hyperkeratosis of the overlying epidermis. They are relatively common on the scrotum of elderly men and, rarely, develop in children or young adults as discrete or clustered lesions over bony prominences, particularly of the fingers and toes.

Angiokeratomas may also be inherited as part of a complex disorder of glycolipid metabolism, associated with vasomotor disturbances and progressive renal disease (Anderson–Fabry disease). In this rare disorder, the angiokeratomas are often concentrated over the lower trunk and genital region.

Lymphangioma

Cutaneous lymphangioma is an uncommon congenital malformation of lymphatic vessels, which may occur at virtually any site but is most frequently found on the proximal parts of the limbs and adjoining areas of the trunk and neck.

Superficial lymphangioma

Small semi-translucent vesicles, mostly filled with clear fluid, are clustered within a circumscribed area of skin. The lesion is usually skin-coloured, but may be red or black due to an admixture of blood. A few vesicles are often noticed soon after birth, but the number increases and the area enlarges as the child grows. It is likely that most, if not all, superficial lymphangiomas are connected to a deeper lymphatic cistern, so that attempts at superficial surgical excision result in recurrence.

Deep lymphangioma

The more deeply situated naevus forms a soft, poorly defined mass, usually associated with other defects of lymphatic drainage.

Connective tissue naevi

Connective tissue naevi are hamartomas containing an abnormal proportion of collagen and elastic tissue. They are present at birth, or develop in childhood, and may be solitary or multiple. Lesions most frequently occur as skin-coloured or creamy white plaques, composed of firm, closely set papules, imparting a roughness to the surface. Common sites are the arms, trunk and buttocks.

Connective tissue naevi occur as isolated defects or in association with several hereditary syndromes, especially tuberous sclerosis.

Cutaneous mastocytosis

Abnormal numbers of mast cells may accumulate in the dermis as a solitary localised naevus, in multiple discrete deposits, or as a diffuse infiltration. Each of the various presentations affects a favoured age group and bears a relationship to the number of mast cells within the lesions.

Histology

All forms of cutaneous mastocytosis demonstrate a dermal infiltrate of mast cells, but these are difficult to recognise without the use of special stains to demonstrate the characteristic cytoplasmic granules. Degranulation is easily provoked by trauma, so the biopsy needs to be taken with care, after injection of the local anaesthetic well clear of the biopsy site. It is necessary to inform the pathologist of the suspected diagnosis, so that the appropriate staining is performed.

Clinical features

■ *The mast cell naevus* is a solitary pink to brownish nodule or plaque that contains huge numbers of mast cells and presents at birth or soon after. Friction or other minor trauma releases histamine from the large number of mast cells, leading to itchy swelling of the lesion. Occasionally there may be sufficient oedema to cause blistering. Wealing may be followed by a refractory period lasting a day or two, during which urtication cannot be elicited. The prognosis for solitary mast cell naevi is excellent, spontaneous resolution being almost invariable before the age of 10 years.

■ *Urticaria pigmentosa* is a more common presentation, usually commencing during childhood with the development of multiple yellowish-red macules, papules or nodules, scattered irregularly over the body. Lesions urticate with rubbing, and within a few months develop brown pigmentation. Large numbers of mast cells are present within the superficial and mid dermis. Resolution can confidently be anticipated for the great majority of patients, persistence into adult life being very uncommon. Pigmentation remains for a few years after the lesions have ceased to urticate, but this too, ultimately fades.

■ *Telangiectasia macularis eruptiva perstans* is a less common pattern of discrete deposits that presents in adults. As the name indicates, the lesions are mildly telangiectatic macules that are reddish-brown, and do not urticate. The lesions persist unchanged throughout life. Within each macule there is only a moderate increase in the number of mast cells within the superficial dermis so it is uncommon for the pathologist to diagnose this variant without the clinician's notes indicating the need for special stains.

■ *Diffuse cutaneous mastocytosis* is a rare disease that is seen in older adults. The diffusely thickened skin has a doughy consistency and may be red or yellowish-brown in colour. Pruritus is usually severe and blistering may follow minor trauma to the skin, which contains enormous numbers of mast cells. Occasionally mast cells may be found in the circulation.

Complications

■ *Systemic symptoms* of generalised pruritus, vomiting, diarrhoea and even syncope from hypotension may be produced if enough histamine is released. These features are more likely to occur in patients with multiple or diffuse lesions. Attacks are usually precipitated by ingestion of histamine-releasing substances such as aspirin or codeine, or traumatisation of lesions by heat or other physical stimuli.

■ *Visceral deposits* may occur but the frequency of the association is uncertain. The incidence is higher in patients with late onset of cutaneous lesions and may then approach 15 per cent. Deposits may occur in almost any organ, but are most often found in the gastro-intestinal tract, liver, spleen and bones. These lesions very rarely cause any symptoms.

Diagnosis

▶ **Suspect** the diagnosis in any pigmented macule or plaque where there is associated telangiectasia or a history suggesting urtication.

▶ **Consider and exclude**

■ *Melanocytic naevi.* These do not urticate with light rubbing.

■ *Xanthomas*, which differ in distribution, are yellowish, and do not urticate.

■ *Histiocytosis X* is a rare disease, which may produce lesions resembling cutaneous mastocytosis. However, lesions do not urticate and the histology is different.

▶   **Confirm the diagnosis** by histology, although this is usually not required for the solitary mast cell naevus, where urtication with minor trauma is readily evident.

Treatment

There is no satisfactory treatment for the disease, although those forms which begin early in life are likely to resolve during childhood. For patients in whom systemic symptoms are a problem, H_1 antihistamines, alone or in combination with H_2 antagonists, may rarely provide some relief. Oral disodium cromoglycate may also be useful, particularly when gastro-intestinal symptoms predominate, but very large doses are required.

Known histamine-releasing agents may provoke urtication, and are better avoided. These include morphine, codeine, aspirin, alcohol, and vigorous use of the towel after bathing.

PUVA can temporarily cause clearing of lesions and reduce urtication and systemic symptoms. Although mast cell numbers usually remain unchanged, this treatment transiently produces mast cells with non-functional granules.

12

Diseases of genetic origin

1. Disorders of keratinisation
   (a) ichthyosis
   (b) keratosis pilaris
   (c) Darier's disease
   (d) hyperkeratosis of palms and soles
2. Disorders of collagen and elastic tissue
   (a) pseudoxanthoma elasticum
   (b) Ehlers–Danlos syndrome
   (c) cutis laxa
3. Congenital ectodermal dysplasia
4. Neurocutaneous syndromes
   (a) neurofibromatosis
   (b) tuberous sclerosis
5. Xeroderma pigmentosum

Changes in the skin are a feature of many genetic diseases and several of these, such as diseases of hair and nails, blistering diseases, and psoriasis, are discussed in the relevant section.

This chapter discusses the commoner, well defined structural disorders of the skin that are genetically determined.

Disorders of keratinisation

Ichthyosis

After prolonged soaking, normal skin becomes soft and wrinkled. Abnormally dry skin, by contrast, is taut and inelastic. If the dryness is severe, fine cracks develop in the surface and may extend to form a crazy-paving pattern, isolating 'islands' of stratum corneum which are seen as scales.

The abnormal skin of ichthyosis resembles that produced by excessive dryness. The skin feels dry and taut, and scales form in the stratum corneum. Ichthyosis is worse in dry, windy weather and improves during the humid months of summer. After bathing, the scales may temporarily disappear, only to reappear as the skin dries. Ichthyotic skin has greater than normal transepidermal water loss. Whether this is due to defective water binding in the stratum corneum, or to an ineffective barrier formed by abnormally keratinised cells, is unknown.

Although there are many varieties of ichthyosis, the most common are an autosomal dominant, an X-linked recessive and two types that present with erythroderma in the neonatal period.

Ichthyosis vulgaris (autosomal dominant)

Clinical features (Colour plate 45)

The skin is normal at birth, but becomes dry and rough within a year or two. Mildly affected patients progress no further than this and may improve during childhood. Others develop thin polygonal scales that are firmly attached, except at the edges.

Most of the skin is affected, but there is considerable regional variation of severity. Scaling is most pronounced over the back and the extensor surfaces of the limbs, often with discrete areas of thickening over the elbows knees and ankles. The scalp tends to be dry and scaly, and there may be a little roughness over the forehead and cheeks. Markings are exaggerated on the palms and soles, but the larger flexures are usually normal.

Histology

Moderate thickening of the stratum corneum is associated with an inconspicuous stratum granulosum, which contrasts with hyperkeratosis from other causes, in which the stratum granulosum is broad and prominent.

Pathogenesis

The keratohyaline protein filaggrin is reduced or absent.

Associations

■ *Atopic eczema*, hay fever and asthma occur more common than in the general community. However, although the patient with routine atopic eczema often has dry skin, that is very rarely true ichthyosis vulgaris.

■ *Keratosis pilaris* is accentuated.

X-linked ichthyosis

Clinical features

Patients showing the full range of signs are males. As in ichthyosis vulgaris, the skin is normal at birth, but there are the following differences:

The onset is usually within the first few months. The scales are larger and darker and tend to be more pronounced over the ventral surface. There is less sparing of the flexures and more marked involvement of the face and scalp.

The female heterozygote often has a generally dry skin, although there may be localised zones showing the typical large dark scales.

Histology

The keratin layer is thickened, as is the epidermis, but the granular cell layer looks normal.

Pathogenesis

The basic genetic defect is a deficiency in the enzyme steroid sulphatase. Large amounts of cholesterol sulphate are found in the keratin layer but how this produces the clinical changes observed is unknown.

Associations

■ *Unusual maternal pregnancy.* Urinary oestriol, which is normally a guide to foetal well-being, cannot be utilised in mothers pregnant with an affected child because this substance requires foetal steroid sulphatase within the placenta for normal formation. For reasons that are unknown, the labour is often long and difficult.

■ *Corneal opacities.* These can also be seen in the female carriers.

Bullous ichthyosiform erythroderma (autosomal dominant)

Clinical features

The disease begins soon after birth, with bullae and widespread scaling. The early bullous phase may be of life-threatening severity or relatively mild, with inconspicuous bullae which quickly evolve to raw, weeping erosions. Blisters become less troublesome during childhood, but secondary infection of the erosions is a common problem, and the child may present with recurrent impetigo, usually over the limbs.

Thick hyperkeratotic ridges gradually form in the flexures, and over the hands and feet, occasionally becoming generalised.

Histology

The granular layer of the epidermis is thickened and the cells in this zone show vacuolation of the cytoplasm, with large keratohyaline granules.

Pathogenesis

The basic defect is unknown but keratinisation is affected in that tonofilament formation is very irregular and desmosome function reduced. Secondary infection with bacteria seems to promote blister formation.

Association

Ectropion, which is a measure of severity, is not specific and can occur in any erythroderma.

Non-bullous ichthyosiform erythroderma (autosomal recessive)

Clinical features

The onset, usually at birth, is of a generalised erythroderma with fine large scales. The redness persists through to middle life, when it may improve but the scaling worsen. The flexures are involved and there is usually diffuse hyperkeratosis of the palms and soles.

Histology

There is epidermal acanthosis and parakeratosis with a prominent granular layer. An inflammatory infiltrate is present within the upper dermis.

Pathogenesis

There is marked increase in the rate of epidermal cell production and the keratin formed has large amount of n-alkanes.

Associations

- Ectropion
- Corneal dystrophy
- Short stature is often a feature.

Diagnosis of the ichthyoses

▶ **Suspect** the diagnosis in the patient with extensive dry scaly skin.

▶ **Consider and exclude**

- *Hypothyroidism* in young children. This is suggested by large tongue, coarse features, poor muscle tone and retarded development.

- *Acquired ichthyosis of neoplasia* in adults. Lymphomas are the commonest cause but visceral carcinoma can also be responsible.

- *Severe nutritional deficiency*, especially essential fatty acids.

- *Xerosis*, which is seen in those with atopic eczema and in the elderly during the winter months.

- *Asteatotic eczema* is usually localised to the anterior lower legs.

▶ **Confirmation of diagnosis** is usually based on family history and clinical features. Biopsy is occasionally required for exact classification and genetic counselling.

Treatment of the ichthyoses

The skin is made softer and more pliable with the regular use of emollients which contain lanolin or petrolatum. These are best applied after bathing when the skin is hydrated. Bath oils are convenient but more expensive and less effective. Creams containing 3 to 6 per cent salicylic acid help to control scaling, but when used over large areas may lead to sufficient percutaneous absorption of the salicylic acid to cause systemic toxicity. Urea, 10 to 20 per cent, or 5 per cent lactic acid are effective alternatives. Retinoic acid ointment (0.1 per cent), or 40 per cent propylene glycol left on overnight, under plastic sheeting, may be used for severe cases, but are rather irritating applications.

Oral retinoids, especially etretinate and its metabolite acitretin, are helpful in the ichthyoses by influencing keratinisation, but in the bullous form the blistering may be worsened and in many, the skin of the soles may be made so thin as to make walking painful. The long-term use in childhood is questionable because of the possibility of effects on bone epiphyses. Taken during pregnancy, these drugs produce characteristic embryopathic effects on the facial skeleton and cardiovascular system.

Keratosis pilaris (autosomal dominant)

This very common disorder of follicular keratinisation is characterised by the presence of horny follicular papules, usually over the arms and thighs.

Histology

A conical plug of keratin is embedded in a dilated follicular pore.

Clinical features

The papules are small, spiky elevations, scattered over affected areas without any tendency to grouping or coalescence. The appearance resembles permanent goose-pimples and the papules are, in fact, more apparent in cold weather. The keratinous plug can be picked out of the follicular pore, but soon regrows.

Distribution is generally confined to the extensor surfaces of the arms and thighs, but may extend to other areas.

Diagnosis

▶ **Consider and exclude**

■ *Darier's disease*. Papules differ in distribution and frequently coalesce.

■ *Pityriasis rubra pilaris*. Palms and soles are hyperkeratotic, psoriasiform plaques form over elbows and knees, and distribution of papules is different.

■ *Lichen planopilaris*. The eruption is composed of itchy acuminate papules with a predilection for the trunk.

Treatment

Temporary improvement follows the daily application of 3 per cent salicylic acid ointment, but treatment is usually unnecessary.

Darier's disease (autosomal dominant)

This is an uncommon disturbance of keratinisation in which discrete papules coalesce to form crusted plaques, typically over the scalp, neck, and upper part of the trunk. Many patients give no family history of the disease, and probably represent new mutations.

Histology

A defect in synthesis or maturation of the tonofilament–desmosome complex produces a characteristic microscopic appearance. Individual cells are prematurely and abnormally keratinised, and are conspicuous in the stratum spinosum because of their homogenous eosinophilic cytoplasm and deeply staining nuclei. Clefts form above the basal layer from loosening of desmosomal attachments and later extend throughout the stratum spinosum. Older papules show acanthosis, hyperkeratosis and keratotic plugs, sometimes set in follicular pores.

Clinical features

■ *The primary lesion* is a firm, skin-coloured to yellowish-brown papule, which becomes crusted and greasy to the touch. Plaques form from the coalescence of papules, and develop a rough, irregular surface.

■ *Distribution* often involves the sides and back of the neck, the upper back and the presternal region. The scalp, retro-auricular and nasolabial folds are also common sites. The palms and soles are frequently thickened with punctate keratoses, but palmoplantar pits are more specific for this disorder. Wart-like papules may develop on the dorsae of the hands.

■ *The nails* are frequently brittle, with distal subungual hyperkeratosis. However, the most characteristic abnormalities are longitudinal red or white streaks ending in V-shaped nicks at the distal nail margin.

■ *Mucosal lesions* are common in some affected families. White papules on the oral mucosa may coalesce to mimic leukoplakia, and similar lesions may be present on the rectal and genital mucous membranes.

Complications

Infection of the skin with bacteria, most commonly of thickened plaques, is often a problem. Patients are also more susceptible to herpes simplex infection, often developing the widespread form of herpes simplex infection known as Kaposi's varicelliform eruption.

Course

The disease most often begins in children of school age, but may be delayed until middle age or later. Sunburn appears to precipitate new lesions in some, and cause aggravation in others. Lesions may remain localised to relatively small areas, but gradual progression is the rule.

▶ **Consider and exclude** Grover's disease, an acquired transient acantholytic dermatosis of unknown cause in which itchy, keratotic, fleshy papules appear on the torso of middle-aged males. Histology can be very similar to Darier's disease, but all other clinical signs are absent. Treatment is to relieve itch until spontaneous resolution occurs.

Treatment

Although not warranted for minor expressions of the disease, systemic etretinate therapy appears to provide an effective and, in the absence of contra-indications, a relatively safe method of treatment.

Hyperkeratosis of palms and soles

The majority of patients with hyperkeratosis of the palms and soles are suffering from diseases which are acquired, or genetically influenced only in a broad sense. Diffuse hyperkeratosis may be a feature of tinea, psoriasis, pityriasis rubra pilaris or atopic dermatitis. More localised hyperkeratosis may be due to callus, corns, lichen planus, syphilis, Reiter's disease, or the chronic ingestion of arsenic.

Palmoplantar hyperkeratosis is a minor feature of several more generalised genetic disorders, as in Darier's disease, recessive ichthyosis, and congenital ectodermal dysplasia. In one group of genetic diseases, palmoplantar hyperkeratosis is the major presenting feature.

Diffuse type (autosomal dominant or recessive)

The more common dominant form is usually apparent in the first year of life. The palms and soles become red, later thickening to a diffuse yellowish hyperkeratosis. Severity varies from barely perceptible thickening to severe hyperkeratosis with painful fissuring. The abnormal skin is strictly confined to the palms and soles, and is often bordered by a narrow band of erythema. Palmoplantar hyperhidrosis is a common association. A very rare variant is characterised by dominant transmission, and a high incidence of oesophageal carcinoma.

Focal type (autosomal dominant or recessive)

In the relatively common dominant form, which may first appear any time between the ages of fifteen and fifty, discrete keratinous papules are scattered over the palms and soles, sometimes with associated nail abnormalities.

Treatment of palmoplantar hyperkeratosis

There is no really effective treatment. Although discomfort is generally not severe, some improvement can be obtained with creams containing salicylic acid or urea. Painful fissures are best treated with twice daily applications of 1 per cent aqueous silver nitrate.

Disorders of collagen and elastic tissue

These are rare diseases that for purposes of this text can be divided into three syndromes, each with a characteristic skin appearance, thus giving the impression of distinct diseases. However, in reality each syndrome consists of many genetic disorders with different patterns of inheritance and different metabolic defects, that produce a common phenotype.

There is no specific treatment for any of these three syndromes.

Pseudoxanthoma elasticum

Pseudoxanthoma elasticum is a very uncommon disorder of elastic tissue, involving the skin, eyes and cardiovascular system. All three are involved in most patients, but the contribution from each varies considerably and determines the overall severity of the disease. Cutaneous changes are frequently recognisable in childhood, but the disease is usually first detected in young adults. Some varieties are inherited in an autosomal dominant way and others by an autosomal recessive pattern.

Pathology

Elastic fibres of the reticular dermis are swollen, irregular and fragmented. As calcium accumulates on the fibres they become basophilic. In the stomach, intestines and other viscera, small to medium arteries develop calcification of elastic fibres of the intima; elsewhere, in larger arteries, calcium deposits around elastic fibres of the media.

Clinical features

■ *Cutaneous*. The primary lesions are small yellowish papules grouped in a recticulate pattern over the sides of the neck and in the large flexures, or soft rhomboidal plaques bounded by the skin lines. Between the papules the skin has a velvety texture and a yellowish colour, likened to the appearance of a freshly plucked chicken. There is variable involvement of other areas, and in a few patients, much of the skin surface is affected. The altered skin is less elastic than normal, and in older patients may hang in loose folds.

■ *Ocular*. The eyes are affected in most patients. The characteristic lesions are slate grey to reddish-brown streaks over the fundus ('angioid streaks') caused by breaks in the elastin of Bruch's membrane. Haemorrhage from altered retinal vessels may lead to blindness.

■ *Other organs*. Gastro-intestinal haemorrhage is a frequent and sometimes fatal complication, but bleeding may occur in virtually any organ. Hypertension, myocardial or peripheral ischaemia, and subarachnoid haemorrhage are not uncommon.

Ehlers–Danlos syndrome (cutis hyperelastica)

Ehlers–Danlos syndrome is an inherited defect of collagen metabolism, manifested by abnormalities of the skin, joints and viscera.

Pathology

There is a wide range of structural and biochemical abnormalities of collagen, each with its own pattern of inheritance and subtle clinical differences. However, for some types the defect is not known.

Clinical features

■ *Cutaneous*. The skin is soft, pliable, and has an unusual, chamois-like texture. It is hyperelastic and easily pulled away from underlying tissue, but quickly returns to its normal position when released. The skin is fragile and easily bruised. Wounds gape, hold sutures poorly and heal slowly, leaving thin atrophic scars, often with spongy underlying nodules ('pseudotumours').

■ *Other organs*. Joints are hyperextensible and unstable so that subluxation is common. There may be megacolon, inguinal and diaphragmatic hernia or more serious complications which include gastro-intestinal haemorrhage and dissecting aneurysm of the aorta.

Cutis laxa

Cutis laxa is a rare disorder of elastic tissue, in which distinctive cutaneous changes are associated with variable visceral manifestations. In some cases, transmission appears to be autosomal dominant, but the more severe forms of the disease are probably inherited as a recessive trait.

Pathology

The amount of elastic tissue in skin and other organs is decreased, and the elastic fibres present are abnormal in size and shape.

Clinical features

■ *Cutaneous*. There is a defective elasticity of the skin which may be apparent from infancy or may begin in adult life. The skin is extensible but, in contrast to the Ehlers–Danlos syndrome, when pulled away from underlying tissue, returns only slowly to its previous position. It becomes inelastic, lax and pendulous, and tends to hang in loose folds from the face, neck and abdomen. The facial expression develops an aged look, rather like that of a bloodhound.

■ *Other organs.* Emphysema is common and may lead to cor pulmonale. Less frequent associations include rectal prolapse, inguinal hernia, sexual immaturity, aortic aneurysm and pulmonary stenosis.

Congenital ectodermal dysplasia

The term 'congenital ectodermal dysplasia' includes a group of hereditary syndromes which are characterised by abnormal development of the skin and its appendages and are often associated with changes in other ectodermally derived tissues such as teeth and nails.

The two most common representatives of this group of disorders are described below.

X-linked (anhidrotic)

The eccrine and sebaceous glands are markedly reduced in number and size, and may be almost completely absent. In some patients there is also hypoplasia of the salivary, lacrymal and mucous glands. The complete syndrome occurs only in males, but female heterozygotes may have patchy eccrine dysplasia.

The skin is soft, dry and smooth, and the facial appearance characteristic. The brows are prominent, the ears large, the lips thick, and the nose depressed. Teeth may be absent or malformed, and those present are often conical and prone to caries. Scalp hair is fine and sparse, and the nails thin and brittle. Impaired sweating leads to fatigue and pyrexia in warm weather or with exercise, while even minor infections may cause dangerous elevation of body temperature.

Autosomal dominant ('hidrotic')

Eccrine glands function normally, but there is a mixture of other cutaneous abnormalities. The nails are dystrophic and frequently lifted by subungual hyperkeratosis. They may be discoloured, thick, and grow slowly.

There is diffuse hyperkeratosis of the palms and soles and the skin over the joints tends to be thick and hyperpigmented. The teeth are generally normal, but the hair is sparse, thin and fragile.

Neurocutaneous syndromes

Neurofibromatosis (autosomal dominant)

Neurofibromatosis is a relatively common group of clinically and genetically distinct syndromes which share an association of characteristic cutaneous lesions with abnormalities of the peripheral and central nervous system. There is a wide range of clinical expression, but all patients display an inexorable progression: an increase in the number or size (or in both), not only on cutaneous lesions, but also of the tumours at all sites.

At least half of all patients with classical neurofibromatosis give no family history of the disease, but many mild cases are probably unrecognised.

Gene location

The variant which has predominantly central nervous system neuro-fibromas, such as acoustic neuromas, is coded for by a gene on chromosome 22, whereas the long arm of chromosome 17 contains the gene for the more common classic form in which peripheral neurofibromas predominate.

Clinical features

■ *Cutaneous*. Neurofibromas are benign tumours formed by various combinations of neurons, Schwann cells, fibroblasts, mast cells, and vascular elements. The dermal tumours are soft sessile elevations, which sometimes become pedunculated. There may be a few, or there may be hundreds, and no site is exempt, although palms and soles tend to be spared.

Most are from 2 cm to 4 cm in size but, occasionally, tumours are very much larger. Subcutaneous neurofibromas are firmer and may be grouped along peripheral nerves. Pruritus may occur over existing neurofibromas or at sites of recent trauma, and is occasionally severe. Relief with H_1 antihistamines suggests that the pruritus is mediated by histamine release from the large number of mast cells in neurofibromas.

Areas of hyperpigmentation are present in almost every patient. There are evenly pigmented, light or dark brown macules, ranging from a millimetre to many centimetres in size. They are usually round or oval, with a well-defined border (café au lait spots). Multiple small, freckle-like macules in the axillae and perineum are less common, but virtually pathognomonic.

■ *Other organs*. Tumours of the central nervous system including, particularly, acoustic neuromas occur in 5 to 10 per cent of patients and account for a major proportion of the severe morbidity and mortality of the disease. Neurofibromas may also be associated with other cranial nerves, or may develop in the gastro-intestinal or urinary tracts.

Pigmented iris hamartomas are present in 95 per cent of patients over the age of six years. They bear no relation to severity, nor to other manifestations of the disease, but are helpful in establishing the diagnosis. Uncommon features include frank mental retardation, epilepsy and kyphoscoliosis. Acromegaly, Addison's disease and other endocrine disorders are occasional associations.

Course

Pigmented macules may be recognisable at birth, but become more obvious as they increase in size and number during childhood and adult life. Neurofibromas are generally noticed in the first decade and have a tendency to rapid growth during adolescence and pregnancy. Pain and swelling of a neurofibroma should arouse suspicion of sarcomatous change, which occurs in 2 per cent of patients.

Treatment

Epileptic patients are investigated in the hope of finding a remediable lesion. Excision of cutaneous tumours is usually impractical because of the large number present.

Tuberous sclerosis (autosomal dominant)

Most patients with tuberous sclerosis do not reproduce, and the disease would disappear if it were not for new mutations. However, as with neurofibromatosis, clinical expression varies widely, and careful examination of apparently normal parents or siblings may reveal minor features of the syndrome. Those with minor signs carry the gene and even though they are not severely affected, if they transmit the gene, the child is usually more severely affected.

Gene location

Although the exact gene has not been isolated, current evidence indicates the gene is located on the short arm of chromosome 9.

Clinical features

The typical syndrome is a triad of epilepsy, mental retardation and cutaneous lesions formed by fibrovascular proliferation. The triad is frequently incomplete, and the classical cutaneous lesions are usually preceded by pigmentary changes which are useful in early diagnosis.

■ *Cutaneous*. More than 90 per cent of affected infants have characteristic leafshaped areas of white skin. Up to 3 cm in size, the hypopigmented macules are found on the trunk and legs, and are usually multiple. In fair-skinned babies, they may be difficult to recognise, but are more apparent when illuminated by a Wood's lamp. There may be one to two café au lait macules and other less distinctive pigmentary changes.

By the age of five, facial angiofibromas (sometimes incorrectly referred to as adenoma sebaceum) are generally apparent as firm pink or reddish papules over the centre of the face. The nasolabial folds and sides of the nose are common early sites. Rough, skin-coloured plaques may develop, usually over the lumbosacral region and, at puberty, firm fibromas may emerge from beneath the nail folds to grow out over the adjoining nail plate.

■ *Other organs*. The earliest manifestation is usually focal or Jacksonian epilepsy, caused by cerebral gliomas. Mental retardation and, occasionally, hydrocephalus may follow. Retinal gliomas are common, but cause little or no disturbance of vision. Other malformations include pulmonary cysts and hamartomas of the heart and kidneys. Tooth enamel may be affected by a distinctive pattern of pitted defects, but deciduous teeth do not usually show this defect.

Treatment

Apart from anticonvulsant therapy, little can be done for these patients. Surgery may be necessary for hydrocephalus, and the cautery can be used to reduce disfigurement from facial lesions. However, the disease is frequently progressive and many patients die from neurological complications before the age of thirty.

Xeroderma pigmentosum (autosomal recessive)

Xeroderma pigmentosum is a group of rare inherited disorders, manifested as a progressive and accelerated degeneration of the skin, eyes and nervous system, with its most prominent features directly attributable to the basic defect, which is an inability to repair DNA that has been damaged by ultraviolet light.

Clinical features

■ *Photosensitivity* is usually apparent before the second birthday, as severe and persistent erythema after moderate exposure to sunlight. The skin becomes dry, freckled and develops small areas of atrophy and hypopigmentation. Telangiectases and small haemangiomas develop not only on exposed and unexposed skin, but also on mucosal surfaces.

■ *Benign and malignant tumours* begin to develop by the fourth or fifth year. There are solar keratoses and kerato-acanthomas, basal cell and squamous cell carcinomas, and melanomas. Severely affected children may die in the first decade from melanoma or metastasising squamous cell carcinoma.

■ *Photophobia* is usually a prominent early feature. With time, severe damage to conjunctiva and cornea occurs.

■ *Neurological symptoms* such as mental retardation, spasticity and ataxia are more likely in those patients with the most marked in vitro sensitivity of fibroblasts to ultraviolet-induced damage, but the reason for this correlation is not known.

Diagnosis

▶ Consider and exclude

■ *Rothmund–Thomson syndrome*, which includes photosensitivity and poikiloderma, but also features dwarfism, hypogonadism and sparse scalp hair. Keratoses may develop on exposed areas, with later carcinomatous change, but the early onset of multiple cutaneous tumours seen in xeroderma pigmentosum is lacking.

■ *Bloom's syndrome* may present in infancy with photosensitivity and facial erythema, but is accompaniend by dwarfism and immunological aberrations.

■ *Ataxia telangiectasia* may also produce dry erythematous facial skin with telangiectases, but has other features, including cerebellar and mental disease, and recurrent infections of the respiratory tract.

Treatment

The child should be protected from sunlight by every available means. Premalignant lesions are treated as they arise, and malignant tumours excised as early as possible.

13

Reactions to physical agents

1. Actinic
   (a) sunlight and the skin
   (b) sunburn
   (c) chronic solar degeneration
   (d) photosensitivity
2. Mechanical
   (a) callus
   (b) corns
   (c) bedsore
3. Cold and heat
   (a) chilblains
   (b) Raynaud's phenomenon
   (c) frostbite
   (d) burns

Actinic

Sunlight and the skin

The sun emits a wide spectrum of electromagnetic radiation. Wavelengths range from the very short cosmic and gamma rays, through the medium band of ultraviolet radiation (UVR), to the longer wavelengths of visible light–infrared and beyond. Wavelengths of UVR shorter than 290 nm (UV-C) are filtered off in the ozone layer of the upper atmosphere, so that the shortest wavelengths reaching the earth's surface are between 290 nm and 320 nm (UV-B). Most of the effects the layman recognises as being caused by the sun are produced by UV-B.

After irradiation by UV-B, normal skin develops an initial erythema, which fades quickly when exposure ceases. With sufficient irradiation, a delayed erythema develops within a few hours, and increases in intensity to a maximum at twelve hours, before fading during the next twenty-four hours. The delayed erythema is accompanied by histological evidence of epidermal damage which shows as epidermal cells with shrunken pyknotic nuclei and are known as sunburn cells. There is also increased vascular permeability, oedema, and an infiltrate of polymorphs in the upper dermis.

Exposure to UV-B induces new pigment formation. Approximately two days after exposure there is increased synthesis and increased transfer of melanin, which reaches a maximum at two to three weeks and fades gradually over several months.

Oxidation of existing pigment to melanin of a darker colour is produced by UV-A (320–400 nm). This occurs within minutes of exposure and lasts about 12 hours before returning to the non-oxidised paler form. Although UV-A can induce new pigment formation, it is one-thousandth as potent as UV-B in this respect.

UV-A enhances the erythema-producing effect of UV-B but on its own UV-A can produce a different sort of erythema that appears 24 to 48 hours after exposure, reaches its maximum at 72 hours and lasts for about one week. Ordinarily this is not a problem because very large amounts of UV-A are required to produce erythema. However, the presence of abnormal substances (such as drugs or porphyrins) which sensitise the skin to sunlight usually do so by sensitising to UV-A.

Unlike UV-B, the longer wavelengths (UV-A) can penetrate window glass and are only partially absorbed by the chemically acting sunscreens. UV-A penetrates more deeply into the dermis than UV-B and may have a significant role in the induction of long-term changes characteristic of solar degeneration.

Sunburn (acute solar toxicity)

Because melanin provides a measure of protection against UVR, sunburn is more frequent early in summer before pigmentation has been stimulated. Damage occurs more quickly in fair-skinned people with a poor ability to tan but, with sufficient exposure, even the blackest of skins are affected. Sunburn is normally caused by UV-B and, as thin clouds filter UV-B poorly, severe sunburn may develop on relatively dull days. Sunburn is less likely in smoky industrial areas, where the smoke and soot filter a significant proportion of UV-B.

Clinical features

Minor degrees of sunburn produce a mild erythema with little or no discomfort, which lasts three or four days and is followed by increased pigmentation. With more severe damage, erythema begins within a few hours of first exposure and increases in intensity for a day or two. The skin is painful, tender and oedematous, and may develop vesicles and bullae. The blisters rupture to leave raw erosions, which become crusted. In very severe reactions, there may be necrosis with subsequent scarring. The crusts dry and separate, while scaling develops in other areas and varies from a light branny desquamation to frank peeling of large areas.

With severe involvement of large areas, systemic features are prominent. There may be headache, nausea, fever, delirium and hypotension. Impaired sweating over much of the body may lead to hyperpyrexia.

Diagnosis

▶ **Suspect on basis of**
- Distribution to areas exposed to sun
- History of exposure compatible with diagnosis
- Clinical signs

▶ **Consider and exclude**

■ *Pathological photosensitivity* as caused by drugs or photosensitising diseases such as lupus erythematosus or the porphyrias. In these disorders the severity of the sunburn seems disproportionate to the exposure which caused it.

■ *Photocontact dermatitis* such as those caused by perfumes in after-shave lotion. Photosensitivity is seen only in parts of the sun-exposed skin that have come in contact with the responsible substance.

■ *Airborne contact allergy* that is not truly photosensitive but mimics photosensitivity because parts not protected by clothing are involved. However, areas normally shielded from the sun for anatomical reasons, such as the upper eyelids, under the chin and behind the earlobes, are involved in these patients. Allergens of this type include wood saw dusts and pollens from the compositae group of plants such as Capeweed.

Prevention

Exposure to sunlight should be kept within the limits of individual tolerance. Individuals particularly susceptible to sunburn should minimise exposure during the middle of the day when the intensity of UVR is greatest. They should restrict their swimming to the early morning or late afternoon, avoiding the 'day at the beach'. Because of refraction through the earth's atmosphere, almost no UV-B reaches the earth's surface before 10 am and after 3 pm (true local time). It should be understood that hats and umbrellas protect only against direct overhead irradiation and are ineffective against UVR reflected from sand or water. Even those with a good capacity to tan are well advised to avoid excessive exposure to sunlight, but graduated exposure is good advice, easily forgotten. When excessive exposure is unavoidable, suitable protective applications should be used.

Zinc oxide and titanium dioxide are opaque substances which provide a physical barrier to transmission of ultraviolet radiation. Although extremely effective, zinc oxide cream has to be applied thickly, which limits its acceptability. This has been overcome to a degree in the case of titanium dioxide by having very finely milled titanium dioxide particles incorporated into a vanishing cream base.

More readily accepted are sunscreens that contain substances that react chemically with ultraviolet light of specific wavelengths and so prevent these rays from reaching the surface of the skin. This type of sunscreen needs to be applied generously one to two hours before exposure, with the skin clean and dry at the time of application. As their effectiveness is impaired by sweating and swimming, these sunscreens are least effective when most needed. For adequate protection, people who are engaged in heavy outdoor work should apply UV filters every two or three hours.

Chemically reacting sunscreens give excellent protection against UV-B, letting through less than one per cent of all incident rays within this band. However, currently available chemically reacting sunscreens are a poor barrier to UV-A because they interact well only with the shorter wavelength UV-A rays and even then still allow a significant proportion of this incident radiation to reach the skin.

Commonly used sunscreening chemicals are cinnamates, derivatives of para-aminobenzoic acid, benzophenones and butyl methoxydibenzoyl-methane, with the last two providing some protection against shorter wavelength UV-A. As UV-B has one thousand times the ability of UV-A to induce cutaneous erythema and presumably the other features of acute actinic damage, UV-B screens therefore provide adequate protection against acute damage in most instances. However, around midday in summer the greatest intensity of UV-A is sufficient to have a significant acute effect upon the skin and in this situation it is helpful to use sunscreens with some activity against UV-A because these rays may be very important in inducing changes within the dermis that are a consequence of sun damage.

Treatment

Topical steroids are helpful in suppressing the erythema of mild sunburn. Although systemic steroids are used in severe sunburn they seem more effective in suppressing the constitutional toxicity than the erythema. The erythema and other changes of acute sundamage are mediated by prostaglandins and therefore some of the non-steroidal anti-inflammatory prostaglandin synthetase inhibitors such as indomethacin have some effect in reducing severity. The main treatment is prevention.

Chronic solar degeneration

Aetiology

Early this century a suntan acquired by holidaying on the French Riviera became a symbol of the leisurely moneyed society rather than a sign betraying time spent performing unskilled outdoor labour. Also, although now forgotten by most, the awarding of the Nobel prize for work showing that ultraviolet light had beneficial effects on cutaneous tuberculosis (which was closely followed by the discovery that rickets was prevented by sunlight-induced Vitamin D) did much to foster the belief that a suntan was a sign of good health.

Our society has therefore developed an ingrained desire to achieve a suntan. Unfortunately this desire often outweighs advice concerning the dangers of prolonged sun exposure.

After thirty to forty years of sun exposure, degenerative and neoplastic effects become evident on the epidermis, dermal connective tissue, blood vessels and hair follicles. Exposure during early childhood is important in initiating the process but continued exposure also has a promoting effect. It is therefore never too early or too late to protect the skin from excessive sun exposure. UV-B is most important in production of epidermal skin cancers but UV-A has a facilitative effect and, because it penetrates through the skin much deeper than does UV-B, UV-A may be responsible for much of the changes within the dermis and adnexa.

Clinical features

The skin is thinner, drier and less elastic than normal. The wrinkled appearance is described as 'aged', but is due to the cumulative effect of solar damage rather than to age itself. Skin markings are exaggerated, especially over the back of the neck, where the skin tends to be thick and leathery.

The sides of the neck are wrinkled, often with telangiectases and spotty pigmentation. Venous lakes may be seen on the lips and the ears. Linear telangiectases are often present on the cheeks. There may be a netlike pattern of small yellowish papules over the cheeks or forehead, while yellowish nodules may form over the back of the neck and around the eyes. Large comedones are frequently found in the lateral periorbital regions.

Circumscribed areas become scaly, and slowly thicken to form horny papules (keratoses) which may sometimes progress to squamous cell carcinoma.

Histology

The epidermis is thin, with localised areas of thickened stratum corneum. The dermo-epidermal junction is flattened and overlies an atrophic dermis. The upper third of the dermis consists of fragmented thickened basophilic fibres except for a narrow band of normal collagen adjacent to the dermo-epidermal junction which in localised areas may also change from a loose network of fibres to homogenous eosinophilic zones.

Treatment

The dry inelastic skin is more comfortable with regular application of an emollient, such as 10% glycerine in sorbolene cream. Prolonged application of retinoic acid can cause collagen to return towards normal histologic staining and morphology, and clinically can improve minor degenerative changes provided further sun exposure is avoided. Keratoses are treated as they arise.

Photosensitivity

Acute photosensitivity in which there is severe erythema confined to light-exposed areas is a feature of photocontactants such as tars and perfumes; photosensitising drugs such as thiazides and griseofulvin; the collagen diseases lupus erythematosus and dermatomyositis; and the biochemical disorders pellagra and most of the porphyrias.

An exaggeration of the normal physiological response to sunlight occurs in disorders with defective pigmentation such as albinism, vitiligo, hypopituitarism and phenylketonuria.

Many diseases are aggravated or precipitated by sunlight. Examples of these are lupus erythematosus, pemphigus erythematosus, and varicella.

The onset of Darier's disease may be associated with an episode of sunburn, as are recurrences of herpes simplex and erythema multiforme in some patients. Psoriasis is usually improved by sunlight but may appear as a Koebner phenomenon within an area of sunburn about ten days after the exposure.

An early onset of chronic degenerative and neoplastic effects caused by sun exposure can be seen in Rothmund–Thompson syndrome and xeroderma pigmentosum, in which there is defective repair of ultraviolet-induced damage to DNA.

Polymorphous light eruption

This is a very uncommon disorder, in which patients develop lesions on areas exposed to sunlight in the absence of any known cause. Lesions are usually papules or plaques, but may be noduclar, eczematoid or frankly vesicular. The commonest variety consists of itchy red papules that appear about three days after a sudden increase in sun exposure during late spring, early summer or a winter holiday in a summer climate. However, once lesions are present, further exposure to light causes worsening within a few minutes. Episodes settle if further sun exposure is avoided for approximately one week and do not reappear once ultraviolet intensity begins to taper. Gradual exposure seems to be protective and therefore the face and hands are often spared. Many cases are caused by UV-A and in those patients sunscreens are of no benefit. Surprisingly, melanin offers little protection as very darkly pigmented races may also suffer from this disorder. Some patients, previously classified as having polymorphous light eruption, are now known to have erythropoietic protoporphyria. It is likely that specific causes will be found for other patients in the future.

Mechanical

When an area of skin is rubbed repeatedly, there may be necrosis of cells in the stratum spinosum. The degenerate cells separate from their neighbours, and a split forms in the epidermis. Accumulation of fluid follows, with bulla formation. Friction of less intensity, applied over a longer period, may lead to increased cohesion between cells with delayed shedding from the surface. The epidermis then becomes thicker and hyperkeratotic. Scratch papules and plaques of lichenification develop in this way, as do calluses and corns.

Callus

The localised area of acanthosis and hyperkeratosis which constitutes a callus may develop in many ways, all of which involve some form of pressure and friction. Calluses are common on the palms from the use of hand-tools, and on the soles as a result of foot deformities or badly fitting shoes.

Many lesions are asymptomatic and require no treatment. Painful calluses are relieved by daily applications of 10 per cent salicylic acid in soft paraffin, but permanent resolution occurs only after removal of the cause. When this is irreversible, as with some orthopaedic problems in elderly people, it may be necessary to combine careful regular paring with the use of salicylic acid ointment.

Corns

The corn is a small, well-circumscribed, conical, keratinous thickening, usually on the sole or the dorsum of a toe. A common site is the outer surface of the fifth toe, where the appearance is characteristic. On the soles, corns are depressed by weight-bearing and may resemble a plantar wart. Paring of the surface, however, reveals a seed-like body of keratin, in contrast to the pinpoints of bleeding from the surface of a pared

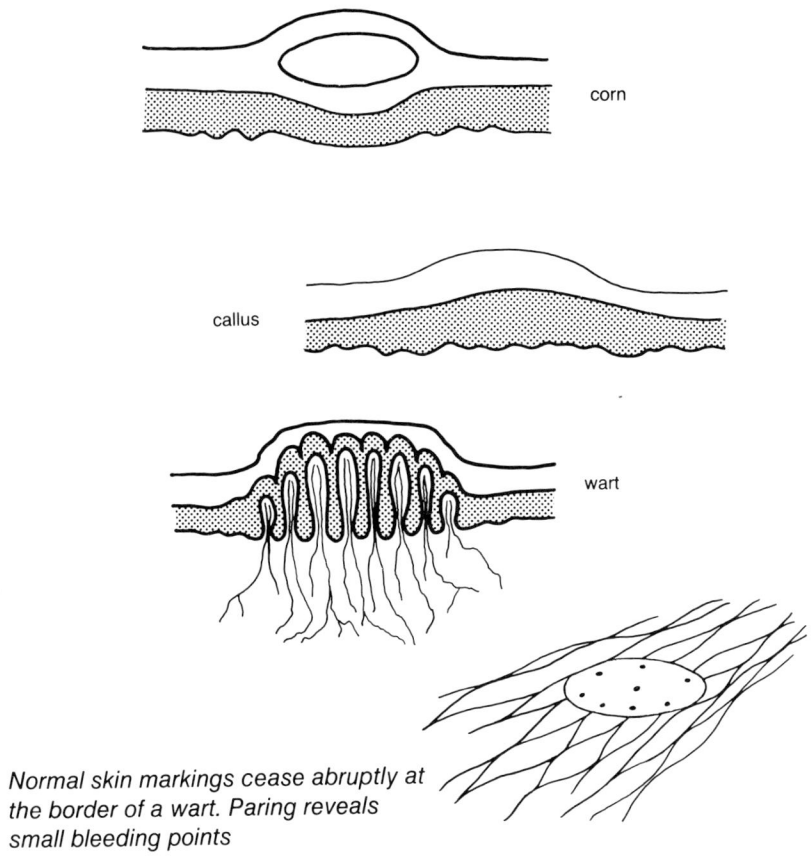

corn

callus

wart

Normal skin markings cease abruptly at
the border of a wart. Paring reveals
small bleeding points

wart. Corns may form between the toes, especially between the fourth and fifth, overlying an osteophyte at the proximal interphalyngeal joint of the fourth toe. Here maceration alters the appearance, and secondary infection is common. At all sites, pressure on corns produces pain.

Removal by paring provides temporary relief, but the cause of friction must be removed if recurrences are to be avoided. Paring is facilitated if the corn is first softened by a few daily applications of 15 per cent salicylic acid in collodion. Diabetics and those with peripheral vascular disease should be warned against inexpert paring of corns.

Bedsores (pressure sores)

The bedsore is an ulcer which involves the skin and subcutis, sometimes with extension to deeper tissue, and occurs in immobilised patients at sites of pressure over bony prominences. Coma, paralysis, diminished sensation, incontinence, obesity, and severe debility are predisposing factors, but the essential cause is inadequate circulation in an area compressed by sustained pressure. As the skin resists ischaemia better than underlying tissue, pronounced undermining of the borders is frequent.

Clinical features

A firm area of fixed erythema develops at the site of pressure and, often quite suddenly, becomes necrotic and ulcerates. The ulcer is undermined at the edges, and may extend rapidly, both laterally and in depth. A slough forms and secondary infection is soon added. Common sites in the bedridden are the lower back, heels, hips and buttocks.

Prevention

Unnecessary sedation should be avoided, and early ambulation encouraged. The patient confined to bed or chair needs careful nursing, with frequent changes of position. Areas at risk should be handled gently; there is no merit in the traditional rubbing with alcohol after bathing. Ripple beds and similar devices are invaluable for the immobilised patient. Regular inspection of pressure areas allows early recognition of premonitory signs, and prompt remedial measures.

Treatment

The general health of the patient should be reassessed, and such contributing factors as anaemia and hypoproteinaemia corrected. The affected area is relieved of further compression, and only bland applications are used. Weak solutions of eusol or aluminium acetate are suitable. An appropriate systemic antibiotic should be prescribed for secondary infection, but antibiotics generally are of limited value. The circulatory changes which precede the formation of bedsores also impede adequate penetration of the antibiotic to the site of infection. Debridement of necrotic tissue may be required, sometimes with subsequent grafting.

Cold and heat

Chilblains

Chilblains are itchy, tender nodules, which develop as an abnormal vascular reaction to cold. With rewarming, there is an exudate into the dermis and subcutaneous tissue, probably caused by the persistence of venular constriction after arterioles have begun to dilate. Although occurring at any age in either sex, chilblains typically affect children and young women.

Lesions are small, doughy, poorly circumscribed, red or purplish nodules, which blanch with pressure. They are most common on the fingers and toes, but may occur on the ears, nose, heels and legs. Chilblains may be vesicular or pustular, and occasionally ulcerate. Healing takes about ten days, but new lesions may continue to form throughout the winter months.

Treatment

The most useful measure is protection from cold with woollen socks and gloves. Improvement can sometimes be achieved using cutaneous vasodilators such as the oral calcium channel blocker nifedipine or nitroglycerine ointment.

Raynaud's phenomenon

Raynaud's phenomenon is a characteristic sequence of vascular changes, which begins with severe vasoconstriction, usually after exposure to cold. Only the fingers may be involved, but the hands and feet are frequently affected simultaneously.

Aetiology

Raynaud's phenomenon may be a manifestation of an underlying disorder (Raynaud's syndrome), but usually occurs without discoverable cause (Raynaud's disease) more often in young women.

Underlying causes of Raynaud's syndrome include occlusive vascular disease, cryoproteinaemia, cervical rib and scalene syndrome; intoxication with vinyl chloride, ergot and heavy metals; and the connective tissue diseases, particularly scleroderma.

Clinical features

Attacks are usually precipitated by cold and begin with marked pallor which lasts several minutes. The skin of affected digits becomes cyanotic and there is typically a reactive hyperaemia as the episode passes. The idiopathic type is bilaterally symmetrical, but the secondary forms may be unilateral. Repeated attacks may cause small areas of gangrene at the tips of the digits, but persistent or pronounced ulceration strongly suggests an underlying disease, most often scleroderma.

Treatment

Reassurance, protection from cold, and avoidance of cigarette smoking are sufficient for many patients with the idiopathic form. Vasodilator drugs are usually unnecessary and not always helpful. More severe forms are seldom idiopathic, and symptomatic relief is less important than elucidation of the underlying disease. Sympathectomy should be reserved for the few patients with severe disease but no demonstrable cause, who do not respond to conservative management.

Frostbite

Frostbite is a localised injury of skin and underlying tissue, caused by freezing.

Clinical features

Mild frostbite produces marked and prolonged vasoconstriction, which is followed by desquamation during the recovery period. With more severe injury, blistering may be accompanied by frank necrosis of skin and deeper tissue.

Treatment

Rewarming should be rapid, and is best accomplished by immersion in water at a temperature of 40°C to 42°C. Massage and rubbing of the damaged area are harmful, and movements should be minimised until normal temperature has been restored. Analgesics are necessary during the painful thawing period, and the administration of systemic antibiotics may be necessary later. Surgical treatment is better deferred until demarcation of ganrenous tissue has occurred. This often takes two or three months, but secondary infection may force early intervention.

Burns

Minor burns, which damage only the epidermis and papillary dermis, produce erythema, swelling and pain. Healing occurs within a week, and there is no scarring. More severe burns blister the skin, and heal by restoration of the epidermis from appendageal epithelium and fragments of surviving epidermis. There may be altered pigmentation in the healed area, but scarring is not usually severe, unless the dermis is destroyed.

Burns which destroy the full thickness of the skin can heal only from the edges of the wound. Unless the burned area is small, skin grafting is necessary. Full thickness burns are suggested by deep coagulation of tissue, with insensitivity to touch and absent superficial blood flow.

Treatment

Minor burns need only protection from trauma and infection. Extensive burns, or those involving the full thickness of the skin, require careful management by experienced personnel.

14

Bacterial infections

Bacterial flora

There is a permanent surface flora resident in the stratum corneum and in the more superficial portions of hair follicles, which regularly includes micrococci and coagulase-negative staphylococci, as well as aerobic and anaerobic diphtheroids. In addition, transient organisms are constantly arriving at the skin surface but are prevented from multiplying by the normal defence mechanisms. When these are impeded, organisms which are normally transient may multiply and colonise the altered skin. Such colonisation may not proceed to infection, but predisposes to it. On the moist skin between the toes, Gram-negative bacilli are frequent colonists without any evidence of disease. If, however, the macerated interdigital skin is further compromised by fissuring of the toe web, frank infection easily follows.

Some individuals have potentially virulent bacteria as part of the resident flora at certain sites. *Staphylococcus aureus* is seldom found in significant numbers on normal skin, but is a fairly common commensal of the nostrils and may be found in areas which are easily contaminated from the nose. Perineal carriage of the organism occurs in others. In infants, *Staph. aureus* is a relatively frequent colonist of the umbilicus, groins and axillae. *Streptococcus pyogenes* is rarely cultured from normal skin, in contrast to the frequency of its pharyngeal carriage.

There is considerable variation of the bacterial flora with age. The skin of infants is more moist than at other ages, and supports greater colonisation by more virulent organisms. During childhood, the skin lacks sebum, is exposed to a wide variety of transient organisms, and has the most variable resident flora. Gram-negative bacilli frequently colonise the toe webs of adults and the large flexures in old age. Streptococci are very uncommon at any age, but are more often cultured from the skin of elderly people than from younger individuals.

Staphylococcal and streptococcal infections

These are the bacteria that most commonly infect the skin. Infection is usually seen as a complication of everyday causes of a damaged epidermal barrier such as minor wounds, scratched insect bites or areas of dermatitis. However, these bacteria may also produce primary infection of otherwise normal skin.

1. Impetigo
2. Folliculitis
3. Erysipelas
4. Cellulitis

Impetigo *(Colour plate 46)*

This is a contagious, superficial infection of the skin characterised by the presence of honey-coloured crusts. Impetigo may occur at any age, but is more frequent in children. Being infectious, the disease often affects more than one member of a household, and may be epidemic in schools and nurseries. Although it occurs throughout the year, impetigo is considerably more common in summer.

In some parts of the world, impetigo arising on normal skin (primary impetigo) is due to *Strep. pyogenes* but in Australia, and many other countries, *Staph. aureus* is by far the commonest organism responsible for primary impetigo. However, when impetigo complicates another skin problem (secondary impetiginisation), the organism is always *Staph. aureus*, no matter in which country the infection is acquired.

Staphylococcal impetigo

A distinctive variant of impetigo caused by special types of *Staph. aureus*, to which children are particularly susceptible, is bullous impetigo. The primary lesion is a relatively thick-walled superficial blister, which may last two days and reach two centimetres or more in diameter before breaking. The blister fluid is at first clear, but soon becomes turbid. When the bulla ruptures, a thin yellowish crust forms and spreads peripherally, with a tendency to central clearing, often producing an appearance like a miniature of the 'scalded skin syndrome', which is no coincidence because in both conditions the blistering is caused by the same epidermal splitting toxin released by specific strains of *Staph. aureus*. Lesions usually remain discrete and, even when numerous, generally cause little systemic disturbance until late in the course, when fever and lymphadenopathy may be added.

Non-bullous staphylococcal impetigo is more common than the bullous form and the clinical features are similar to streptococcal impetigo described below.

Streptococcal and mixed infection

The early lesion is a small, thin-walled blister surrounded by a narrow band of erythema. The vesicle, which is not commonly seen because it ruptures quickly, leaves a superficial erosion which is soon covered by a honey-coloured crust and expands peripherally. Individual lesions are usually only a centimetre or two across, but satellite lesions erupt nearby and may coalesce to produce large, oozing, crusted areas with little tendency to central clearing. Regional lymphadenopathy is frequently evident early in the course, even when only two or three lesions have developed.

When there is mixed infection, the condition has usually commenced as streptococcal impetigo and become secondarily infected with *Staph. aureus.*

Distribution and course

Impetigo most often occurs on the face, especially around the nose and mouth. The legs of children are also a common site. Any area may be affected, but the palms and soles are rarely involved. Untreated, new lesions may continue to erupt for months. Scarring does not occur, except with badly neglected lesions. Post-streptococcal glomerulonephritis is a possible complication but has been a rare sequel in Australia. The streptococci that produce rheumatic fever do not colonise the skin.

Diagnosis

▶   **Suspect** impetigo with:
- bullous eruptions in children
- dermatitis not responding to steriods
- presence of honey-coloured crusts

▶   **Consider and exclude**

- a secondarily impetiginised underlying dermatosis such as *scabies* or *lice*;

- *tinea*, which sometimes may only be excluded by examination of skin scrapings;

- *herpes simplex*, which should be suspected if there is a history of recurrent impetigo in the same location;

- *discoid eczema*, which lacks the steady extension but may be secondarily infected.

▶   **Confirm** the diagnosis by

- bacterial culture, which also ensures that the correct treatment is given.

Treatment

Impetigo responds best to systemic antibiotics. For the streptococcal type, either erythromycin or penicillin is generally effective. Difficulty is more likely to be encountered with staphylococcal impetigo, for which it is desirable to culture the organism for sensitivity testing. A penicillinase-resistant penicillin, or trimethoprim-sulphamethoxazole, may be prescribed pending determination of antibiotic sensitivity, and continued for seven days if found suitable. During an epidemic it is sufficient to culture the organism from a sampling of patients.

Topical mupirocin is probably as effective as oral antibiotics in treatment of primary impetigo. However, its use in secondary impetigo is not recommended because persistence of the underlying dermatosis means prolonged treatment, which in turn encourages the emergence of resistant strains of bacteria, irritation of the underlying dermatosis, and the consequences of absorption.

When treating impetigo with oral antibiotics, gentle removal of crusts with soap and water is the only topical antibacterial therapy required.

Folliculitis

Inflammation which begins in and around hair follicles may involve only the superficial portion, or may extend to the full depth of the follicle.

Superficial folliculitis

The organism most commonly cultured is *Staph. aureus*. Predisposing factors include maceration induced by sweating, adhesive strapping and plastic dressings; occlusion caused by oils, greases, coal tar, ointments and oily creams (especially those containing steroids); and abnormalities of the follicular lining, such as keratosis pilaris.

Clinical features

Lesions are small, itchy, follicular or perifollicular papules or pustules, which are often pierced by a hair and surrounded by a narrow band of erythema. The pustules rupture, leaving small crusts which heal without scarring.

Diagnosis

▶ **Consider and exclude**

■ *Other non-bacterial folliculitis*

— *Tinea* produces a localised area of involvement. Hairs are usually loose and broken and the inflammation is more acute.
— *Candida* typically induces white pustules around the periphery of a red zone. The pustules evolve to small papules with a collarette of scale.
— *Pityrosporum* folliculitis occurs on the trunk, usually in the presence of typical pityriasis versicolor.

■ *Miliaria* can become secondarily infected. The pustules are not follicular.

■ *Acne* has comedones present.

■ *Pseudofolliculitis* is associated with ingrown hairs.

Treatment

Superficial folliculitis will usually respond to removal of the cause. Occasionally oral flucloxacillin may also be required.

Deep folliculitis

Inflammation which extends to the deepest part of hair follicles frequently results in scarring with destruction of the follicle. When a number of follicles are destroyed, particularly on the scalp, the resulting cicatricial alopecia makes deep folliculitis a most disfiguring disease.

Acute forms of deep folliculitis include styes, boils and carbuncles. Subacute and chronic forms may be confined to the scalp (folliculitis decalvans), the beard area of men (sycosis barbae) or the nape of the neck (folliculitis cheloidalis).

Stye

An acute pustular infection of an eyelash follicle with *Staph. aureus.*

Clinical features

A tender red nodule develops around an eyelash, with inflammation and swelling of surrounding tissue. The nodule enlarges, becomes pustular and discharges onto the lid margin, often with crust formation.

Treatment

Bathing in warm saline solution may be followed by the application of an antibiotic ointment as the stye begins to discharge. Nasal carriage of staphylococci is common in patients with multiple or recurrent styes, and regular application of a suitable antibacterial cream to the nostrils should then be advised. The administration of systemic antibiotics is sometimes necessary.

Boil (furuncle)

A boil is a staphylococcal abscess of a hair follicle and may occur at any site, except the palms, soles and mucocutaneous junctions.

Boils most often affect young adults but, although uncommon in children, no age is exempt. Many patients with recurrent boils have nasal or perineal carriage of the same strain of *Staph. aureus* found in the boil. Furunculosis is more common in uncontrolled diabetes, but the vast majority of patients have no disturbance of carbohydrate tolerance. Trauma may have a role in the localisation of boils, which often occur at such sites as the belt line or the area of the neck in contact with a collar.

Clinical features

Boils may be solitary or multiple, and tend to occur in crops. The early lesion is a small, tender, inflamed nodule around a hair follicle. As the nodule enlarges, the skin becomes bright red and shiny. Within three or four days, the mass becomes fluctuant and develops a central yellowish punctum. The necrotic centre discharges as a 'core' of thick yellow pus tinged with blood, leaving a purplish crater which heals with scarring. Occasionally, the boil begins to regress before discharge occurs, forming a cystic subcutaneous swelling ('blind boil') which persists.

Boils are painful, especially at sites where the skin is tightly bound to underlying structures, as on the nose or ear. Staphylococcal bacteraemia occasionally occurs, but is usually transient. Osteomyelitis and other metastatic lesions are rare sequelae. Cavernous sinus thrombosis is another rare but dangerous complication of boils involving the cheek or upper lip.

Treatment

Obtain pus for bacterial culture. Until sensitivities are known, commence an appropriate antibiotic such as flucloxacillin, or erythromycin for the patient allergic to penicillin. Exclude an underlying predisposing cause such as diabetes, leukaemia or HIV infection. Relieve the pain using analgesics. If the lesion is fluctuant, the pain may be relieved by surgically assisting drainage, using simple incision.

Recurrent episodes are commonly due to asymptomatic colonisation and persistence of bacteria in locations relatively protected from systemic antibiotics such as the nose and perineum. Culture of bacteria from the boil and these 'carriage sites' so that infection and antibiotic sensivity can be confirmed is followed by a very prolonged course of an appropriate antibiotic and the application of topical antiseptics to the carriage sites. Predisposing causes should be looked for again.

Carbuncle

The carbuncle is a cluster of small abscesses, involving a group of adjoining hair follicles and caused by *Staph. aureus*. Carbuncles tend to occur later in life than boils, and men are more commonly affected. Most patients are otherwise healthy, but the incidence is higher in diabetics.

Clinical features

The lesion begins as a hard, round, red lump, most often on the back of the neck, the shoulders, buttocks or over the hips. The swelling is smooth, painful and tender, and, within a week, progresses to suppuration, with discharge of pus through multiple follicular openings. A large slough forms and separates, leaving a granulating crater which heals slowly with scarring.

Lymphadenopathy is the rule, and constitutional disturbance may be severe. There is a greater tendency to embolic complications than with furunculosis.

Treatment

Immobilise the part and treat as for boils. The deep cruciate incisions formerly used to promote drainage are of doubtful value and may be harmful.

Sycosis barbae

A subacute or chronic infection of the beard or moustache follicles of adult men.

The disease is more common in those who do not shave, and seborrhoeic dermatitis is a frequent association. The infecting organism is usually the staphylococcus, but other bacteria may be involved.

Clinical features

Individual lesions are perifollicular papules or pustules which may coalesce to produce an irregular, swollen red area, studded with pustules. The disease waxes and wanes, but spontaneous clearing is unusual. In severe cases, scarring with cicatricial alopecia may occur.

Diagnosis

▶ **Consider and exclude**

■ *Rosacea*, in which the pustules are not perifollicular.

■ *Tinea barbae*, which is very localised, the inflammation is more acute and usually more intense around the periphery. Hairs are often broken.

■ *Pseudofolliculitis*, which occurs only in those who shave and is relieved by allowing the beard to grow. Ingrown hairs can be seen easily.

Treatment

Remission generally follows a course of systemic antibotics effective against staphylococci. In most patients, recurrences soon follow when the antibiotic is discontinued and prolonged administration may be necessary to maintain suppression. Shaving may have to be suspended during acute exacerbations, and lotions or wet packs used for a few days.

Sterile folliculitis

Keratin lying free within the dermis can produce a severe acute sterile inflammatory response. This happens when the hair lies in the dermis unsheathed by the hair follicle epithelium.

Pseudofolliculitis

The disorder is common and occurs where there are strongly curved hairs. Close shaving cuts the hairs so short that they retract below the surface; then, because they are curved and have a sharp bevelled tip, they penetrate the follicle wall, enter the dermis and produce severe inflammation. Waxing may cause similar distortion of follicles, producing the same course of events.

Clinical features

Perifollicular itchy papules and pustules appear. Curved hairs are often seen growing just below the skin surface. Long ingrown hairs can sometimes be withdrawn from lesions. In males the changes are seen in the sides of neck and jaw line whereas in women the problem is usually on the inner thighs and margins of the pubic region. Individual papules may resolve but the course is protracted and significant scarring can occur.

Treatment

The only effective treatment is to stop shaving or waxing. The patient should be taught to shave with the direction of hair growth rather than against the grain and not to try for as close a shave. Chemical depilatories have been used but the hairs are usually too strong. Topical retinoic acid may help by making the keratin of the inner root sheath more able to resist penetration by the hair shaft. If secondary bacterial infection is present, that component will be helped by oral antibiotics.

Folliculitis cheloidalis

A characteristic chronic inflammation of hair follicles on the nape of the neck. The disease occurs only in men and progresses to thick cheloidal scarring.

Clinical features

Clusters of follicular papules and pustules form on the nape of the neck just below the hairline and extending a short distance into the hair-covered portion. Individual lesions tend to coalesce, and form boggy nodules or plaques with discharging sinuses. Scarring eventually follows, usually as a thick, cheloidal band. Within close proximity, follicles may be seen where two to three hairs emerge from a single follicular orifice. This may be responsible for the rupture of hairs into the dermis, which is the initiating event in this condition.

Treatment

In the early papulopustular stage, oral tetracycline as used for acne may sometimes be helpful in supressing new lesion formation. Nodules and hypertrophic scars can be flattened with intralesional injections of steroid. However, some badly affected patients respond only to excision and surgical reconstruction of the whole involved area.

Infection of the dermis

Erysipelas

A distinctive, acute infection of the skin with *Strep. pyogenes*, involving particularly the superficial lymphatic vessels.

Erysipelas may complicate any lesion which allows penetration of β-haemolytic streptococci into the skin. Minor injuries, surgical wounds, ulcers and the neonatal umbilicus may all be sites of the infection, but erysipelas frequently occurs with no apparent portal of entry. It more easily develops when lymphatic drainage is already impaired, and is more common in those whose resistance is compromised by malnutrition, diabetes, or other systemic illness.

Clinical features *(Colour plate 47)*

Any area may be affected, but common sites are the face, the anterior abdominal wall, and the legs of children. When the infection follows a definite injury, there is an incubation period of a few days which is followed by an abrupt onset of fever and malaise. Systemic disturbance may be marked, especially in children. The infected skin becomes red, swollen and tender. The extending borders are sharply demarcated and sometimes vesicular. Most untreated cases settle slowly over a week or two, usually with light scaling from the surface as the infection subsides.

Complications

As a consequence of patchy damage to small lymphatic vessels within the area, persistent lymphoedema may develop at sites of recurrent erysipelas, but is generally prevented by prompt and adequate treatment. An acute, febrile onset in young children may be accompanied by convulsions and vomiting. Bacteraemia, endocarditis, metastatic abscesses, and glomerulonephritis are infrequent but serious complications of untreated erysipelas. Rare cases progress to gangrene and ulceration.

Diagnosis

▶ **Suspect** the diagnosis in the febrile patient who has a sharply defined, red hot region of skin.

▶ **Consider and exclude**

■ *Acute allergic contact dermatitis.* This is vesicular and is not accompanied by fever and systemic disturbance.

■ *Acute rosacea,* which is not painful; the patient is neither ill nor febrile.

■ *Direct invasion of breast cancer* into the overlying skin. This has a more gradual onset and lacks the really acute inflammation of typical erysipelas.

■ *Irritant contact dermatitis* should be suggested by a history of exposure to the causative agent.

▶ **Confirmatory testing** is not required unless the disease is not responding to appropriate treatment and the patient is predisposed to bizarre infections by an underlying disease such as lymphoma or AIDS. In those situations diagnosis is achieved by culture of biopsied skin.

Treatment

The disease responds well to adequate doses of systemic antibiotics, the parenteral administration of penicillin being the most appropriate.

Cellulitis

There is no sharp distinction between cellulitis and erysipelas, but the term 'cellulitis' implies inflammation of loose connective tissue, particularly of the deep dermis. Cellulitis usually develops as a complication of an ulcer or wound, and oedema is often a factor. Streptococci and, less commonly, *Staph. aureus* are the usual causative organisms, but occasionally other bacteria are responsible.

Clinical features

A red, swollen and often painful area spreads out from the ulcer, without the well defined border of erysipelas. Lymphadenopathy, fever and malaise are common accompaniments. Untreated cellulitis may progress to suppuration and necrosis. Occasionally the site of entry of the bacteria may be distant from the zone of redness. This is often seen with cellulitis of the leg secondary to fissures between the toes. In young children, perianal streptococcal cellulitis produces the characteristic clinical picture of a sharply defined, bright red, extremely painful perianal zone from the surface of which streptococci can be readily cultured.

Diagnosis

▶ **Suspect** the diagnosis when redness appears around an ulcer, and in the patient who has a red, hot, swollen area of skin.

▶ **Consider and exclude**

■ *Contact dermatitis* due to treatment of the ulcer. This does not produce the local heat of cellulitis and does not produce lymphadenopathy or malaise.

▶ **Confirm the diagnosis.** Bacterial culture of the ulcer or any regional areas of impetigo will usually recover the organism responsible.

Treatment

Until results of culture are available, penicillin should be administered. For the patient allergic to penicillin, erythromycin is a useful alternative. The affected part should be immobilised and elevated. Cellulitis of the face carries the risk of thrombophlebitis of the cavernous sinus and warrants aggressive antibiotic therapy.

Bacillary infections

1. Erythrasma
2. Anthrax
3. Erysipeloid
4. Gram-negative infections

Erythrasma

A chronic superficial infection of the skin by the Gram-positive *Corynebacterium minutissimum*. Erythrasma is favoured by maceration and is usually confined to the groins, axillae, submammary folds and interdigital skin of the feet. Incidence rises sharply in tropical climates.

Clinical features

Lesions are slowly spreading, pink to reddish-brown, lightly scaling patches with well defined borders. There is little or no pruritus and the infection usually remains confined to the skin folds, although rare disseminated forms occur. In the groins, erythrasma often corresponds well with the area in contact with the scrotum. Lesions fluoresce a bright coral pink when illuminated by a Wood's lamp, which allows clinical differentiation from intertrigo and tinea. However, the presence of erythrasma does not preclude a co-existing tinea or candidiasis.

Treatment

Most patients are cleared by a week of erythromycin or tetracycline therapy, at a dosage of 1 g daily. The frequency of recurrences is reduced by the regular use of an antibacterial soap.

Anthrax

An acute infection, usually of the skin, with the Gram-positive *Bacillus anthracis*.

Aetiology

Spores of the bacillus are particularly hardy and may survive for years in dry paddocks. In Australia, anthrax is mainly a disease of men who handle sheep and cattle, or their hides. Infection is generally at a site of trauma on the hands or forearms, but may be acquired by inhalation (woolsorter's disease) and, rarely, by ingestion.

Clinical features

A reddish papule forms at the site of inoculation, after an incubation period of only a few days. The papule rapidly enlarges, becomes oedematous and develops a central bulla which is frequently haemorrhagic. The blister quickly ruptures to leave a dark crust. The lesion is neither painful nor tender. Despite the appearance of inflammation, with erythema and infiltration around the crusted area, the skin does not feel hot to the touch. There may be regional lymphadenopathy, but constitutional disturbance is not usually severe.

The pulmonary and systemic forms are very serious infections with a high mortality rate.

Treatment

Procaine penicillin, 10^6 units daily for one to two weeks, is sufficient for most patients. Systemic anthrax necessitates the administration of large doses of crystalline penicillin intravenously. Tetracyclines, streptomycin and chloramphenicol are less reliable alternatives.

Erysipeloid

An acute infection which is caused by a specific Gram-positive bacillus, and usually contracted by inoculation of minor wounds on the hands or forearms of those handling infected fish, meat, or poultry.

Several days after inoculation, a dark red swollen area develops, often with regional lymphadenopathy. The cellulitis spreads peripherally, with a well-defined border and a tendency to central clearing. Constitutional symptoms are not severe, except with the rare generalised form. The infection responds to penicillin or tetracyclines, but otherwise may persist for weeks or months.

Gram-negative infections

Gram-negative bacilli are not normally resident on the skin but under favourable conditions, especially of moisture or suppression of Gram-positives, they may colonise the skin. The majority of infections are secondary to some primary moist lesion such as otitis externa, paronychia, leg ulcers in the elderly, or the umbilical cord remnant in the newborn. There is usually no distinctive morphology to indicate Gram-negatives are responsible although there are some characteristic pictures.

Pseudomonas infections may sometimes be distinctive if the characteristic greenish pigment these bacteria produce stains the nail plate in paronychia or the pus in wound infections.

Folliculitis

Pseudomonas folliculitis develops within forty-eight hours of exposure to contaminated water in hot spa pools. Pustules and papules occur on parts that have been submerged, with accentuation beneath the bathing costume. Often there is associated malaise and fever. The disorder is usually self-limiting over 10 to 14 days, but more rapid clearing occurs with oral trimethoprim-sulphamethoxazole.

Gram-negative folliculitis secondary to oral tetracyclines and topical antiseptics for treatment of acne produces papules and pustules that are typically centred around the nose and mouth.

Cellulitis

Haemophilus influenzae is an occasional cause of cellulitis, particularly in young children, and may be suggested by the distinctive purplish or dusky red colour sometimes present in affected areas. The inflamed skin is warm, tender and frequently firmer towards the centre of the swelling. The cutaneous disease is generally accompanied by serious systemic illness which is frequently respiratory and, less often, septicaemic.

Klebsiella and other Gram-negative species may also be associated with cellulitis, especially in diabetic or debilitated patients. There may be crepitus from gas production, with progression to necrosis and gangrene.

Mycobacterial infections

1. Leprosy
2. Tuberculosis
3. Other mycobacteria

Leprosy

Leprosy is a chronic infectious disease caused by *Mycobacterium leprae*, a slightly curved bacillus which resembles *Mycobacterium tuberculosis* but is less acid-fast. The incubation period is long, and it seems that children are more susceptible than adults.

After infection, spontaneous resolution may occur. If the infection persists, the subsequent course is largely determined by host resistance. When this is low, the bacilli multiply freely and there are many lesions (lepromatous leprosy). When host resistance is high, bacilli are scarce and lesions are few or solitary (tuberculoid leprosy). Between these two extremes there is a broad spectrum of disease.

Histology

In lepromatous leprosy there is an extensive dermal infiltrate with many swollen histiocytes, in which numerous bacilli are demonstrable with the Ziehl-Neelsen stain. In tuberculoid leprosy, bacilli are few and difficult to demonstrate, and the infiltrate is granulomatous, with epithelioid and giant cells. All gradations are seen between these two histological poles.

Early lesions that have not developed towards either the lepromatous or tuberculoid pole (indeterminate leprosy) show a non-specific dermal infiltrate of lymphocytes, histiocytes and plasma cells. A few mycobacteria are usually demonstrable.

Clinical features

The clinical spectrum of leprosy, like the histological spectrum, shows all gradations between lepromatous and tuberculoid. In urban areas of this country, most new cases are found among migrants from the

Mediterranean region, south-east Asia, and from the islands to the north of Australia. However, there are endemic regions in northern Australia.

■ *Lepromatous leprosy*. Early lesions are mucocutaneous. Ill-defined, red or hypopigmented macules appear on the skin, without altered sensation. Particularly in dark-skinned patients, they are at first barely perceptible. They are multiple, more or less symmetrical in distribution, and tend to spare the warmer skin of the large flexures. The macules become infiltrated to form papules, nodules and plaques, or the infiltration may be more generalised, with diffusely thickened skin. Irregular thickening of the face produces the characteristic leonine facies, with loss of eyebrows and lashes.

The nasal mucosa is involved early. Erosion causes epistaxis and may progress to destructive ulceration of the nose. Neural lesions lead to severe trophic changes, with deformities caused by injury and secondary infection. The eyes, larynx, lymph nodes, liver and testes are all eventually involved.

■ *Tuberculoid leprosy*. Only skin and nerves are affected. The changes may be entirely neural, being apparent only because of anaesthesia or loss of motor function. Peripheral nerves may be palpably and visibly thickened—a change most easily detected in the great auricular, ulnar or peroneal nerves.

Cutaneous lesions are solitary or few, asymmetrical in distribution, and are invariably partially or completely anaesthetic. They may be macules or plaques, and are red, purplish or brown, often with central hypopigmentation. The plaques have an irregular surface and well-defined, elevated borders. Skin over the lesions is dry, incapable of sweating, and devoid of hair.

■ *Indeterminate leprosy*. Typically, there is a solitary, smooth, poorly defined, hypopigmented macule. There may be partial loss of sensation over the lesion.

Diagnosis

■ *Lepromatous leprosy* is confirmed by identification of bacilli in biopsy specimens, or dermal smears of tissue obtained by gently scraping the base of a scalpel incision wound. The smears are usually taken from the eyebrow, earlobe or nasal mucosa.

■ *Tuberculoid or indeterminate leprosy* is diagnosed after microscopic examination of biopsies from involved skin or an affected superficial nerve.

■ *Lepromin test*. In treating leprosy, the duration of treatment is determined by the patient's immune response to the bacillus. There are many instances where, clinically and histologically, it is not obvious whether the disease is at the lepromatous or the tuberculoid end of the spectrum. The lepromin test, which provokes a delayed hypersensitivity reaction to intradermal injection of an extract made from killed lepra bacilli, provides a helpful guide to immune status and therefore to treatment duration. This test is of no value in diagnosis, as patients with lepromatous leprosy are negative, and many Mantoux-positive people who do not have leprosy give a positive lepromin skin test.

Treatment

The sulphone drug *dapsone*, which in the past has been the standard treatment for leprosy, is bacteriostatic. If used as the sole treatment in lepromatous leprosy, a severe inflammatory response to slow destruction of the bacilli may be induced which can cause marked tissue swelling, with resultant damage to involved structures. Also, monotherapy with dapsone can induce drug-resistant bacilli. *Rifampicin* is rapidly bacillicidal, which therefore minimises the inflammatory reaction. *Clofazamine* has inherent anti-inflammatory properties as well as antileprotic activity. Treatment of lepromatous leprosy is therefore with these three drugs in combination. Duration of treatment is for a minimum of two years and is continued until smears are negative.

In patients with very few bacilli and a positive lepromin test, the inflammatory reaction and drug resistance are not practical problems. However, the addition of rifampicin to dapsone reduces the duration of treatment of tuberculoid leprosy to six months.

Tuberculosis

Cutaneous tuberculosis is a rare disease in this country. As with leprosy, the clinical pattern which results from infection with *M. tuberculosis* is profoundly influenced by host resistance to the bacillus. When a person who was never previously infected with tuberculosis develops a primary lesion by inoculation, bacilli are at first plentiful in the lesion, and the inflammatory infiltrate is non-specific. Weeks later, as immunity rises and the tuberculin test becomes positive, the number of bacilli falls sharply and the infiltrate becomes granulomatous, with lymphocytes, epithelioid cells, and Langhans giant cells.

When a person with good immunity to the bacillus is inoculated, host resistance may be sufficient to confine the infection to a few granulomatous foci in the dermis, with a verrucoid thickening of the overlying epidermis (warty tuberculosis). If resistance is less effective in localising the infection, typical tuberculoid granulomas may develop and the infection becomes more chronic, with progression and healing occurring simultaneously in different parts of the same lesion. There are areas of granulomatous infiltration side by side with areas of scarring and atrophy. Bacilli are very scanty in such lesions (lupus vulgaris).

Clinical features

■ *Primary inoculation tuberculosis*, in a person with no past tuberculous exposure and poor immunity to the bacillus, may be quite nondescript but typically begins as a reddish-brown papule which enlarges to a firm nodule or plaque. Necrosis may produce an indolent ulcer with purplish, undermined borders. Regional lymphadenopathy is an invariable sequel and, if the ulcer has healed, may be the presenting complaint. Spontaneous healing usually occurs over a few months, but occasionally there is persistence, with evolution to lupus vulgaris.

■ *Warty tuberculosis* develops when there is exogenous cutaneous inoculation in a person with past tuberculous exposure and good immunity. An infiltrated papule or pustule thickens and extends peripherally to form a brown or purplish plaque. After a period of enlargement, the lesion slowly regresses over months or years to heal with scarring. Lymphadenopathy is not a feature.

■ *Lupus vulgaris* is the most common form of cutaneous tuberculosis. It is the outcome of infection in a person with moderate immunity. The bacilli may arrive by direct exogenous inoculation, spread directly from underlying structures or by reactivation of latent bacteria spread at the height of previous infections.

The disease is chronic and progressive, and usually begins as a solitary brownish plaque on the head or neck. As the lesion extends the colour deepens, often with tiny nodules set in the semitranslucent active areas. The nodules are more apparent when diascopy reduces the background colour. Progression is slow and complete spontaneous resolution is exceptional. Thin atrophic scars form in areas of healing, while the plaque extends in other areas. Ulceration and scarring may lead to severe mutilation.

■ *Other rare forms* of cutaneous tuberculosis include extension of infection from underlying lymph nodes or bone (scrofuloderma), orificial tuberculosis (which is produced by auto-inoculation in a patient with active disease), and disseminated lesions due to haematogenous spread in a patient with poor immunity and overwhelming disease.

Treatment

Antituberculous triple drug therapy in the same doses as used for visceral tuberculosis is effective and impedes the emergence of bacterial resistance. Drugs used include isoniazid, streptomycin, rifampicin, and ethambutol. Whichever drug combination is prescribed, treatment should continue uninterrupted for a year or more depending on clinical and bacteriological response.

Small lesions of lupus vulgaris or warty tuberculosis may be excised, provided that removal is combined with chemotherapy. Successful rehabilitation often requires the use of plastic surgery for correction of the mutilating results of longstanding lupus vulgaris.

Other mycobacteria

In addition to the organisms responsible for leprosy and tuberculosis, there is a large group of poorly classified mycobacteria, some of which are regularly found in association with human disease. Cutaneous infection with these 'atypical mycobacteria' may produce a rapidly spreading necrotic ulcer with extensively undermined edges (*M. ulcerans*), or indolent warty papules or ulcerated plaques (*M. marinum, M. kansasii, M. chelonei, M. avium intracellulare*). The papules are often seen in a row up the arm or leg where they have been inoculated by lymphatic spread.

The 'swimming pool granuloma' is one clinical pattern of infection with atypical mycobacteria, usually acquired at the site of an abrasion from a swimming pool or fish tank. Most lesions occur on the hands, forearms, elbows, knees or face. A reddish-brown papule or pustule forms at the site of inoculation and evolves to a crusted ulcer or verrucoid plaque. Spontaneous healing is the rule, but may take many months.

In patients with HIV-induced acquired immunodeficiency syndrome, widespread ulcerated cutaneous nodules may appear as a result of atypical mycobacteria being disseminated from a primary infection within the lung.

The atypical mycobacteria are somewhat unpredictable in their response to chemotherapy. When possible, sensitivity testing should be done before commencing treatment. Tetracycline, minocycline and trimethoprim-sulphamethoxazole have all been reported successful in some patients, while rifampicin in combination with ethambutol has been effective in others.

Syphilis

Syphilis is a systemic infection with *Treponema pallidum*, almost always acquired by intimate contact with an infected person or as a congenital infection. The organism is a thin, corkscrew-like spirochaete which withstands drying poorly, but is easily transmitted under the moist conditions of genital or oral contact. The disease may be acquired by the foetus of an infected mother, generally from the fifth month of pregnancy onwards, the risk being greater with maternal syphilis of less than two years' duration.

Infection by other means is rare. Inoculation of minor wounds is occasionally reported in medical or nursing personnel after careless handling of infectious lesions. Indirect transmission with spoons and similar objects must be extremely rare, except under the most primitive conditions of hygiene. Despite the availability of effective therapy, the reported incidence of syphilis has continued to rise. Changing patterns of sexual behaviour, the oral contraceptive, and an altered attitude to homosexuality are likely to have contributed to the increase.

There are four recognisable clinical stages of syphilis. The primary lesion is followed by a secondary eruption, after which an asymptomatic period of variable duration (latent phase) may be succeeded by a tertiary stage of cutaneous and visceral disease. The first two years of infection are regarded as 'early' syphilis, and include the highly contagious primary and secondary stages.

Histology

In all stages, cutaneous lesions are characterised by endothelial swelling and proliferation in dermal vessels, with a perivascular infiltrate in which lymphocytes and plasma cells predominate. In primary lesions, the infiltrate is more dense and compact, and spirochaetes are demonstrable with silver stains or by the fluorescent antibody technique. The infiltrate may be less typical in secondary lesions, and organisms are generally difficult to find. In tertiary lesions, there is caseation necrosis and a granulomatous component is added to the infiltrate. The treponeme is not demonstrable in sections of the tertiary stage.

Clinical features

It is convenient to describe the succeeding phases of syphilis as primary, secondary, latent and tertiary. However, the primary lesion is still present in many patients when the secondary eruption begins, and a quarter of all patients with secondary syphilis give neither history nor clinical evidence of a primary stage. There may be no tertiary stage at all; more than half of those who enter the latent phase suffer no serious sequelae.

Primary syphilis

The earliest lesion is a firm red papule which develops about two to four weeks after infection. The surface becomes eroded and may ulcerate, but there is neither pain nor tenderness unless secondary infection is added. The typical primary chancre is a firm, round or oval erosion with a raw oozing surface. However, chancres are frequently atypical and occasionally multiple.

The most common site in men is in or close to the coronal sulcus, but any part of the penis and even the pubic region may be affected. In women the chancre is most often on the labia, but may occur on the cervix or anywhere in the anogenital region. Around the anus, a chancre is often painful and may present as a firm fissure or nondescript ulcer in either sex. Extragenital chancres are occasionally encountered on the lip or inside the mouth, on the nipple or areola and, rarely, at other sites.

Regional lymphadenopathy is invariable, but may be occult, with cervical or rectal lesions. The enlarged nodes are firm, discrete, mobile and painless. With extragenital lesions, the lymphadenopathy is often more pronounced.

Secondary syphilis

The untreated primary lesion persists for a month or two, and is often incompletely healed when the secondary eruption appers. The rash is frequently accompanied by malaise, headache, arthralgia and mild fever. There may be hoarseness, splenomegaly and, less often, iritis or hepatitis. Lymphadenopathy is generalised but modest, and standard serological tests for syphilis are invariably positive.

The eruption may be of several types, but in a typical patient begins insidiously as a faint macular rash on the trunk. Pruritus is unusual and the duration inconstant. The rash may last for only a few days, but more often persists for weeks or months, deepening in colour and extending to involve the face and limbs, including the palms and soles. Individual macules are generally less than a centimetre across and have poorly defined margins. They may be barely perceptible at first, but become more conspicuous as the colour darkens from light pink to reddish brown. There is often a little surface scale as the macules eventually resolve and, in brunettes, there may be a residual mottling of pigmentation over the neck and chin, sometimes dappled with spots of hypo-pigmentation.

Secondary syphilis may be papular from the outset, but the papular rash frequently follows the macular phase, papules arising on macules to produce a distinctive mixture of lesions. Individual papules are firm, round or lenticular, reddish or coppery-brown elevations up to half a centimetre or more in diameter. Palmoplantar lesions are suggestive, and are usually firm palpable thickenings rather than elevated papules.

Around the anus and in body folds, the papules tend to be macerated and eroded; they may become hypertrophic, forming large soft masses, particularly in the anogenital region of women. Papules may evolve to annular lesions or to scaly psoriasiform plaques. Crusting and ulceration are rare.

Some temporary hair loss is common. There may be a patchy, 'moth-eaten' pattern of bald areas on the scalp and eyebrows, or a more generalised shedding may produce diffuse thinning over the whole scalp. Mucosal erosions are characteristic but inconstant, usually developing when the secondary stage is well advanced. They are flat, greyish white erosions about half a centimetre across and occur on the pharynx, buccal, labial or vaginal mucosa.

Untreated, the secondary stage may last up to two years. A latent period follows with only serological evidence of the disease, although the patient may remain infectious for a variable time into the latent phase. The duration of this asymptomatic period varies widely and it may be many years before evidence of the tertiary stage becomes apparent.

Tertiary syphilis

The cutaneous lesions of tertiary syphilis may arise as dermal nodules, or more deeply as the classic gumma. The lesions tend to be painless, solitary or few, and asymmetrical. Partial healing is not uncommon, but complete spontaneous resolution is exceptional. Tertiary syphilis is not infectious.

The more superficial lesions are grouped, reddish-brown nodules, frequently arranged in circles or arcs. There is often a firmly adherent scale and there may be superficial ulceration with crusting. Individual nodules are a centimetre or so across, but the annular groups may be several centimetres in diameter and extend slowly to involve very large areas. Progression is serpiginous, with healing in one area while extension proceeds in another. As a rule, scarring is slight.

The deeper lesion begins as a firm, ill-defined subcutaneous thickening with dull red overlying skin. As the gumma enlarges, necrosis proceeds to ulceration. There may be multiple small ulcers, or the whole area may break down. The ulcer floor may be clean and red, or covered with a stringy yellow slough. The walls are steep and in large ulcers the border is often scalloped. Serpiginous extension may produce arched, reniform, or irregular shapes.

Cutaneous lesions of late syphilis favour the legs, extensor surfaces of the knees and elbows, the face and scalp, but any site may be affected. A gumma in the centre of the tongue may form a painless punched-out ulcer, or the tongue may be affected more diffusely, with irregular fibrosis and lobulation. Necrosis of the hard palate or nasal septum may lead to perforation. Patients with tertiary syphilis of the skin often have bone lesions as well, frequently without evidence of the cardiovascular, neurological or other visceral disease usually seen with tertiary syphilis. Longevity is not affected, and the association has been called 'late benign syphilis'.

Diagnosis

Primary syphilis is established by identification of the treponeme in smears taken from the chancre, either by dark ground microscopy or with fluorescein-labelled specific antibodies. In the mouth, where other spirochaetes are present, the dark ground method is less reliable. Organisms can also be identified in aspirate from enlarged draining lymph nodes. Serological tests should be performed at the first visit. When a chancre has been present for weeks, the serology is often positive and, even if negative, provides a baseline for follow-up.

Overt secondary syphilis is always accompanied by positive reactions to the standard serological tests for syphilis, and the organism can often be identified in smears taken from exudative lesions. Tertiary syphilis of the skin is also reflected by a positive serology, often in high titre. However, no serological test does more than indicate past or present treponemal infection.

Congenital syphilis

Positive serological tests in a newborn child may indicate active infection, or merely the presence of antibodies passively acquired from the maternal circulation. If the antibodies are only maternal, the titre falls over two or three months; a steady or rising titre indicates the need for active treatment.

■ *Early congenital syphilis*. The infant is often underweight, with an aged, wrinkled appearance. There may be anaemia, and a prominent abdomen due to enlargement of the liver and spleen. A profuse nasal discharge, sometimes bloodstained, may precede septal perforation. Skin around the mouth and anus may be infiltrated, become fissured, and heal with radial scars.

Usually within six weeks of birth, a rash develops. It generally resembles the secondary eruption of adult syphilis, but may be bullous. Laryngeal involvement is common and causes hoarseness. There is generalised lymphadenopathy, and there may be epiphysitis and phalangeal periostitis.

■ *Late congenital syphilis*. The facial appearance may resemble that of a person suffering from anhidrotic ectodermal dysplasia, with frontal bossing and a saddle nose. The six-year-old molars may be malformed with dwarfed cusps and the permanent upper incisors thickened, barrel-shaped and notched at the biting edge.

Nerve deafness is uncommon but characteristic, beginning around adolescence. Retinal changes resemble those of retinitis pigmentosa, and corneal opacities are common. Interstitial keratitis may develop in the second decade. Involvement of the central nervous system occurs in about 20 per cent, often with associated optic atrophy. Cardiovascular and late cutaneous lesions are very rare.

Serological tests for syphilis

1. Non-treponemal antigen ('reagin') tests
2. Treponemal antigen tests

■ *Non-treponemal antigen tests* demonstrate antibodies which are formed after the interaction of *T. pallidum* with tissue. As the antigens (reagins) involved are present in many normal tissues, the tests lack specificity.

However, because they are easy to perform and titres fall rapidly with effective treatment, non-treponemal antibody tests are still used as initial screening tests and as a guide to therapeutic response or recurrence.

− The original non-treponemal test was the ***Wassermann reaction***, which demonstrates complement fixation during antigen–antibody interaction. Other simpler methods have now replaced the Wassermann as the standard non-treponemal test.

− The ***Venereal Disease Research Laboratory (VDRL) test*** uses flocculation of antigenic rods on a glass slide as an index of non-treponemal antibodies in the test serum. The test lacks specificity and may give a false-negative result when only undiluted serum is tested. However, the VDRL and its modifications (such as the ***Rapid Plasma Reagin test (RPR)***) provide a cheap and sensitive procedure for rapid screening and quantitative serial testing.

The non-treponemal antigen tests must be interpreted with the knowledge that individuals without syphilis may be serological rectors. False-positive reactions not due to laboratory error (*biological false-positives*) may follow immunisations and infections and are then of relatively brief duration. Reactions lasting six months or more ('chronic BFP') are important, not only because of confusion with syphilis, but because of their frequent association with serious systemic disease, particularly the connective tissue diseases. False-positive reactions may occur during pregnancy but, as with BFP due to other causes, the titre of antibodies is generally low and more specific treponemal antigen tests are negative. Although apparently normal people may develop BFP, any false-positive reactor should be investigated for associated disease.

■ *Treponemal antigen tests* demonstrate antibodies to treponemes and are therefore more specific. They are used to confirm a positive reagin test but, because the titres fall only slightly and slowly with treatment, are not used as a guide to response.

− The ***Treponema pallidum immobilisation (TPI) test*** measures the ability of the patient's serum, in the presence of complement, to immobilise live *T. pallidum*. The positive reaction is slow to develop after infection, one-third of patients with secondary syphilis being non-reactive. The test is cumbersome, expensive and difficult to bio-assay, but distinguishes individuals with non-specific BFP to the standard tests.

− Two treponemal antigen tests that are almost as specific as the TPI are the ***Treponema pallidum haemagglutination test (TPHA)*** and the ***fluorescent treponemal antibody-absorption test (FTA-ABS)***, which is an indirect fluorescence technique that uses lyophilised *T. pallidum* as the antigen and pretreatment of the test serum with other spirochaetes to absorb and remove antibodies to non-specific group antigens. These tests are cheaper and easier to perform than the TPI and become reactive earlier in the disease. Infrequent false-positive reactions may occur, particularly in patients with lupus erythematosus.

Differential diagnosis

■ *Primary*. Any eroded or ulcerated lesion of the anogenital region warrants exclusion of syphilis. Extragenital chancre should be considered in the differential diagnosis of any erosion or ulcer of less than three months' duration which is accompanied by painless enlargement of the regional lymph nodes. Non-syphilitic causes of anogenital ulceration include trauma, herpes simplex, erythroplasia, Bowen's disease and carcinoma.

There are three other venereally transmitted infections which may cause genital lesions and lymphadenopathy, but all of these are rare in Australia. *Chancroid* is characterised by a painful, undermined ulcer, often associated with enlarged regional nodes which may suppurate. The ulcer of *granuloma inguinale* is painless, but is destructive and progressive. The draining lymph nodes are not enlarged unless secondary infection is added. The genital lesion of *lymphogranuloma venereum* is minor and transient. The regional nodes enlarge and become matted together. The fused mass becomes fixed to the skin and breaks down to form discharging sinuses.

■ *Secondary*. The macular eruption may be mistaken for rubella, pityriasis rosea, drug eruptions, guttate psoriasis and the rash associated with infectious mononucleosis. It should be remembered that viral infections can also cause BFP.

The papular and papulosquamous eruptions may resemble lichen planus, pityriasis lichenoides, psoriasis, drug eruptions and arsenical keratoses. A routine VDRL is a wise precaution for any undiagnosed generalised rash.

■ *Tertiary*. The clinical diagnosis of tertiary lesions may be very difficult and a reactive TPI or FTA-ABS does not necessarily mean that a cutaneous lesion is syphilitic. It may be necessary to give a therapeutic trial of penicillin, to which cutaneous syphilis quickly responds. Diseases which may be misdiagnosed for late syphilis include stasis ulcers, severe rosacea, pyoderma gangrenosum, mycosis fungoides, lupus vulgaris, leprosy and a granulomatous reaction to bromides and iodides.

Treatment of syphilis

Penicillin remains the most effective drug for the treatment of syphilis in all its stages. However, its limited penetration of the blood-brain barrier and the relative frequency of cerebrospinal fluid abnormalities in patients with early syphilis suggest the need for doses higher than those previously prescibed. For primary, secondary and early latent syphilis, satisfactory schedules are:

1×10^6U of procaine penicillin daily for 10 days, or
2.4×10^6U of benzathine penicillin given as a single dose.

When the patient cannot be depended upon to return daily for treatment, benzathine penicillin should be used. For patients allergic to penicillin, erythromycin (0.5 g four times daily for 15 days) or tetracycline hydrochloride (0.5 g four times daily for 15 days) may be substituted.

Patients treated in the primary and secondary stages should be followed with progress serological testing for two years. A rising titre, or one remaining at the same level for six months, is an indication for retreatment. When early syphilis is treated with penicillin, rapid destruction of the organisms may produce fever and intensification of lesions. The reaction begins within a day of the first injection and passes within 24 hours.

Contact tracing is an essential part of the management of early syphilis. If the attending physician is unable to cope with this difficult task, the patient should be referred to those equipped to handle the problem. Notification of syphilis is a legal obligation in this country.

Syphilis of greater than 12 months' duration requires more intensive therapy. Recommended schedules are:
1.5×10^6U of procaine penicillin daily for 15 days or
7.2×10^6U of benzathine penicillin given as three doses of 2.4×10^6U once per week for three consecutive weeks.

A persisting titre with repeated serological testing does not carry the same significance in patients treated for the late disease as it does in patients treated for early syphilis. In the treatment of late syphilis, the efficacy of drugs other than penicillin has not been established. Those allergic to penicillin should be treated with tetracycline hydrochloride 0.5 g four times daily for 30 days. It is desirable to examine the cerebrospinal fluid of patients in whom syphilis has been present for more than a year. Neurosyphilis requires inpatient treatment with very high-dose aqueous penicillin given intravenously.

Infants with congenital syphilis are best treated with aqueous or procaine penicillin to a total dose of 500,000 U per kg of body weight, which should be divided into ten consecutive daily doses. Late congenital syphilis is treated in the same way as acquired syphilis in an adult.

Syphilis and HIV infection

Syphilis and any other cause of genital ulceration is associated with a higher risk of developing HIV infection. The immunological abnormalities in patients with HIV infection cause special problems in both diagnosis and management. Serological tests may be negative, which means that, in patients with HIV infection where syphilis is suspected but serology is negative, diagnosis of syphilis is made by demonstration of the spirochaete within tissues. Daily procaine penicillin is the recommended treatment regimen, because other antibiotics are not effective and even benzathine penicillin may not be sufficient. Syphilis has a very rapid progression in HIV-infected patients, and therefore any neurological symptoms should be considered as possible neurosyphilis. Post-treatment serological testing to confirm therapeutic efficacy should be more frequent than in the usual patient with syphilis, and CSF examination should also be arranged.

15

Viral infections

1. Papulonodular
   (a) warts
   (b) molluscum contagiosum
   (c) milker's nodules
2. Maculopapular
   (a) measles
   (b) rubella
   (c) roseola infantum
   (d) erythema infectiosum
   (e) infectious mononucleosis
   (f) Ross River virus
   (g) pityriasis rosea
3. Vesiculopustular
   (a) varicella and herpes zoster
   (b) herpes simplex
   (c) orf
   (d) hand, foot and mouth disease
4. Acquired immunodeficiency syndrome

Viruses may be classified on the basis of size and morphology, nucleic acid content, antigenic and other criteria. To the clinician, viral infections of the skin are more usefully grouped according to the type of lesion produced. The great majority fall into three groups. Acquired immunodeficiency syndrome (AIDS) will also be discussed in this chapter, because of the frequent presence of skin signs.

Infections with papulonodular lesions

Warts

A wart is a circumscribed thickening of the skin or adjoining mucous membrane, caused by infection with the human papilloma virus. Based on patterns of DNA content, there are many identifiable subtypes of this virus, some of which have particular clinical associations and others which can be isolated from several varieties of wart. The virus has been successfully transmitted to human volunteers, with an incubation period which averages four months but may be as short as a month or as long as a year.

214

Warts occur in all races and at all ages, with a peak incidence around adolescence. They can be auto-inoculated from one part of the skin to another, or transferred from one person to another, either by direct contact or by an intermediate object. Transmission appears to be favoured by communal baths and swimming pools, and trauma is a factor in localisation. Genital warts are often, but not always, transmitted by sexual contact.

Warts are more frequent and more persistent in individuals whose immune function is defective. The spontaneous regression of warts in otherwise normal people is accompanied by immunological changes involving, particularly, cell-mediated mechanisms.

Histology

The appearance varies to some extent with the size and type of wart, but acanthosis and hyperkeratosis are characteristic. With common, plantar and plane warts there are large vacuolated cells in the stratum spinosum and there may be inclusion bodies. Typically, the rete ridges are elongated, flattened and curve inwards at the base of the lesion.

Clinical features

■ *Common warts* are skin-coloured or brownish elevations with a rough, uneven surface. Size varies from a pinhead to a thumbnail, but large masses may result from coalescence. They are most common on the fingers, elbows, knees, and sites of minor trauma. Warts are normally painless, but may be painful and tender at sites of pressure. Around the nail folds, warts are usually multiple and may disturb nail growth.

■ *Plane warts* tend to be more uniform in size, often about three or four millimetres in diameter. As the name implies, they are flat-topped and only slightly raised. They are almost invariably multiple and are particularly prone to form linear clusters along scratch lines. Plane warts are frequently brownish in colour and the majority occur on the face, neck, and limbs. They are most common in children, in whom the prognosis is excellent. Persistence beyond a year or two is very unusual in normal children.

There is, however, a rare, recessively inherited disorder (*epidermodysplasia verruciformis*) in which very large numbers of warts, mostly plane warts, develop particularly over the face, neck and the peripheral parts of the limbs. Lesions resembling Bowen's disease are present in some of these patients, and frankly-invasive SCC is a frequent complication, especially over light-exposed areas. Despite epidermodysplasia verruciformis being an inherited disorder, viral DNA is regularly recovered from the skin of these patients and is of a subtype of human papilloma virus found only in this condition.

■ *Filiform warts* are fine, elongated outgrowths, frequently solitary, and usually on the face or neck. Although firm and keratinous, the filiform wart lacks the spiky hardness of a cutaneous horn.

■ *Digitate warts* are clustered, finger-like projections, most often on the scalp or neck. They are most commonly seen in the elderly as a solitary lesion.

■ *Plantar warts* are firm, rounded thickenings of the sole, with a rough, granular surface. The border is well-defined and often surrounded by a smooth callus-like epidermal hypertrophy. There may be solitary or multiple discrete lesions, or a group of warts may be clustered into a tightly packed mosaic. Plantar warts are usually painful and tender, particularly on the heel or under a metatarsal head. The duration is unpredictable. They may disappear spontaneously within a few months, especially in children, or they may persist for years.

■ *Genital and perianal warts* may range in size from small, barely perceptible papules to large, fleshy, accuminate warts. Although warts in these locations may be transmitted through sexual activity, not all warts in the anogenital region are acquired this way. Children with warts of this type should therefore not be assumed to have been the subject of sexual abuse without other corroborative evidence. Some of the subtypes of wart virus that produce genital warts are particularly prone to produce neoplastic change in the epithelium of the female cervix. This occurs not only in those females with genital warts, but also in females who are the sexual partners of males with warts on the penis. Visualisation of small warts in these locations may be enhanced by the application of 5 per cent acetic acid for five minutes. Warts treated in this way become white, unlike the surrounding skin, which is not altered. An important part of the management of at-risk females is the regular microscopic cytological examination of Papanicolaou smear tests. This not only detects the atypia of neoplasia, but can also reveal the vacuolated cells indicative of active warts. Females with this type of wart should also ensure the male sexual partner is examined for genital warts, which should be treated if present.

In both males and females the genital area may be affected with small brownish papules that are not warts but are caused by the human papilloma virus. The histology of these lesions is of dyskeratosis and cytological atypia (which resembles Bowen's disease) and the disorder is called Bowenoid papulosis. Because DNA from the same wart viruses that produce carcinoma of the cervix is found in Bowenoid papulosis, females with this disorder, and those who are the sexual partners of males with Bowenoid papulosis, should be managed as if the lesions were warts.

Diagnosis

▶ **Suspect** warts when papules are present in sites of predilection, especially if the patient is a child and the lesions Koebnerise.

▶ **Consider and exclude**

■ *Granuloma annulare.* Lesions tend to form an annulus and there is no hyperkeratosis.

■ *Molluscum contagiosum.* Papules are pearly and umbilicated.

■ *Corns, callosities and punctate keratoses* of the palms and soles can be excluded by gentle paring.

■ *Lichen planus* differs from mulitple plane warts in colour and distribution. Pruritus is the rule, and mucosal lesions are frequent.

- *Anogenital papules of secondary syphilis* are accompanied by positive serology, generalised lymphadenopathy and other mucocutaneous lesions. Typically, the anogenital lesions are broad-based and flat.

▶ **Confirmatory tests** are seldom required.

- *Acetic acid application* may be helpful in doubtful genital lesions.

- *Paring of overlying keratin* on palms and soles will reveal that the skin lines stop abruptly at the edge of the wart and may produce pinpoint bleeding characteristic of the wart vasculature.

- *Histology* is usually required to exclude other conditions rather than for confirmation.

Natural history

Untreated, in approximately 65 per cent of people, warts will disappear within two years. Spontaneous resolution produces no residual mark. The commonest history is that one day the warts were present, the next day they were not. This rapid resolution is via apoptosis of epidermal cells. Less commonly, as a result of lymphocyte-induced occlusion of blood supply, the warts become haemorrhagic, then keratotic and within a few weeks fall off. This is seen most commonly with warts of the hands and feet. Plane warts often involute by first becoming red, slightly swollen and associated with a tingling feeling. These changes correspond to the onset of infiltration of the wart with lymphocytes.

Treatment

The ideal treatment is with a viruscidal antibiotic but currently there is not one effective against the human papilloma virus. Treatment is therefore to destroy the lesion with the aim of destroying the virus. When choosing treatment, one should bear in mind the high rate of spontaneous resolution that leaves no scar.

- *Topical chemotherapy.* Salicylic acid is widely used as a paint (10 to 20 per cent in collodion), or in stronger concentrations as a paste, particularly on the sole; 10 per cent formaldehyde or 15 per cent lactic acid may be added to the paint, which is applied twice daily and left uncovered. As a paste, up to 70 per cent salicylic acid is applied to the wart after protection of surrounding skin with adhesive strapping. The paste is covered by an occlusive dressing, and left in place for a week. The macerated, necrotic surface is then pared away, and the paste is reapplied. Three or four weekly applications are often sufficient.

For multiple plantar warts, daily soaks with 3 per cent formaldehyde solution, combined with regular paring, are often effective. The formaldehyde is irritating, and should not come in contact with the more sensitive skin between the toes and on the dorsum of the foot.

Cantharidin is a vesicant which may be carefully applied to a wart, as 0.7 per cent solution in equal parts of collodion and acetone. A part or all of the wart is lifted with the roof of the blister, which is trimmed off two days later. Repeated applications are usually necessary. Trichloracetic acid can be used if applied carefully, but more destructive acids cause pain and scarring. Retinoic acid is often helpful for large numbers of plane warts. Podophyllin, 10–25 per cent solution in spirit, or in tincture of benzoin compound, is most useful for acuminate warts. Two or three weekly applications may suffice. However, podophyllin is a cytotoxic agent and significant amounts may be absorbed through the skin. It should not be applied to large areas, and should be used with caution, if at all, during pregnancy.

■ *Physical methods*. Freezing of warts may be accomplished with liquid nitrogen or a solid pencil of carbon dioxide. Cryotherapy is somewhat painful, particularly on the sole, and is unsuitable for young children. Destruction with the cautery, diathermy, or carbon dioxide laser necessitates local anaesthesia, causes scarring, and has a substantial recurrence rate. The method is unsuitable for cosmetically significant sites, for the sole, where the residual scar may be more troublesome than the wart, and for the proximal nail fold, where damage to the germinal nail matrix will produce a permanent nail dystrophy. However, when warts are few or solitary, carefully softening the wart by electrodesiccation, so that gentle curettage will then remove it, is followed by minimal scarring.

Scalpel excision should not be used. Scarring is unavoidable, and the recurrence rate unacceptably high.

■ *Topical immunotherapy* is often used in difficult cases. An agent to which the patient is allergic is applied to the wart to induce lymphocytes into the wart tissue. Warts cleared in this way heal without a scar but the contact dermatitis produced locally or at distant sites of accidental transfer may prove troublesome.

Molluscum contagiosum

Molluscum contagiosum is a common and characteristic lesion, caused by infection with a specific poxvirus. The disease is usually contracted by direct contact, but indirect transmission may also occur. Incidence is highest in school-age children.

Histology

The microscopic appearance is pathognomonic. Hypertrophy and hyperplasia of infected cells in the stratum spinosum produce a characteristic lobular acanthosis. Eosinophilic cytoplasmic inclusion bodies are visible just above the basal layer and, passing up the stratum spinosum, become larger and basophilic. By mid-epidermis, the basophilic inclusions dominate the appearance of the swollen epidermal cells.

Clinical features *(Colour plate 48)*

■ *The typical lesion* is a shiny, round, pink or off-white papule, often with a small central depression. Starting as a tiny elevation, the papule slowly enlarges and may reach a centimetre or more in diameter over two or three months. Most lesions are about 3 mm to 5 mm across, with well-defined borders and a smooth, semitranslucent surface. They persist for months, and new lesions may continue to erupt for years. Large mollusca are easily traumatised and may become inflamed, then burst and resolve. Eventually all lesions resolve, usually within a year.

■ **Distribution** may be generalised or remain confined to a single region. The trunk, large flexures such as axillae, cubital and popliteal fossae, and the anogenital area are common sites, but lesions may occur anywhere except on the palms and soles, which are rarely affected. Mucosal lesions are very uncommon and are mostly confined to the conjunctivae. There may be no more than a few papules in one axilla or on the eyelids, but in most patients lesions are numerous. Even with many mollusca, the disease has an unexplained tendency to localise in a single region, leaving the rest of the skin unaffected.

Diagnosis

With multiple lesions, clinical diagnosis is not difficult, and may be confirmed histologically. Solitary lesions may be confused with milia, syringoma, basal cell carcinoma, granuloma telangiectaticum and, when inflamed, with styes and other inflammatory lesions.

Treatment

Lesions can be very easily dislodged using a sharp curette. Using this method, there is a distinct zone of cleavage between the lesion and surrounding skin. This method is usually not suitable for young children because of the discomfort.

Liquid nitrogen application is useful when there are large numbers of lesions and is usually tolerated well by children.

Chemical destruction of lesions can be achieved using iodine solution or 15 per cent podophyllin in tincture of benzoin compound but for these to be reliably effective, the lesions should be punctured at time of application. Other methods include the careful application of 1 per cent phenol or 30 per cent trichloracetic acid.

Whichever form of therapy is used, the patient should be reinspected regularly for six to eight weeks, because the variable incubation period means new lesions may still appear.

Milker's nodules

The infection is caused by a poxvirus, which is acquired by handling infected cows or calves. About a week after infection, one or more red papules develop, usually on the fingers or hand. The papules enlarge to become tender, crusted nodules. Lymphagitis is common, but constitutional disturbance is minor. Spontaneous resolution occurs in five or six weeks.

Infections with maculopapular lesions

Measles

Measles is a highly contagious viral disease, transmitted by droplet infection. It occurs predominantly in young children and is followed by a lifelong immunity to reinfection.

After an asymptomatic incubation period of 10 days, the child develops fever, cough, nasal discharge, and conjunctivitis. The soft palate becomes suffused and, a day or two later, small white spots surrounded by a red halo appear on the buccal mucosa. On the fourth day, a characteristic rash begins behind the ears as a spotty macular erythema and spreads to the rest of the body over the next 24 hours. The macules evolve to flat red papules, which may coalesce before fading in three to five days.

Complications

- *Otitis media* and **bronchopneumonia**.
- *Purpura, bullous erythema multiforme* and *toxic epidermal necrolysis* are uncommon complications.
- *Encephalitis* occurs in 0.1 per cent of patients.
- *Subacute sclerosing panencephalitis* is a rare, late sequel.

Rubella

Rubella is spread by the respiratory route and is most commonly acquired by schoolchildren and young adults. The disease is most contagious towards the end of the incubation period, which averages between 16 and 18 days. Infection is generally followed by lifelong immunity to the disease.

The brief prodromal illness is generally mild and may pass unnoticed in children. Lymphadenopathy, most apparent in the posterior occipital, postauricular and cervical nodes, is often evident. In adults, a few days of headache, malaise, and mild conjunctivitis are followed by an eruption of pink macules on the face. The rash may be faint and transient, or there may be no rash at all. Typically, the macules spread to the rest of the body within 24 hours, thickening a little before fading over the next two days.

Complications

- *Arthralgia* and *arthritis* may begin in the prodromal phase and persist for two or three weeks.
- *Abortion, stillbirth, prematurity, neonatal thrombocytopenia* and the various malformations of the congenital rubella syndrome may be complications of rubella in the first 16 weeks of pregnancy.
- *Purpura* and *encephalitis* are rare.

Roseola infantum

Human herpesvirus-6 causes this common febrile illness, which is almost exclusively confined to children less than four years old. A high fever, which lasts three to five days, ends abruptly with the appearance of a bright pink, maculopapular eruption on the neck and trunk. The rash may become generalised, usually with relative sparing of the face. Clearing occurs within two days. Convulsions may complicate the prodromal phase, but the disease is otherwise benign.

Erythema infectiosum

Erythema infectiosum is a distinctive cutaneous eruption of children and young adults, caused by the human parvovirus. There is a mild prodromal fever in occasional patients, but generally there are no constitutional features.

The rash develops in two stages. Sharply circumscribed, symmetrical areas on both cheeks become red and raised above the level of surrounding skin, contrasting with unaffected skin around the mouth and eyes to give a 'slapped face' appearance. Two days later, as the facial erythema begins to fade, a reticulate erythematous thickening develops over the extensor aspects of the arms and thighs, and extends peripherally. The trunk may also become involved before the rash subsides in one or two weeks. One attack confers permanent immunity. Infection during pregnancy may cause intra-uterine death. Infection of patients with chronic haemolytic processes (such as sickle cell anaemia) may induce an aplastic crisis.

Infectious mononucleosis

Mucocutaneous lesions are a common manifestation of infectious mononucleosis, and a sore throat is frequently one of the early symptoms. Discrete bright red petechiae at the junction of the hard and soft palate are characteristic, but noted in only 25 per cent of cases. Other oral changes are non-specific and range from erythema, superficial erosions and mild exudate, to necrotic sloughing areas.

A macular or maculopapular eruption develops in more than 10 per cent of patients, usually between the fourth and sixth days of the illness. The rash may be scarlatiniform or may resemble measles, but lasts for only a few days before fading. Urticarial lesions may follow, and oedema of the upper eyelids occurs in 50 per cent of patients. A bright maculopapular eruption almost invariably complicates ampicillin therapy in patients with infectious mononucleosis, and generally develops six or seven days after beginning the drug.

Ross River virus

Despite its name, which implies a very localised geographical distribution, this virus is very widespread throughout Australia, occurring in every state and territory, as well as Papua New Guinea, Indonesia and the Pacific Islands. The virus is carried by mosquitoes and is the commonest insect-borne virus in Australia.

Clinical features

Approximately one week after being bitten, a rash appears that is accompanied or closely followed by arthritis and transient constitutitonal symptoms such as mild fever, myalgia and fatigue.

The rash consists of erythematous papules and macules from 1 mm to 5 mm in diameter which are distributed on the trunk and limbs. On the lower limbs, lesions may be purpuric. Resolution of the rash usually occurs over one week, to leave normal skin, although sometimes there is an intermediate stage of fine desquamation. Polyarthritis evolves quickly and is often accompanied by extra-articular manifestations such as tendinitis or fasciitis. Wrists, knees and ankles are the most frequently affected joints. Unlike the rash and the constitutional symptoms, which resolve quickly, the arthritis persists for a period ranging from many months to a few years, but eventually resolves completely to leave no residual disability.

Diagnosis

▶ **Confirmation** is by serological testing demonstrating rising titre of specific virus antibodies.

Pityriasis rosea

The cause of pityriasis rosea is unknown. The course suggests an acute infection, and a viral aetiology is suspected. Although unusual in the very young and very old, the disease has been recorded from infancy to old age.

Histology

The changes are those of a mild dermatitis with slight spongiosis. In addition, there is usually slight papillary oedema and a few extravasated red blood cells, even though purpura is rarely a clinical feature.

Clinical features *(Colour plate 49)*

■ *The initial lesion* (herald patch) is usually a solitary, rounded, slightly infiltrated plaque, from 2 cm to 8 cm in diameter, with a well-defined, slightly raised border. The plaque is reddish-pink, with light surface scaling, and generally occurs on the trunk or on the more proximal part of a limb.

■ *The secondary eruption* develops after a variable interval, usually five to seven days from the appearance of the herald patch. The secondary lesions resemble the herald patch, but are oval and smaller, being only a centimetre or two across. They appear in crops which may continue to erupt for a week or more.

The colour deepens from pink to fawn as lesions develop a fine, branny scale. The scaling has a characteristic appearance, peeling outwards from the centre to form a peripheral collarette. Distribution is largely restricted to the trunk and proximal parts of the limbs. On the sides and back of the thorax, lesions often lie parallel to the ribs, producing a distinctive pattern. The rash disappears in three to eight weeks without sequelae. Mild pruritus occurs in about fifty per cent of cases but severe pruritus is exceptional. There are no complications.

■ *Atypical cases.* The herald patch may be followed by the secondary eruption in a matter of hours, or the herald patch may be absent. Rarely is there more than one herald patch. A few patients have an inverse distribution, with lesions which are concentrated on the limbs and with relative sparing of the trunk. Sunlight promotes resolution of pityriasis rosea and, in summer, patients may present with lesions confined to the area covered by the swimming costume. A few reddish papules are not uncommon among the more typical lesions but, particularly in children, the entire secondary eruption may be papular, or even vesicular. When older patients are affected, lesions of the secondary eruption may be very large and confined to the axillae and inguinal regions.

Diagnosis

Pityriasis rosea is usually so characteristic that mistakes are unlikely and special tests are usually not required. Papular or vesicular variants are suggested by the distribution and later evolution to more typical lesions. The inverse pattern differs only in distribution, and individual lesions retain the features of pityriasis rosea, especially the scaly collarette.

▶ **Consider and exclude**

■ *Drug eruptions*, which are often itchy, and are unlikely to follow the distribution of pityriasis rosea.

■ *Secondary syphilis* warrants exclusion by serological testing of patients with 'atypical pityriasis rosea'.

■ *Tinea* may be suggested by the raised border, scaling and erythema of the herald patch.

■ *Guttate psoriasis* differs in distribution and has a more adherent silvery scale.

■ *Seborrhoeic dermatitis* may have a similar distribution, but lesions are yellowish-pink or dull red, with a soft, soggy scale. There is no herald patch, and the scalp and face are often affected.

Treatment

Resolution is accelerated by exposure to sunlight or to artificial sources of ultraviolet radiation, but, for most patients, nothing more than reassurance is necessary.

The application of a cream containing menthol is adequate for the mild pruritus in most patients. When the itch is more severe, dilute topical steroids usually provide relief.

Infections with vesiculopustular lesions

Varicella and herpes zoster

Herpesvirus varicellae is responsible for two diseases in man, varicella (chickenpox), and herpes zoster (zoster, shingles). Primary infection with the virus is manifested as chickenpox, while zoster is believed to be a reactivation of latent infection in a person with partial immunity to the virus. Zoster may cause chickenpox in a susceptible contact, but a history of exposure to either zoster or chickenpox is exceptional in patients with zoster.

Varicella

Chickenpox is highly contagious, most city children being infected by the age of nine. The incubation period averages 15 days and second attacks are rare. Although normally a minor infection of childhood, chickenpox acquires a special significance in immunosuppressed patients, for whom the disease may be a serious threat to life.

Histology

Both in varicella and in zoster, an intra-epidermal vesicle results from degeneration and separation of infected epidermal cells. Many cells contain intranuclear inclusions, and multinucleated giant cells may form.

Clinical features

In children, there may be a day or two of mild prodromal fever and headache, but the initial manifestation is often an eruption of itchy pink papules on the trunk. The papules quickly develop central vesicles, which soon become turbid, forming tense pustules surrounded by a halo of erythema. The pustules rupture, leaving crusts which separate in seven to fourteen days. There is no scarring, unless bacterial infection is added.

The eruption develops in several crops during the first few days so that the early rash is a polymorphic mixture of papules, pustules, and crusted lesions. Distribution is most dense on the trunk, face and scalp, with some extension onto the limbs. The palms and soles are rarely affected. Mucosal lesions are common, and form superficial ulcers on the palate, pharynx and conjunctivae.

In adults, the disease is more serious, with considerable systemic disturbance and sometimes varicella pneumonia. Immunodeficient patients may develop a severe, generalised haemorrhagic variant, which is frequently fatal. However, it is not uncommon to see larger haemorrhagic vesicles in sun-exposed areas of normal immunocompetent children with varicella.

Diagnosis

▶ **Suspect** the diagnosis in a patient with a papulovesicular eruption distributed mainly on the trunk.

▶ **Consider and exclude**

■ *Disseminated herpes simplex*, which usually develops as a complication of a primary skin disease, most often atopic dermatitis. Early lesions are depressed in the centre and systemic features are more pronounced.

■ *Impetigo* lacks the abrupt onset and steady evolution of chickenpox, the crusts are larger, and the distribution is asymmetrical.

■ *Vesicular insect bites* are usually monomorphic and most commonly seen on the legs.

▶ **Confirmation** that the vesicles are due to a virus is important in immunodeficient patients, and can be rapidly achieved using cytodiagnosis.

Treatment

Applications of 0.5 per cent menthol in aqueous cream is sufficient for most children. Oatmeal baths are soothing if required, and an appropriate systemic antibiotic should be prescribed if bacterial infection develops. For those at special risk, zoster-immune globulin should be administered as soon as possible after exposure to the virus.

Herpes zoster

Zoster occurs at all ages, but is very uncommon in children. The incidence is increased in patients with leukaemia or lymphoma, especially those with Hodgkin's disease. In immunodeficient patients, zoster is more severe and is frequently atypical with widely separated dermatomes being involved or severely ulcerated and haemorrhagic lesions being prominent.

Recurrent herpes zoster or the co-existence of varicella also suggest the patient is immunodeficient. The disease may be precipitated by radiotherapy or tumours which involve the dorsal nerve root. Nevertheless, the great majority of patients with zoster are otherwise healthy.

Clinical features

■ *Pain* is the first and may be the only manifestation. It can be burning, stabbing or dull, but is seldom absent. It is accompanied by hyperaesthesia in the affected dermatome, and usually precedes the eruption by three or four days. There may be prodromal headache and fever, but systemic disturbance is generally minor.

■ *The eruption* may be confined to all or part of the distribution of a single dorsal nerve root or may spread to adjoining dermatomes. Over a few days, crops of clustered red papules form in a discontinuous band and quickly evolve to clear vesicles surrounded by erythema. The vesicles slowly become pustular, and rupture to form crusts which separate in two to four weeks, often with scarring. The regional lymph nodes are enlarged and tender.

Complications

■ *Persistence of pain* is increasingly common with advancing age, especially when the trigeminal nerve is involved. Post-herpetic neuralgia may persist for many months.

■ *Haemorrhagic and necrotic lesions* are a frequent complication of Hodgkin's disease and other serious underlying disorders.

■ *Generalised zoster* is a dangerous but rare sequel in healthy people. A few aberrant vesicles are not uncommon but, in immunodeficient patients, zoster may be succeeded by a varicella-like dissemination and varicella pneumonia.

■ *Serious ocular complications* are frequently caused by zoster of the first division of the trigeminal nerve. If the nasociliary branch is involved, as indicated by vesicles on the side of the nose, changes that are of potential danger are definitely happening inside the eye.

■ *Motor involvement* most often affects the facial nerve, but is uncommon; urinary and faecal retention may complicate zoster which involves sacral dermatomes.

Treatment

The presence or likelihood of complications determines the appropriate treatment.

The young healthy patient usually requires no more than simple analgesia, menthol creams or bland wet dressings, plus measures to prevent secondary bacterial infection.

Acyclovir given orally in the high dose of 800 mg five times per day is an effective treatment that is used in immunosuppressed patients to prevent dissemination. This regimen is also used in the elderly to prevent post-herpetic neuralgia, which is otherwise very common in this age group.

Post-herpetic neuralgia can be made less likely by the prompt use of adequate analgesia. Narcotic analgesics are occasionally required but use should be judicious to avoid the possibility of addiction. In the over fifty age group, prednisolone 50 mg per day for ten days will also reduce the risk of post-herpetic pain.

Should post-herpetic neuralgia occur, capsacin cream applied frequently is helpful because of effects on substance P. Also of benefit as oral medications are the tricyclic antidepressants and carbamazepine.

Pain which persists for longer than three months warrants neurosurgical consultation. Specialist supervision should be arranged for patients with opthalmic zoster.

Herpes simplex

Herpes simplex is a very common infection caused by *Herpesvirus hominis,* of which there are two major antigenic types. Although type I is usually associated with labial and ocular disease and type II is more frequently responsible for genital herpes, there is considerable overlap. Apart from likely patterns of distribution, the two infections are clinically indistinguishable.

The primary infection occurs in those with no demonstrable immunity to the virus. However, the presence of specific antibodies does not prevent recurrences. Most infants are born with an effective passive immunity to the disease, but the incidence rises sharply after the first year. The virus can be recovered from lesions in both primary and recurrent infections and is easily transmitted by close contact. Transfer by intermediate objects probably occurs, and genital herpes is frequently acquired by sexual intercourse.

Recurrences vary in frequency from weeks to many months and appear to be due to reactivation rather than reinfection. The mechanism of recurrence is unknown, but attacks are common with fever of any cause. Other common triggers include respiratory infections, exposure to sunlight, menstruation, emotional factors and, with genital herpes, sexual intercourse.

Primary herpes simplex

Many patients with recurrent herpes simplex give no history of primary infection. When recognised, the initial infection is most often an acute gingivostomatitis. Less frequently, primary herpes simplex presents as vulvovaginitis, balanitis, keratoconjunctivtis, or inoculation herpes.

Primary herpetic gingivostomatitis is most common in preschool children and begins abruptly with fever and stomatitis. Vesicles erupt over the gums, tongue and pharynx, and may extend to the lips and skin around the mouth. The mucosal vesicles quickly rupture to form painful white plaques and superficial ulcers. The gums are red and swollen, and there is tender regional lymphadenopathy. Dysphagia is often severe, and even fluids may be refused by young children. Healing generally occurs within 10 to 14 days.

At other mucocutaneous junctions, the course is essentially the same. With ocular herpes, painful conjunctival and corneal erosions are accompanied by photophobia, lachrymation, and swollen lids. The erosions normally heal within two weeks, but important ocular complications may occur. Primary herpes simplex may also follow inoculation of a minor wound, as on the finger of a dentist or anaesthetist. The vesicles and pustules which follow are easily mistaken for bacterial infection.

Recurrent herpes simplex

Recurrent herpes is a very common disorder, most often affecting the lips. Other parts of the face, the anogenital region, and the buttocks are also relatively frequent sites. Any area may be involved, but there is a marked tendency for herpes to recur repeatedly at the same site.

Tingling or itching is usually noticed for a few hours before one or more clusters of small, discrete vesicles form on an erythematous base. The vesicles are smaller and more closely grouped than with the primary infection, and there is no systemic disturbance. They may last a day or two and often become pustular before breaking to form crusted erosions. Lymphadenopathy is exceptional, and healing follows within a week or so.

Histology

The changes are not substantially different from those of varicella and zoster.

Complications

- **Corneal ulcer** may complicate either primary or recurrent ocular herpes.

- **Disseminated herpes simplex** (Kaposi's varicelliform eruption) is a very uncommon variant, which usually develops as a complication of the primary infection in a patient with a pre-existing dermatosis, particularly atopic dermatitis, or in one with defective immune responses. Crops of vesicles, sometimes haemorrhagic, erupt over several days. They may be generalised or restricted to areas altered by dermatitis. There is lymphadenopathy, fever and considerable malaise. Death may result from visceral involvement, especially in young children.

- **Neonatal herpes simplex** may be acquired by an infant born to a mother suffering from genital herpes. The high infant mortality associated with neonatal herpes justifies delivery by caesarean section for women with active genital herpes at the onset of labour.

- **Erythema multiforme** may follow three to fourteen days after herpes simplex, but is an uncommon complication. However, patients who develop erythema multiforme after one attack, often do so with recurrences.

- **Significant scarring** may complicate repeated attacks at the same site.

- **Secondary lymphoedema** is a rare complication in areas affected by recurrent herpes.

- **Persistent herpes simplex** is a rare entity largely confined to immunodeficient individuals. In the male homosexual, persistent severe perianal herpes simplex may be the presenting feature of HIV-induced acquired immunodeficiency syndrome.

Diagnosis

▶ **Suspect** herpes simplex in the patient with an episodic vesicular eruption continually recurring in the same location.

▶ **Consider and exclude**

■ *Bullous erythema multiforme*, which may resemble primary herpes simplex in the mouth, but other mucocutaneous junctions are almost always affected and typical lesions of erythema multiforme are usually present in other areas.

■ *Aphthous ulcers* are painful, occur anywhere in the mouth and individually may resemble the ulcers of herpes simplex. However, they are few in number, are not clustered, and occur mainly in adults.

■ *Herpangina* is a painful eruption of the pharynx caused by a Coxsackie virus. The gums and front of the mouth are unaffected, while papules, vesicles and small ulcers occur on the fauces, soft palate and posterior part of the tongue.

■ *Zoster* may be simulated by a dermatomal distribution of recurrent herpes simplex. 'Recurrent zoster' usually proves to be recurrent herpes simplex.

■ *Monilial vulvovaginitis* has only a superficial resemblance to herpetic vulvovaginitis; the patient is troubled by pruritus and discharge rather than by an acute eruption of painful erosions, although superficial erosions may be present.

■ *Fixed drug eruption* may cause confusion because of the history of recurrent episodes in the one location. However, blistering is typically unilocular rather than the clustered small vesicles of herpes simplex; the blistered skin is initially a bluish-red colour instead of pink; post-inflammatory hyperpigmentation is usual; and there is a history of specific drug ingestion prior to each episode.

■ *Disseminated herpes simplex* should be considered in the differential diagnosis of any generalised vesicular or pustular eruption, particularly when the patient suffers from atopic dermatitis or when the lesions are umbilicated.

Treatment

For most patients, herpes simplex is no more than a minor inconvenience which can be allowed to resolve spontaneously, while treatment is directed against discomfort and secondary bacterial infection. There are no commercially available topically applied preparations that alter the natural history of cutaneous herpes simplex even though corneal infection can be minimised if acyclovir or idoxuridine are used this way.

Acyclovir taken orally is very helpful. Primary infection and reactivation episodes can have duration shortened and severity minimised if acyclovir is given as 200 mg five times per day for five days at the first signs. Severe primary gingivostomatitis also requires attention to fluid intake and may need antibiotics for secondary infection. Patients with frequent recurrences may have attacks suppressed using acyclovir 200 mg two to three times per day for three to six months, by which time the natural history is for reduced frequency of attacks. Erythema multiforme secondary to reactivation herpes simplex is very effectively prevented in those predisposed, by prompt treatment of the herpes simplex with acyclovir. This agent has markedly improved prognosis in disseminated herpes simplex so that those with dissemination secondary to an underlying dermatosis can often be managed at home. However, skilled management in hospital by experienced staff is still required when treating the neonate and the immunosuppressed with this complication of herpes simplex.

Orf

Orf is caused by the poxvirus responsible for 'scabby mouth' of lambs and is largely confined to those handling infected sheep. About a week after inoculation, a reddish papule forms, usually on the hand or forearm, and becomes pustular within 24 hours. The pustule collapses in the centre to form a crust which heals in three to four weeks. Lesions are generally solitary or few, and lymphangitis is slight or absent.

Hand, foot and mouth disease

The disease is caused by several strains of Coxsackie virus, and most patients are children. The infection is a mild one, with little systemic disturbance.

After an incubation period of three to six days, small vesicles erupt on the tongue, gums and pharynx. Unlike herpes simplex, lesions do not extend to the vermilion border of the lips. The vesicles quickly break down to form painful superficial ulcers with a yellowish base and surrounding erythema. Within 24 hours, most patients develop a sparse, vesicular eruption on the hands and feet. Greyish vesicles with a red areola form on the fingers, toes, dorsum of the hands and feet, and often on the palms and soles. Lesions in other areas are uncommon. The vesicles may become crusted or may resorb without rupture within a week.

Acquired immunodeficiency syndrome (AIDS)

This is caused by the human immunodeficiency virus (HIV) which has a very long incubation period that can range up to ten or more years. Transmission occurs during sexual activity with an infected partner (especially homosexual males), during the perinatal period in children born to infected mothers, or via infected blood. There are at least two varieties of this RNA retrovirus, which binds to CD4 positive cells and induces changes that eventually result in cell death. The cell with the greatest density of CD4 molecules on the surface is the helper T lymphocyte which, although primarily involved in cellular immunity, also has a central orchestrating role in the overall immune response of humans. Profound immunodeficiency after an initial period of impaired cellular immunity is therefore the eventual outcome of infection with this virus.

Clinical features

AIDS most commonly begins as fever, diarrhoea and lymphadenopathy, but as the immunodeficiency progresses, the lymph nodes involute, wasting becomes prominent and opportunistic infections such as pneumocystis carinii pneumonia appear. In those with persistent lymphadenopathy, there commonly develops a poorly differentiated B cell non-Hodgkins lymphoma with a predilection for the brain. HIV encephalopathy often manifests during the end stages of the disease.

The skin and mucous membranes are prominently involved at all stages of AIDS, with most of the signs the result of the induced immunodeficiency.

Non-bacterial infections

As expected from the effects of the virus on helper T lymphocytes and the prominent role these cells play in combating non-bacterial infections, common viral and fungal infections occur with increased frequency. However, it is the unusual extent, severity and persistence that are the hallmark of these infections in patients with AIDS.

■ *Herpes simplex* produces persistent, non-healing ulcers. In males, the perianal region is a common location.

■ *Herpes zoster*, in addition to being severe and extensive, is characterised by the very marked scarring that remains.

■ *Warts* are often numerous and widespread, but the characteristic variety in AIDS is anogenital warts that form extensive vegetating aggregates.

■ *Molluscum contagiosum* may produce large lesions that mimic keratoacanthoma but, more commonly, it presents as many lesions over a wide distribution, with the face and scalp being a common location. However, patients with AIDS are prone to cutaneous cryptococcus which also appears as small waxy hemispherical umbilicated papules, but is associated with potentially fatal central nervous system involvement that can be cured with appropriate early treatment. Histology is therefore required if molluscum contagiosum is suspected in patients with AIDS.

■ *Tinea and pityriasis versicolor* may show no special features apart from being very extensive.

■ *Candida* of the mouth is very refractory to treatment and may progress to candida oesophagitis with dysphagia. Candida infection is almost invariable in children with AIDS. As well as the mouth, common sites in children include the napkin area, flexures and the nails, which usually become severely dystrophic.

■ *Oral hairy leukoplakia* is a change induced by the Epstein–Barr virus. White villous, corrugated plaques appear on the sides of the tongue. It is exceptional to see this disorder in a person without AIDS.

Bacterial infections

Unusual manifestations of uncommon infections characterise bacterial infections in adults with AIDS. However, children more typically develop severe infections with common bacteria because early in the disease, this age group develop defects in humoral response despite an associated hypergammaglobulinaemia.

■ *Impetigo and cellulitis* due to *Staph. aureus* are usually very severe and common in children with AIDS.

■ **Periorbital cellulitis** due to *Haemophilus influenzae* may be seen in these children but is rare in any other setting.

■ **Syphilis** if untreated, progresses very rapidly from the secondary to the tertiary stage and syphilis serology may be negative.

■ **Atypical mycobacteria**, especially avium intracellulare, may manifest as widely disseminated painful ulcerated plaques and nodules.

Vascular lesions

■ **Kaposi's sarcoma** in AIDS differs from the disease that Kaposi described. In the classic form, slow growing purple nodules and plaques occur on the lower legs and the patient is typically an elderly male who is most commonly Jewish and of Eastern European descent. In AIDS, Kaposi's sarcoma manifests as widely disseminated reddish-purple macules that are oval in shape and tend to be aligned along Langer's lines. Asymptomatic lesions may also be found on examination of the oral mucosa or, during endoscopic examination, on the mucosa of other organs. With both varieties of Kaposi's sarcoma, the lesions do not bleed or bruise very readily in response to trauma, the histology is identical, and death is usually due to other causes. Kaposi's sarcoma is most commonly found in homosexual men with AIDS but is rare in patients with AIDS contracted by blood transfusion or intravenous drug use. This suggests that Kaposi's sarcoma in patients with AIDS may be produced by another sexually transmitted agent, a hypothesis which is supported by the falling incidence of this tumour since the introduction of 'safe sex' practices.

■ **Bacillary epithelioid angiomatosis** is characterised by reddish papules that may also involve the gastro-intestinal tract. Lesions (which may be few or many) resemble pyogenic granuloma but do not bleed readily. Histology (unlike in Kaposi's sarcoma, which is characterised by bizarre shaped vessels and slit-like spaces) reveals lobules of capillaries with plump endothelial cells and an interstitial infiltrate of neutrophils mixed with collections of bacilli that can be demonstrated in special stains. The condition responds readily to orally administered erythromycin.

Erythematous and papulosquamous eruptions

■ **The acute exanthem** of AIDS has been recognised as a result of observing health workers who have developed AIDS following accidental needlestick injury. About two to six weeks after infection, small erythematous macules and papules appear on the trunk accompanied by fever, myalgia and malaise. This lasts a few days then spontaneously resolves. Antibody tests become positive several months later.

■ **Acquired ichthyosis** is the severe progression of the dry itchy skin that is frequently seen in patients with AIDS.

■ **Scabies** can produce generalised scaling with prominent palmar involvement. Large numbers of mites are often recovered from patients so affected.

■ **Seborrhoeic dermatitis**, although common, is usually very distinctive in patients with AIDS. The scale is thicker, the redness more intense and, as well as extensive facial rash, extra-facial involvement is very widespread.

■ *Psoriasis*, although not occurring more commonly in patients with AIDS than in the general population, will often undergo severe sudden exacerbation or, if appearing for the first time, will do so with dramatic onset and rapid progression.

■ *A generalised papular eruption* is recognised in AIDS. Small skin-coloured papules with granulomatous histology mimicking granuloma annulare appear on the trunk and face. The cause is not known.

■ *Drug eruptions* are much more common than in the general population. Often seen is a morbilliform reaction to trimethoprim-sulphamethoxazole that appears about seven to ten days after commencement of the drug and then resolves quickly.

■ *Nutritional deficiencies* appear as a result of the wasting and malabsorption. Pellagra, kwashiorkor, and the zinc deficiency, acrodermatitis enteropathica, can all cause red scaly rashes.

Diagnosis of viral infections

■ *Clinical diagnosis* is relied upon in pityriasis rosea, where there is no definitive diagnostic test, and in conditions such as erythema infectiosum and hand, foot and mouth disease where signs are typical, and the infection is transient and of little significance.

■ *Microscopy*. Cytodiagnosis may be applied to vesiculopustular eruptions which are suspected of being viral. Cells obtained by gently scraping the base of a lesion are stained, and examined microscopically. Herpesvirus infections can often be distinguished by the characteristic multinucleated giant cells with ballooned nuclei. However, an appropriately stained biopsy sample is always superior to a smear and allows provisional diagnosis of herpesvirus infections, molluscum contagiosum and warts. Light microscopy does not differentiate varicella, zoster and herpes simplex, but electron microscopy provides rapid identification of *H. varicellae*.

■ *Immunoperoxidase techniques*. Labelled monoclonal antibodies may be employed to demonstrate viral antigens in tissue sections or samples of body fluids.

■ *Specific antiviral antibodies* may be looked for in the blood. In some diseases, such as acquired immunodeficiency syndrome, it is sufficient to merely show presence of the antibody. However, in other diseases, such as rubella, diagnosis requires demonstration of a rising titre by comparison of serum taken during the acute phase with a later sample.

■ *Culture and identification of the specific virus*. Virus may be recovered from fluid which is aspirated from vesiculopustular lesions and used to confirm infection with herpesvirus, poxviruses, milker's nodules, and orf. Throatwashings or samples of body fluids are used to culture the virus of measles, rubella, and Coxsackie infections. Most viruses can now be grown on cell cultures.

16

Fungal infections

1. Tinea
2. Other superficial mycoses
3. Deep mycoses
4. Fungus-like infections

Tinea

The keratinophilic fungi that cause tinea are called the dermatophytes. They consist of filamentous chains of cells called hyphae which, in vivo, grow by branching and terminal extension. Only dead keratinised structures are directly involved. In the epidermis, hyphae lie parallel to the surface in the stratum corneum, reaching no more deeply than the outer cells of the stratum granulosum. Infection of hair is restricted to the shaft beyond the zone of keratinisation, and nails are invaded only distal to the matrix.

Although spores are a regular feature of infected hair, they are very rarely seen in skin and then only as a special type (arthrospores) that is able to survive for long periods without keratin. However, when grown in the laboratory, spore formation is common and the morphology of these spores (aleuriospores) is used to group the dermatophytes into three different genera—*Microsporum, Trichophyton* and *Epidermophyton.*

Microsporum seldom penetrates nails and *Epidermophyton* rarely, if ever, invades hair, but all three are capable of infecting the epidermis.

Dermatophytes are also grouped according to their natural host. Species confined to humans are anthropophilic fungi. These tend to cause milder, less inflammatory but more persistent tinea.

Zoophilic species are those which usually infect animals. When contracted by humans, zoophilic infections are generally more inflammatory, with some tendency to spontaneous cure. Geophilic species are normally found in soil, but may cause tinea in animals or humans.

The factor most important in modifying the pattern of clinical signs is the part of the body involved and therefore the clinical classification of tinea is based on the site involved.

233

Tinea corporis

This term is used to describe tinea which affects any part of the body except the scalp, face, groins, hands and feet. On the trunk and limbs, the classic inflamed annulus which is responsible for the layman's term 'ringworm' is usually conspicuous, whereas in other locations increased peripheral inflammation is a subtle feature or may be absent.

Causative fungi

■ *Microsporum canis* acquired from cuddling infected kittens or puppies is a very common cause. Lesions therefore tend to be on the neck and chest.

■ *Other zoophilic fungi* such as *Trichophyton verrucosum* from cattle and *Trichophyton mentagrophytes*.

■ *Anthropophilic fungi* transferred from other parts of the body, especially the feet, produce chronic tinea corporis. In Australia the most common isolates of this type are *Trichophyton mentagrophytes interdigitale*, *Trichophyton rubrum* and *Trichophyton tonsurans*.

People at risk

Tinea corporis occurs at all ages and in all races, but is more common in warm humid climates. Among patients who are taking corticosteroids or cytotoxic drugs and among diabetics the incidence is higher, particularly with *T. rubrum*. Chronic infection with *T. rubrum* is also more frequent in atopic individuals, in whom persistence of the infection is associated with altered immunological reactions to fungal antigens. A particular variety known as the granular strain of *T. rubrum* is commonly isolated from Australian Aborigines with tinea corporis.

Clinical patterns

■ *The classic annular lesion* ('ringworm') begins as a reddish papule, which enlarges centrifugally. There is a relative clearing of the central portion, producing a ring-like lesion. The border is raised, reddish and well defined. Small papules or vesicles are usually present in the advancing edge, while a variable mixture of erythema and scaling remains in the older, central area. The lesion continues to enlarge for weeks or months and may reach 10 cm or more in diameter before entering a stable phase, which persists for a variable time before resolution occurs. Lesions are often solitary or few, but may be very numerous. Pruritus is common.

■ *Large sheets* with little or no central clearing are particularly seen in patients with diabetes and those who are immunosuppressed. *Trichophyton rubrum* is the usual cause.

■ *Crusted lesions*, which may be vesicular or pustular, are usually seen with zoophilic or geophilic fungi.

■ *Pustular folliculitis* is particularly seen in women who shave their legs and often evolves to small inflamed nodules on the lower legs which persist for months.

Diagnosis

▶ **Suspect** any lesion enlarging in diameter that has erythema, scaling or a definite border. Despite the varying clinical patterns, most cases retain enough of the classic features at least to suggest the possibility of tinea.

▶ **Consider and exclude**

■ *Impetigo*, which is crusted rather than scaly, often begins with bullae, and lacks the raised border of tinea.

■ *Nummular dermatitis*, which is generally bilateral and peripheral in distribution, begins with plaques of clustered papules and vesicles and is intensely itchy.

■ *Pityriasis rosea*, which has a characteristic distribution, and lesions that rapidly reach a maxium, stable size and are more uniform in appearance.

■ *Psoriasis*, which is unlikely to be confused, except when it is acute and guttate.

■ *Seborrhoeic dermatitis*, which has a characteristic distribution frequently involving the scalp and major flexures.

▶ **Confirm** the diagnosis by:

■ *Microscopic examination* of skin scrapings looking for long branching septate hyphae and *culture* of the dermatophyte from skin scrapings.

Examination of scrapings is a simple procedure and should be a routine for any doubtful scaling or vesicular lesion.

Tinea capitis

Special features of this location

■ *Children* are much more susceptible than adults because, following androgenic stimulation at puberty, sebaceous glands manufacture fungicidal lipids and the scalp has a very dense supply of large sebaceous glands.

■ *Hairs* are the primary target of infection which then spreads onto the surrounding skin. Hairs are therefore required for testing.

■ *Kerion* (a boggy swelling produced by a strong response to fungi when humans are not the true host) may be a prominent feature.

■ *Microsporum canis* acquired from cats or dogs is by far the most common fungus causing scalp tinea in Australia.

■ *Topical treatments* are NOT effective.

Causative fungi

The frequency with which the various fungi produce scalp tinea varies from country to country. In Australia virtually all cases are caused by the following fungi.

■ *Microsporum canis.* This zoophilic fungus, which is responsible for most tinea capitis in Australia, is generally acquired from cats or dogs. Limited transmission occurs from child to child but, after about three human-to-human transmissions, the fungus seems to lose pathogenicity.

■ *Trichophyton tonsurans.* This anthropophilic fungus is usually transferred by transmission of material on brushes, combs and caps.

Australian Aborigines seem particularly prone to this infection, which is reasonably common in adults as well as children.

■ *Microsporum gypseum*. This geophilic fungus is seen in children no matter what part of the body is infected. Presumably this is because of children's playing habits exposing them to infected soil.

■ *Microsporum audouinii*. This anthropophilic fungus used to be responsible for large outbreaks of tinea capitis but is now very uncommon.

Clinical features *(Colour plates 50, 51)*

■ *Patchy hair loss* with low grade scaling and erythema. This is the commonest pattern and, despite the generalisation that geophilic and zoophilic fungi produce a more severe host reaction, can be seen with all dermatophytes. The scaling and erythema are usually seen very early so that it is very rare to see alopecia with normal skin. The hairs usually break a few millimetres above the skin surface producing a patch of dull, broken, short hairs.

■ *Black dot tinea*. When spores are within the hair shaft, hairs may break beneath the skin surface and the follicles fill with debris producing black dots. This pattern is seen with *Trichophyton tonsurans*.

■ *Pustular folliculitis*. The zoophilic and geophilic fungi evoke this more inflammatory pattern, in which stubby broken hairs arise from the centre of small pustules.

■ *Kerion*. This is a severe inflammatory reaction appearing as a large, boggy, oedematous mass resembling a carbuncle. Pus oozes from multiple follicular abscesses and the surface becomes crusted. In severe cases, there is fever and lymphadenopathy, and secondary bacterial infection is not uncommon. Hairs are shed from the area and, as the reaction subsides, the kerion evolves to a rounded, smooth or crusted, hairless patch. Spontaneous resolution and regrowth of hair may follow. Significant scarring is unusual.

Course

In untreated patients the course follows a definite sequence. There is an early phase of spread with formation of new lesions, a stable phase during which no further extension occurs, followed by a period of regression. Duration of the infection generally decreases with increasing inflammation. A kerion may last only eight weeks, while indolent, low-grade infections may persist for years. Even with minimal inflammation, however, spontaneous resolution is the rule and persistence into adolescence is rare.

Diagnosis

▶   **Suspect** the diagnosis of tinea in every child with hair loss, especially when scaling and inflammation are present. Broken hairs, pustules and 'black dots' should also arouse suspicion.

▶   **Consider and exclude**

■ *Alopecia areata*, which is characterised by smooth areas of baldness, with neither scaling nor inflammation.

■ *Trichotillomania* is hair loss caused by pulling on normal hairs. Involved areas are poorly defined, with hairs broken off at different lengths. The patches are never completely bald.

■ A *carbuncle* is more painful than a kerion, and is accompanied by greater constitutional disturbance.

▶ **Diagnostic tests**

■ *Wood's lamp*, which emits light of long wavelength, causes fluorescence of hairs infected with dermatophytes that produce small spores on the outside of the hairshaft. Only a few fungi produce fluorescent hairs but these include the important *M. canis* and *M. audouinii*. Positive fluorescence is a bright apple green, not to be confused with the dull bluish fluorescence of exudates and ointments.

■ *Examine hairs and scale*. This provides rapid confirmation of fungal infection and the pattern of spore production on hairs can often indicate the likely causative fungus.

■ *Culture the hairs and scale*. This is the only way of positively identifying the fungus responsible, but it may be weeks until final identification is complete. Knowing the fungus involved plays an important part in identifying and eradicating the source of infection.

Tinea cruris

Special features of this location

■ *Adult males* are particularly susceptible because the apposition of inner thigh and scrotum produces a warm humid environment which favours fungal growth.

■ *Edge* of the inflamed area is often serpiginous rather than a perfect annulus.

■ *Feet* are often also involved because the infection is frequently carried to the groin from the patient's own feet.

Causative fungi

The anthropophilic fungi *E. floccosum*, *T. rubrum* and *T. mentagrophytes* are the dermatophytes most often recovered from tinea cruris.

Clinical features

The infection usually begins on the upper inner thigh as a scaly red patch with a curved, well defined border. The lesion may spread backwards over the perineum as well as laterally onto the groin. Bilateral involvement is common, and pruritus is often severe. Tinea cruris may become quite extensive, spreading out over the buttocks and lower abdomen, but the penis and scrotum are not usually involved. *(Colour plate 52)*

When tinea cruris is caused by *E. floccosum*, there is little central clearing, scaling is pronounced, and satellite lesions are characteristic. With *T. rubrum*, there is a marked tendency to spread beyond the groins. *T. mentagrophytes* causes more severe inflammation; the border is often distinctly vesicular and there may be follicular papules or pustules in the affected area.

Diagnosis

▶ **Consider and exclude**

■ *Frictional intertrigo*, which is limited to apposing skin surfaces and lacks the central clearing and inflamed border typical of tinea.

■ *Seborrhoeic dermatitis* and *psoriasis*, which are usually centred around the folds rather than the inner thighs, almost always have more typical lesions present in other areas.

■ *Flexural candidiasis* is more common in the obese, those with diabetes and patients who have been using antibiotics for other reasons. Small satellite papules with a collarette of scale are typical and, unlike tinea, involvement of scrotum is very evident.

■ *Atopic eczema* invoves the inguinal fossa rather than the inner thigh and has a poorly defined margin.

Tinea pedis

Special features of this location

■ *Annulus formation* is frequently not evident.

■ *Fluctuation* in clinical features is common as a consequence of changing environment and fluctuating host immunity.

■ *Many conditions can look identical* and can only be differentiated by the examination of skin scrapings.

■ *Children* should have other conditions excluded because tinea pedis is rare in this age group.

Causative fungi

Three anthropophilic fungi are responsible for almost all cases of tinea pedis. These are *T. rubrum, T. mentagrophytes* and *E. floccosum.*

Factors involved

■ *Exposure* to the fungus is believed to occur by walking barefoot on fragments of skin or nail, shed by an infected person. Fungi can be recovered from swimming pool surrounds and fungi can survive for years in keratin deposited in carpet. However, tinea of the feet is extremely difficult to reproduce by deliberate inoculation of fungus.

■ *Environmental factors* such as heat and humidity and variety of foot wear are important; however, it is to be noted that during the Vietnam war Vietnamese soldiers wearing the same type of boots and exposed to the same conditions as American soldiers had a very much lower prevalence of tinea pedis.

■ *Host factors* are probably important in explaining susceptibility differences and for the commonly observed phenomenon of infection being confined to one foot for years.

Cell-mediated immunity to trichophyton is the most commonly positive recall antigen found in the Australian community yet, in those with diffuse chronic tinea pedis, cell-mediated immunity to trichophyton antigen is absent.

Clinical features

Tinea is very uncommon on the dorsum of the foot, most patients with tinea pedis presenting with one or more of three clinical patterns.

- *Interdigital scaling* is the most common pattern, and usually involves the third or fourth interdigital space. Sodden macerated scale accumulates between the toes and may extend to the plantar surface, often with fissuring and secondary bacterial infection. Pruritus may be troublesome, especially during summer, and hyperhidrosis is frequently associated.

- *Vesicles and pustules* may occur alone or be combined with scaling. The vesicles are slow to rupture and may enlarge to sizeable blisters with considerable pruritus. The instep and distal sole are common sites. Interdigital tinea is often present on the same foot.

- *Diffuse hyperkeratosis* of the sole is a persistent chronic form with little inflammation, and is usually caused by *T. rubrum*. Fine, dry scaling, with variable erythema, spreads over the sole and may extend onto the sides and, occasionally, the dorsum of the foot. Similar lesions may occur on the palm.

Diagnosis

▶ **Suspect** the diagnosis in any patient with a rash on the soles, especially if there is involvement between the toes.

▶ **Consider and exclude**

- *Pompholyx*, which is more commonly bilateral and symmetrical than is tinea.

- *Interdigital maceration* from hyperhidrosis, which may be indistinguishable except by microscopic examination of skin scrapings.

- *Pustular psoriasis* of the soles, which is usually bilateral and accompanied by palmar lesions. Lakes of pus occur much more commonly in pustular psoriasis whereas, in tinea, purulent lesions are usually vesicles with pustular contents.

- *A soft corn* between the fourth and fifth toes, which can be clinically indistinguishable from interdigital tinea with which it may coexist.

- *Pitted keratolysis*, which is seen on sweaty soles and consists of pits and furrows.

- *Juvenile plantar dermatitis*, which affects the distal sole of children and is not vesicular.

Tinea unguium

Special features of this location

- *Adults* are the people infected. Tinea of the nails is exceptionally rare in children.

- *Chronic* tinea of the feet (or less commonly the hand) is a usual accompaniment. It is very rare to have tinea of the nails with no skin involvement.

- *Oral treatment* is required. The fungus usually involves the undersurface of the nail and, as keratin is a very effective barrier to penetration of applied substances, fungal growth is not retarded by creams or paints.

Causative fungi

The anthropophilic fungi *T. rubrum* and *T. mentagraphytes* which also cause chronic tinea pedis are the usual cause of tinea of the nails.

Clinical patterns

■ *Onycholysis*. This usually begins distally adjacent to the lateral nail fold. The discoloured area usually expands laterally and proximally and may involve the whole nail plate. Subungual keratin may become very thick and produce marked separation of the nail plate from the nail bed.

■ *Nail dystrophy*. The nail plate may become friable and the changes so severe that distally the nail crumbles away to expose the nail bed. Alternatively, the nail plate may become thick and distorted.

■ *White small friable areas* on the convex surface of the nail, which may coalesce and involve the whole of the surface of the nail, represent a very rare pattern of *T. mentagrophytes* infection where the fungus attacks the surface rather than the underneath of the nail plate. This is the only type of tinea unguium amenable to topical treatment.

Diagnosis

▶ **Suspect** tinea of the nails when there is onycholysis and nail dystrophy in the presence of skin changes. In some patients who present with fingernail involvement, the only skin changes may be present on the feet.

▶ **Consider and exclude**

■ *Psoriasis* affecting the nails, which may be clinically indistinguishable from tinea. However, tinea very rarely involves all ten fingernails or toenails. Psoriatic nails are likely to be accompanied by psoriasis elsewhere.

■ *Dermatitis* involving the proximal nail fold may produce nail dystrophy, but the nails are not friable and retain a normal lustre.

■ *Paronychia* may cause discoloration and dystrophy of the nail, but the primary change is in the nail fold.

▶ **Confirm** the diagnosis by microscopy and culture. As most infections begin beneath the nail and involve the nail plate secondarily, it is important to remove subungual debris as well as nail clippings.

Tinea manuum

Special features of this location

■ *Unilateral* involvement is the rule.

■ *Peripheral enhancement* of inflammation evident as papules, vesicles or pustules is usually visible.

■ *Prolonged oral treatment* over many months is required because of the thick keratin layer of the palm.

Causative fungi

T. rubrum and *T. mentagrophytes* are by far the commonest, with *E. floccosum* the next most likely.

Clinical features

One hand is usually involved. The commonest clinical picture is for redness and scaling to begin on the palm, usually near the base of the index and middle fingers, which then extends slowly proximally and towards the ulnar side with slight extension onto the fingers. The rash then spreads in direct continuity on to the dorsum of the hand and fingers. Although not the usual annulus of tinea corporis, increased inflammation of the periphery is usually much more readily discerned than with tinea pedis. The peripheral inflammation often fluctuates markedly as papules, vesicles or pustules.

Diagnosis

▶ **Suspect** tinea of the hand in a person presenting with a unilateral 'dermatitis'.

▶ **Consider and exclude**

■ *Irritant or endogenous hand dermatitis*, which is usually bilateral, shows no enhancement of inflammation at the periphery and is often fissured.

■ *Psoriasis* may often be unilateral but is usually a rich red colour, shows the typical silvery scale and characteristically involves either the central palm or the fingertips and periphery of the palm. Although pustules may be present, these occur diffusely rather than around the edge of the area. Psoriasis is often found elsewhere.

■ *Allergic contact dermatitis* is usually bilateral, involves the dorsum of the hands, and is diffusely vesicular. There is often involvement of the eyelids, face or sides of the neck.

Tinea faciei

Causative fungi

Tinea of the beard or moustache hairs is more common in rural areas, where the zoophilic *T. verrucosum* and *T. mentagrophytes* are most often responsible. Among city dwellers, *T. rubrum* is a more frequent cause.

Clinical patterns

With the more common zoophilic infections, there is an acute inflammatory reaction, which is centred around hair follicles. Follicular papules and pustules may remain discrete, but often coalesce to form a circumscribed boggy nodule or plaque, studded with discharging pustules. Hairs are loose and broken over the affected area, which may become crusted.

With *T. rubrum*, erythema and scaling may dominate the picture. It may resemble tinea in other areas, showing a progressive circinate lesion with little or no folliculitis, or there may be diffuse redness with only very faint evidence of increased inflammation around the periphery.

When topical steroids have been applied, a rosacea-like picture may be induced, making diagnostic signs even less apparent.

Tinea incognita

This term is used to describe tinea which has been treated with topical steroids. The appearance of lesions is considerably modified, with masking of features which normally suggest the diagnosis. The sharp demarcation and the elevated vesicular border are blurred. Erythema is less apparent and scaling is largely suppressed. The whole inflammatory reaction is dampened, while the fungus continues to multiply. Scrapings usually reveal huge numbers of hyphae. The very persistence of 'dermatitis' after adequate treatment should suggest an unsuspected aetiology, especially contact dermatitis or unrecognised tinea.

Laboratory diagnosis of tinea

■ *Direct microscopy*. Skin scrapings are best taken from the active edge of an enlarging lesion or from vesicle tops. If ointments or other applications are present, the area is first cleaned with spirit or washed with soap and water. Although topical steroids increase the number of hyphae seen, topical antifungal creams should be ceased a few days prior to obtaining samples.

With a scalpel blade, fragments are gently scraped from the surface, placed on a slide and covered with a drop or two of 20 per cent potassium hydroxide under a cover slip. Gentle warming accelerates alkaline digestion, to which fungi are relatively resistant, but boiling should be avoided. During microscopic examination, closing the iris diaphragm to its minimum aperture will make the hyphae easier to see by a phase contrast effect.

When present, the hyphae are seen as long, slender, branching filaments, which do not follow cellular outlines.

Infected hairs are loose and easily extracted with forceps. Hair and scale from scalp lesions are incubated with potassium hydroxide in the same way as skin scrapings.

Preliminary examination with a Wood's lamp may disclose fluorescent hairs, which should then be referred for microscopy. Infected hairs show parallel rows or chains of spores, which may surround the hair or lie within the hair shaft, sometimes accompanied by visible hyphae.

For suspected tinea of the nails, clippings and subungual debris are prepared in the same manner, but require longer incubation with the alkali. Fungal elements are more difficult to find in nails, and repeated examinations may be necessary. In taking samples, it is better to choose friable or discoloured areas.

Specimens taken for transport to a mycologist should be folded in paper, or placed between flamed slides and wrapped in paper.

■ *Culture*. Although direct examination confirms the presence of fungi, culture is necessary for species identification; a modified Sabouraud's medium is suitable for all dermatophytes. Colonies may begin to appear in three or four days, but cultures should not be regarded as negative

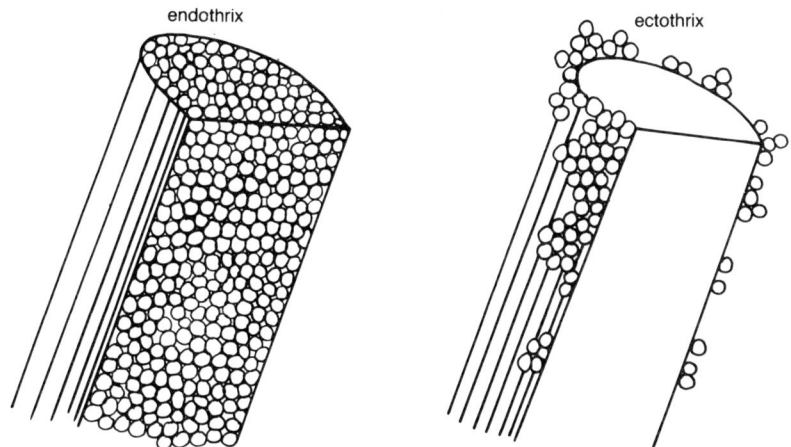

endothrix ectothrix

Spore formation in tinea of hair

in less than three weeks. Inflammatory lesions may contain little living fungus, and repeated cultures may be necessary. A single culture from nail clippings can be particularly misleading. Contaminants easily overgrow dermatophyte colonies, and the fungus may be no longer viable by the time it reaches a position from which samples can be taken. The presence of spores in and around infected hairs ensures a high percentage of positive cultures with tinea capitis.

Complications of tinea

■ *Secondary bacterial infection*

■ *Scarring* is not usually a problem, but may be significant with inflammatory lesions, particularly on the scalp.

■ *Dermatophytide or id reaction* is an uncommon eruption, generally vesicular or papular, which may occur as a distinct complication of acute inflammatory tinea. Kerion of the scalp may be accompanied by a papular eruption on the trunk, and acute tinea pedis may be parallelled by a vesicular eruption on the palms and sides of the fingers. Fungus is not present at the site of the id reaction, which is believed to be a manifestation of allergy to the fungus or its products.

■ *Erythema multiforme* is uncommon and *erythema nodosum* is a rare complication.

■ *Contact dermatitis* from therapeutic applications is relatively common, particularly with tinea pedis.

Treatment of tinea

■ *Topical treatment.* Topical therapy is adequate for many patients with tinea, but does not cure infections of the scalp or nails. It is frequently ineffective for tinea barbae and is unlikely to cure tinea pedis.

Such traditional applications as Whitfield's salicylic and benzoic acid ointment or Castellani's magenta paint are effective, but messy and somewhat irritating. Castellani's paint is most useful for tinea cruris and gives good relief in tinea pedis. For most cases, however, tolnaftate (as a lotion or cream) or the topical imidazoles are just as effective and more acceptable to patients.

Preparations containing nystatin, amphotericin B or clioquinol, although active against *Candida*, have no value in the treatment of tinea.

For acute inflammatory infections of the groins or feet, permanganate soaks give good symptomatic relief. Twice daily application of 1 per cent aqueous solution of silver nitrate relieves the discomfort from fissures between or beneath the toes.

■ *Systemic treatment.* Systemic therapy is necessary for tinea of hair and nails, for many patients with tinea of the groins or feet, and is more practical for the patient with numerous lesions of tinea corporis. There are now two effective drugs available for the systemic treatment of tinea, griseofulvin and ketoconazole. However, the proven relative safety of griseofulvin contrasts with reports of hepatitis and even fatal hepatic necrosis in patients treated with ketoconazole.

Griseofulvin is only sparingly soluble in water and should be taken after food when absorption is better. The oral dose of the microcrystalline form is 10 mg to 20 mg/kg per day, taken as a single daily dose or in two divided doses. An ultramicrocrystalline form is also available and is prescribed in lower dosage, but has not significant advantage over other preparations.

Six weeks' treatment is sufficient for most infections, but tinea capitis may need longer and, for tinea of the nails, griseofulvin therapy needs to be continued until the nail has grown out normally. This may take six months or more for a thumbnail, and more than two years for the first toenail.

When only one or two nails are infected, the duration of treatment can be reduced by avulsion of the involved nail. Even with prolonged therapy, the response of tinea pedis is sometimes disappointing.

Side effects of griseofulvin are uncommon and minor. Headache, nausea and diarrhoea are the most frequent. The headache is a throbbing headache due to the vasodilator properties of this drug. Tachyphylaxis occurs to this vasodilatory effect: by starting with a small piece of a tablet and gradually increasing the size taken over a period of weeks, the drug may be taken without symptoms in those where headache was initially a problem. Photosensitisation can occur but, although rare, is commoner than the other drug eruptions caused by griseofulvin. The drug is reported to be teratogenic in animals and should not be prescribed during pregnancy. Barbiturates reduce absorption of griseofulvin from the bowel. Griseofulvin induces enzymes that metabolise oral anticoagulants, and therefore coumarin dosage needs to be adjusted during and at the completion of griseofulvin treatment.

In some cases of chronic tinea seemingly resistant to griseofulvin, oral ketoconazole may produce a cure. However, there are patients resistant to treatment with oral ketoconazole who respond to oral griseofulvin, and the success rate is roughly similar for both drugs. It should also be remembered that true resistance of dermatophytes to griseofulvin is extremely rare and that apparent resistence to this very safe drug can often be overcome by increasing the dose. Ketoconazole given orally has a greater risk of potentially serious side effects than does oral griseofulvin.

In addition to nausea, pruritus and photophobia, oral ketoconazole can cause disturbance of plasma lipids, an impaired capacity for steroid synthesis (especially androgens) and, most importantly, hepatitis, which is likeliest to occur in patients taking the drug for long periods of time, such as those required in treating tinea of the nails.

Other superficial mycoses

1. Pityriasis versicolor
2. Candidiasis
3. Tinea nigra

Pityriasis versicolor

Causative organism

Pityrosporum orbiculare is a lipophilic yeast present on the skin of all humans. It is found mainly on the chest and back and its growth is most dense in areas of greatest sebum excretion.

Under appropriate conditions it transforms to a hyphal form that is pathogenic and is sometimes given the name *Malassezia furfur.*

The organisms produce lipoxygenases that act on unsaturated fats present in skin surface lipids, to produce lipoperoxides which induce changes in melanin granules.

Clinical features *(Colour plate 53)*

Lesions are asymptomatic macules of altered pigmentation covered by a fine powdery scale often made more obvious by gently scratching the lesions.

At first pink or reddish-brown, the macules generally fade to an area of pallor, but in some areas become hyperpigmented. In general, pale areas are found on dark skin and dark macules on pale skin. Individual macules are usually a centimetre or two in diameter, but may coalesce to form large discoloured patches. Small perifollicular papules are not uncommon in newly affected areas and, in a few patients, the rash is predominantly papular.

The most common site is the front of the chest, but any part of the trunk may be affected. Lesions sometimes extend to the shoulders, arms and neck and, rarely, may become generalised. There is no pruritus, and patients present only because of their appearance, particularly during summer when tanning of unaffected skin contrasts with the pale areas which tan poorly. This contrast can be made even more obvious by examination under Wood's light.

Predisposing factors

Hot humid conditions favour the development of this very common disease. Although the vast majority of patients are healthy, the incidence is increased in those with diabetes, Cushing's disease and those with depressed cellular immunity such as patients with HIV-induced acquired immunodeficiency syndrome.

Diagnosis

▶ **Suspect** pityriasis versicolor in patients with areas of pallor and pigmentation on the trunk and upper limbs.

▶ **Consider and exclude**

■ *Vitiligo*, which is a stark white colour rather than an area of pallor, and which lacks the fine powdery scale. Vitiligo is usually found over the distal hands and feet, bony prominences, anogenital region and around the eyes and the sides of the neck.

■ *Post-inflammatory hypopigmentation*, which usually presents with larger lesions and poorly defined margins, and has a history consistent with a pre-existing dermatosis.

■ *Pityriasis rosea*, which produces lesions that are more uniform in size, with a collarette of scale, and are of limited duration.

▶ **Confirm** the diagnosis by microscopically examining skin scrapings to reveal short, stubby, non-branching hyphae and spores. The organism will not grow on routinely used media.

Treatment

The disease responds well to many applications but, because it is due to proliferation of a commensal in predisposed people, recurrences are common. Although the yeasts are quickly destroyed, it takes a few months until the epidermal cells containing melanosomes altered by yeast products are shed and normal pigmentation reproduced.

■ *All topical treatments* need to be applied from the neck to the wrists to the upper thighs, even when lesions are not visible within all these areas. Tolnaftate and the topical imadozoles are effective although rather expensive for use over large areas and need to be used twice per day for many weeks. Shampoos containing selenium sulphide or zinc pyridinethione are effective if applied overnight, and then washed off in the morning, on each of five consecutive evenings. Sodium thiosulphate 20 per cent aqueous solution applied twice daily for four weeks is also effective but has an odour to which some patients object.

■ *Oral treatment* with ketoconazole is effective but concern regarding liver toxicity limits its use. Despite the sometimes encountered alternative name of 'tinea versicolor', griseofulvin has no effect on this disease.

Candidiasis

Candida is a unicellular fungus, with the ability to reproduce by budding. In cultures, where conditions for growth are optimal, *Candida* exists predominantly in the yeast form. When conditions are less favourable and cell division is impeded, *Candida* assumes a pseudohyphal structure. Pseudohyphae are regularly associated with invasion of tissue by *Candida*.

Various species of the fungus, most often *C. albicans*, are found as harmless colonists of the alimentary canal and vagina of normal individuals. *Candida* is rarely found as a saprophyte on normal skin, but is a frequent colonist of skin which is altered by disease. *Candida* is not a virulent organism, and is probably never pathogenic in normal healthy tissue. When host resistance is impaired by systemic or local factors, the fungus may proliferate and become invasive.

Systemic predisposing factors include diabetes mellitus, antibiotic therapy, idiopathic hypoparathyroidism, general debility, leukaemia and immunodeficiency syndromes. T-cell function appears to be more important than circulating antibodies in preventing candidiasis, and impaired cell-mediated immunity may be associated with severe, chronic infection. Local predisposing factors include obesity, excessive sweating, maceration, and topical corticosteroid therapy. The altered vaginal mucosa of pregnancy and the oral mucosa in infancy are particularly susceptible to candidiasis.

Candidiasis should be accepted as evidence of an underlying abnormality. Usually there will be some obvious local disturbance. When a local cause is lacking, and mucocutaneous candidiasis is chronic or recurrent, careful assessment and investigation are essential.

Clinical features

■ *Candidiasis of the oral mucosa.* Oral candidiasis is very common in infancy, when it most often affects the tongue. Any part of the mouth may be affected and, in severe cases, lesions may extend beyond the pharynx into the oesophagus or trachea. Involved areas are covered by soft white curd-like material which is easily wiped away to leave a raw, red surface. In adults, oral candidiasis is largely confined to the gums of those wearing dentures or to the mucosa of elderly and debilitated people.

■ *Labial candidiasis.* Candidal cheilitis, more often of the lower lip, is a common finding in habitual lip-lickers. There is redness and scaling, which usually correspond well with the area reached by the tongue. Angular cheilitis is common in those with marked infolding at the corners of the mouth. Gum atrophy in elderly, edentulous people leads to overclosure of the mouth and especially with excessive salivation, the commissures are constantly macerated. The affected skin is red and moist, coated with a variable soft, creamy white matter. Angular fissuring is a common sequel.

■ *Genital candidiasis.* The multiple lesions of vaginal candidiasis resemble those of the oral mucosa. There is usually a yellowish white discharge, and the infection may spread to the vulva, perineum, and groins. There is redness, swelling and severe pruritus. Pregnancy, diabetes and antibiotic therapy are common predisposing factors. Genital candidiasis is much less common in men, where it usually presents as balanitis. Small, white, thin-walled pustules form on the glans and quickly rupture to produce small, very shallow erosions with a rim of scale. Healing may be slow in uncircumcised men. Infection may be transmitted between male and female by sexual activity and therefore concurrent treatment of both partners is usually necessary to prevent reinfection.

■ *Flexural candidiasis. Candida* is a common aggravant of any dermatosis which produces macerated flexural skin. Submammary or flexural intertrigo, seborrhoeic dermatitis of the napkin area, and maceration

247

of skin folds in the obese are frequently complicated by candidiasis. The addition of candidiasis is suggested by the presence of broad flaccid pustules, or superficial red erosions with a shaggy white margin. The border is often festooned and satellite pustules are common, producing a very suggestive appearance.

A characteristic pattern of candidiasis often develops in the web spaces of patients who are unable to separate their fingers normally, particularly when the hand is engaged in wet work. The web between the third and fourth fingers is most often affected. The macerated skin becomes itchy, red and glazed, with the characteristic scaling border of candidiasis.

■ *Paronychia*. Candidal infection of the nail folds occurs mainly in women whose hands are frequently wet or who wear rubber gloves for long periods. The nail fold is red, swollen, painful and retracted from the nail plate. Secondary bacterial infection is common. The adjoining nail is frequently discoloured, ridged or furrowed. It is likely that *Candida* infection is merely a minor secondary factor in most cases of inflamed nail folds from which the fungus is recovered.

■ *Extensive cutaneous candidiasis* is seen in special situations. Febrile patients who have been lying in bed while taking antibiotics are frequently seen in hospital with extensive cutaneous candidiasis. The back is often predominently involved. Babies and patients with AIDS are also subject to this pattern. As in other forms of cutaneous candidiasis, the characteristic feature is the presence of very small red papules or shallow erosions surrounded by a collarette of scale. These typical one to two millimetre lesions are most commonly seen around the periphery of the affected area.

■ *Chronic mucocutaneous candidiasis*. Severe, chronic, and recurrent candidiasis of the skin and mucous membranes develops in a small group of patients in the absence of any obvious local or systemic cause. The infection is often atypical, with crusted or hyperkeratotic lesions. Hornlike projections may form on the scalp, face and in other areas. Affected nails become thick and discoloured, with much subungual hyperkeratosis. In other patients, the lesions are more typical of candidiasis, but are extremely resistant to topical therapy. Systemic candidiasis is a surprisingly rare complication.

Patients with chronic mucocutaneous candidiasis belong to two groups. The candidiasis may be only one of many infections in a patient with a well-defined immunodeficiency syndrome. In others, candidiasis is the outstanding clinical feature, and is the reason for which the patient seeks advice. T-cell dysfunction is frequently demonstrable. Some have hypoparathyroidism and other endocrine deficiencies. There is also a sub-group of patients with low iron stores who, when this is corrected, have the candidiasis resolve.

Diagnosis of candidiasis

In its usual forms candidiasis should be a clinical diagnosis. The growth of *Candida* in cultures does not distinguish between primary invasion and secondary incidental colonisation, which is common on abnormal skin due to several causes. The presence of pseudohyphae is of greater significance and is usually associated with invasion of tissue.

Treatment

Most localised forms of candidiasis respond well to topical therapy, provided that predisposing factors have been remedied. Topical steroids are often required to clear underlying skin changes and do not impair the efficacy of the topical antifungal agents. Effective applications include nystatin, amphotericin and natamycin, and the imidazoles. Aqueous gentian violet is effective, but staining and irritation limit its use. Clioquinol is also effective, but it stains clothing and skin yellow and has significant potential for allergic sensitisation.

Chronic mucocutaneous candidiasis rarely responds satisfactorily to topical therapy. Systemic administration of ketoconazole in doses of 200 mg to 400 mg daily is effective in most patients, but the frequency of recurrences and the safety of prolonged therapy have yet to be established. Parenteral amphotericin B is generally successful in eradicating the infection, but requires careful monitoring of the patient during the period of treatment. Toxicity of the drug can be considerably reduced by combining a low-dose regime of amphotericin B with simultaneous flucytosine therapy. Transfer factor has proved helpful in maintaining remission in patients successfully treated with amphotericin B.

Tinea nigra

Presenting as a chronic, asymptomatic, superficial, brown, sharply defined stain on the palm, tinea nigra is caused by *Exophyla werneckii*, which is a saprophyte of rotting vegetation in tropical areas. Most cases have been acquired in northern Queensland. Microscopic examination reveals brown, septate, branching hyphae.

The condition will respond to salicylic and boracic acid ointment (Whitfield's ointment) but does not improve with the use of imidazole creams.

Deep mycoses

1. Sporotrichosis
2. Chromoblastomycosis
3. Cryptococcosis
4. Histoplasmosis

Dermatophytes are capable of infecting only the most superficial layers of the skin and its keratinised appendages. Other fungi are able to infect not only the dermis and subcutaneous tissue, but internal organs as well. Deep fungal infections of the skin are very uncommon in Australia, the only ones encountered with any frequency being sporotrichosis, chromoblastomycosis, and, under special circumstances, cryptococcosis and histoplasmosis.

Sporotrichosis

A rare infection, primarily of subcutaneous tissue, sporotrichosis is caused by a saprophyte of soil and rotting timber. Spores are inoculated into a minor wound, usually of the hand or forearm.

The early lesion is quite non-specific. It may be a papule, nodule or plaque, or may be pustular, resembling a boil or other pyogenic infection. Slow enlargement is followed by ulceration and lymphatic involvement. The draining lymphatic vessels become firm and secondary nodules may ulcerate or remain as persistent painless swellings. Systemic symptoms are not usually marked and haematogenous dissemination is very rare.

Biopsy of the skin reveals a granulomatous abscess in which are seen small numbers of the fungus often surrounded by radiating eosinophilic material shown to be coating antibodies. Culture grows the causative fungus *Sporothrix schenckii*.

Treatment is with oral potassium iodide.

Chromoblastomycosis

A chronic infection of the skin and subcutaneous tissue, chromoblastomycosis can be caused by several fungal species. In Australia the usual organism is *Cladosporium carrionii*. Most patients are male labourers in rural areas; there is a relatively high incidence among sugarcane workers in Queensland.

The primary lesion is a painless warty papule or nodule, which extends slowly to form a pink or brownish plaque with a rough surface. The lesion is generally solitary at first and develops at a site of trauma, usually on a limb. There is steady, painless enlargement of the plaque, and satellite lesions eventually develop. Very large areas may become involved, sometimes with ulceration, but dissemination is rare.

Histology shows the pigmented fungus looking like groups of small copper coins. Treatment is with oral ketoconazole.

Cryptococcosis (torulosis)

An acute, subacute, or chronic infection, cryptococcosis may involve the skin and subcutis. The yeast responsible for the infection is a saprophyte of soil, believed to infect man via the respiratory tract.

Cryptococcosis may remain confined to the lungs or may disseminate to other organs, particularly the central nervous system. About 10 per cent of patients develop cutaneous lesions, most often firm papules or pustules on the head or neck, especially around the nose and mouth. Enlargement and ulceration may produce lesions which resemble basal cell carcinoma. Verrucoid plaques, fixed nodules, and cystic subcutaneous swellings are less frequent manifestations.

Rarely, the infection is acquired by inoculation of the skin, and produces a purely cutaneous, localised lesion. However dissemination occurs quickly. Biopsy of skin shows large numbers of the encapsulated yeasts. Treatment is with flucytosine intravenously.

Histoplasmosis

In many ways, histoplasmosis is comparable to cryptococcosis. The infection is usually confined to the lungs, but the skin may be involved in the uncommon, progressive, disseminating disease. Firm ulcers of the nose and mouth may be suggestive, but cutaneous lesions of histoplasmosis are notoriously non-specific. As with cryptococcosis, there is a rare, localised cutaneous form, acquired by inoculation.

Biopsy shows an intracellular yeast which is confirmed by culture. Treatment requires intravenous amphotericin B.

Fungus-like infections

1. Actinomycosis
2. Mycetoma

Actinomycosis

Actinomycetes are Gram-positive bacteria, composed of fungus-like filaments with a tendency to branching. In tissue, the filaments form felted masses resembling mycelia. In the pus of actinomycotic infections, the 'mycelia' may be visible as tiny granules less than a millimetre in size.

Human actinomycosis is a chronic infection with *Actinomyces israeli*, a normal commensal of the mouth. The organism is anaerobic and infection is encouraged by the low oxygen tension of damaged, devitalised tissue. Actinomycosis most often begins in the cervicofacial region, after dental operations or fracture of the mandible. A hard red lump develops over the lower jaw, and breaks down to form purulent discharging sinuses. The skin may also be involved when ileocaecal actinomycosis burrows through the abdominal wall to the surface, or when the chest wall is eroded by sinuses from underlying pulmonary infection. The diagnosis is suggested by the presence of greyish white 'sulphur granules' in pus, and is confirmed by anaerobic culture.

Actinomycosis requires prolonged therapy with large doses of penicillin. For patients who are allergic to penicillin, tetracycline or erythromycin may be substituted.

Mycetoma

Mycetoma is a clinical pattern of chronic progressive infection which begins in the skin and subcutaneous tissue, and slowly extends to involve deeper structures. Many species of aerobic actinomycetes and filamentous fungi have been recovered from mycetoma, and the progressive course probably depends more on host factors than on the particular organism, which is usually a common saprophyte of low virulence.

The disease is mainly one of labourers in tropical and subtropical regions. Most lesions occur on the foot, but the organism may be inoculated into the hand, knee, buttock or other sites of trauma. The early lesion is a firm papule or plaque, which slowly enlarges to form a subcutaneous nodule.

Suppuration produces chronically discharging sinuses, which may eventually heal as new abscesses form nearby. Slow extension gradually transforms the foot into a large irregular mass, distorted by nodules and sinuses. Underlying bone is eroded away, but dissemination to remote areas is not a feature.

Granules may be recognised in the pus, which on microscopic examination are seen as masses of interwoven filaments. Treatment depends on the particular organism indentifed by culture, but is most likely to be successful when commenced early. Prolonged cases usually require surgery, often with amputation.

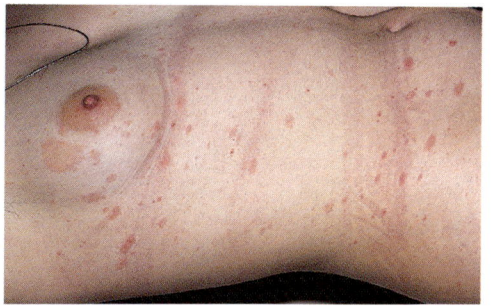

49. Pityriasis rosea

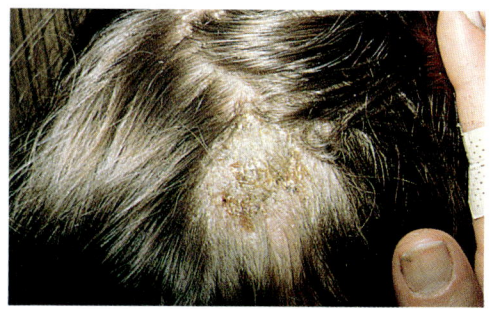

50. Tinea capitis

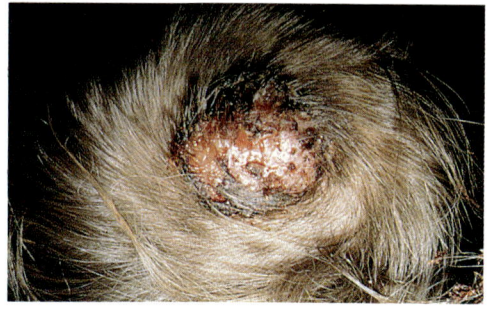

51. Kerion

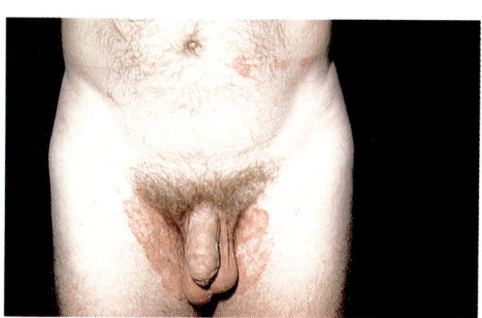

52. Tinea cruris

53. Pityriasis versicolor

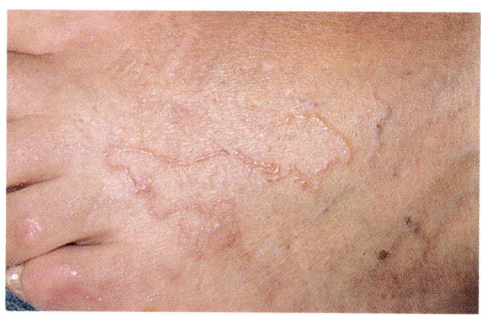

54. Larva migrans

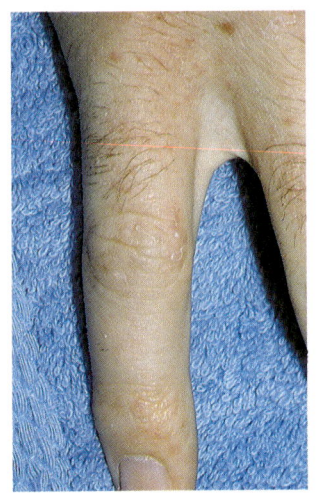

55. Scabies burrows

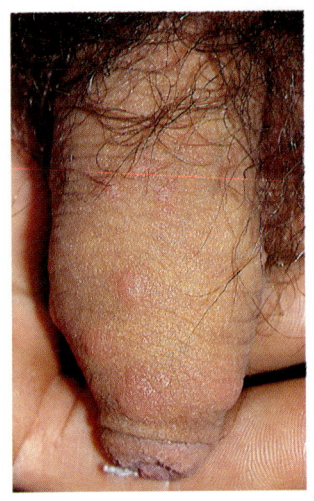

56. Scabies papules

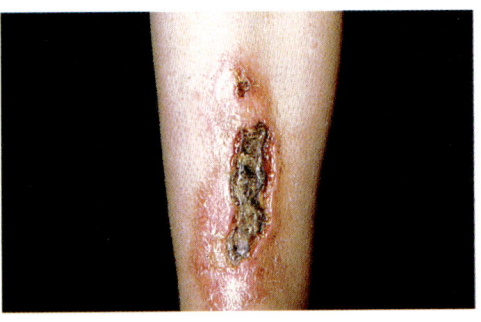

57. Necrobiosis lipoidica, with ulceration

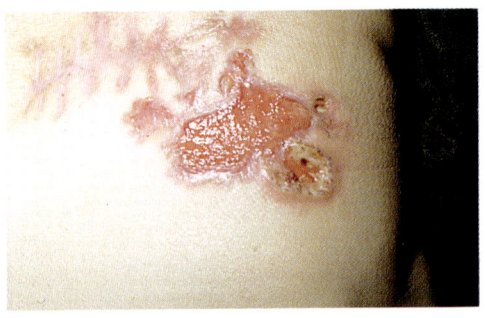

58. Pyoderma gangrenosum

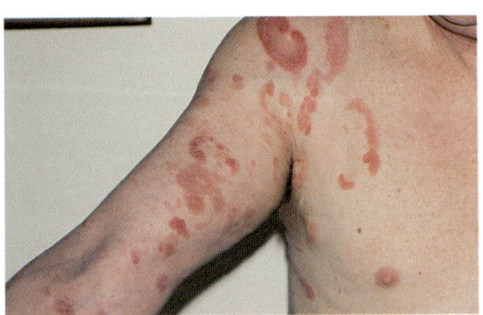

59. Mycosis fungoides

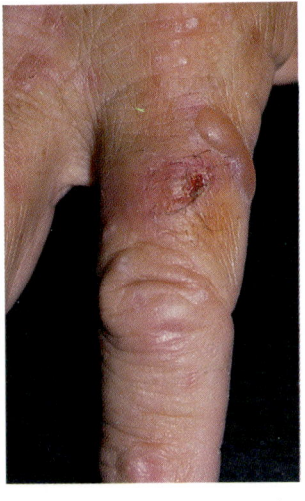

60. Porphyria cutanea tarda

17

Diseases caused by animal parasites

1. Fleas, lice and bedbugs
2. Papular urticaria
3. Mites and ticks
4. Parasitic worms

Fleas, lice and bedbugs

Some arthropods inject injurious substances directly into the skin, but much of what follows an ordinary insect bite is an expression of allergy to antigens present in the saliva of the insect. The newborn child bitten by a mosquito or flea develops no more than a haemorrhagic punctum, sometimes surrounded by a small area of erythema. After sensitisation to salivary antigens, a bite from the same species is followed a day or two later by an itchy papule at the site—a manifestation of the tuberculin-type, cell-mediated immune reaction. After repeated bites, the delayed papule is preceded by an oedematous swelling which develops within minutes of being bitten. The immediate weal is antibody-mediated, and resembles the weal of urticaria.

The period of combined immediate and delayed response is frequently a transient phase, soon followed by disappearance of the delayed papular reaction. Further bites then cause only an immediate weal of brief duration. This phase persists indefinitely, although some individuals become temporarily desensitised with numerous bites so that even the immediate reaction is lacking. The reactions produced in people bitten by even the same species may, therefore, vary considerably both in severity and type, and may be profoundly modified by drugs which suppress the immune response.

Fleas

The flea is a wingless, blood-sucking ectoparasite of animals and humans. The human flea is reddish brown, about 3 mm long, and breeds in gaps between floorboards, around skirting boards, in rugs and beds, or in dust and debris. The fleas of dogs, cats, rats and other animals have low host-specificity and frequently attack humans.

253

Lesions resulting from fleabites vary from small pink macules to papules or weals, but are often distinguished by a deep-red central punctum. In extremely sensitive individuals, lesions may be bullous. The bites are more often on covered areas and asymmetrical in distribution. They are itchy and frequently excoriated, and tend to appear in crops and clusters. The eruption of new lesions may provoke renewed inflammation in others, previously present and partially healed.

Complications
- *Impetigo*
- *Papular urticaria*

Control

Residual spraying of the breeding places with propoxur-dichlorvos aerosol is effective for domestic infestations. Vacuum cleaners are helpful, especially those with disposable dust collectors which may be burned. For infested dogs and cats, malathion wash may be used, but should be handled with care.

Lice

Lice are flat, greyish, wingless insects about 3 mm long. Unlike fleas, they complete their life cycle on skin or clothing, laying eggs which hatch in about a week. The eggs, or nits, are oval grey structures about the size of a pinhead. They are firmly cemented to the side of a hair or, in the case of body lice, to fibres of clothing. Only three types of lice exist as parasites of man, animal lice being unable to survive on human skin.

Head lice

The infestation is much more common in children, and is usually confined to the scalp, although eyebrows and lashes are occasionally involved. Heavy infestations in adults may spread to the beard and other hairy areas. The bites cause severe pruritus, particularly over the occipital and temporal regions. Excoriations may become infected and the occipital and cervical lymph glands are frequently enlarged. A few patients develop a pink macular rash on the trunk, which resembles rubella.

Adult lice are few and easily missed, but nits are usually numerous and are a certain guide to past or present infestation. Eggs are laid close to the scalp, so the distance of nits from the scalp is proportional to the time since deposition. However, the nits persist after hatching and do not imply continuing infestation. Although it is usually true that nits found further than 1.3 cm (0.5 inches) from the scalp can be presumed to be dead or hatched, this is not necessarily the case during hot summer weather, when viable nits can be found three to four times this distance from the scalp. If there is any doubt regarding viability, microscopic examination of nits on freshly plucked hairs will provide the answer. Nits that are still alive contain a well formed nymph, whereas non-viable nits are either empty or contain amorphous material.

Diagnosis

▶ **Suspect** the diagnosis in any patient with an itchy scalp especially if impetigo is present and the patient is a child.

▶ **Confirm** the diagnosis by finding nits on the hairs. For rapid screening in schools this can be aided by use of Wood's light.

▶ **Ensure** that hair casts are not being confused. These are larger than nits and can be moved freely along the hair towards its free end. Pruritus is not a feature.

Treatment

Gamma benzene hexachloride 1 per cent lotion has been a safe and effective treatment. However, although the adult lice are very readily destroyed by this substance, nits are not so uniformly sensitive. Therefore, the most effective method of use is to apply the lotion and leave the hair unwashed for seven days so that any newly hatched lice are destroyed. Unfortunately resistance is now occurring to this substance.

The alternative treatment is 0.5 per cent malathion which is uniformly effective against nits and adult lice. However, because this substance is a cholinesterase inhibitor that can be absorbed through the skin, it is therefore issued as a premeasured single dose application which is left on for twelve hours then washed off. Rarely, a second application may be required seven days later.

Any non-viable nits remaining after completion of treatment are firmly adherent to the hair with a naturally secreted cement-like substance. Removal of the residual nits therefore requires the strong shearing forces generated by combing the hair from base to tip with a fine tooth comb. This job can be made easier by rinsing the hair with an 8 per cent solution of formic acid, which destroys the adhesive bonds of the cement-like substance.

Body lice

The body louse is morphologically indistinguishable from the head louse, but infests clothing, not skin. Eggs are deposited on fibres, particularly along seams, although nits are occasionally found on body hairs. The eggs remain viable up to four weeks, but generally hatch sooner.

The lice attach to skin only to feed, leaving small red macules with a central haemorrhagic punctum. The macules evolve to intensely itchy papules, which may persist for several days. However, most lesions are quickly altered by scratching, and are seen as crusted linear excoriations, particularly over the shoulders, back of the neck, trunk and buttocks. The excoriations are often infected and may heal with scarring. Patches of lichenification are common with longstanding infestation.

The body louse is the vector for several rickettsial diseases, the most notable of which is epidemic typhus. In that disorder, the presence of the rickettsiae in vascular endothelial cells of brain, heart and skin produces fever and malaise, followed by pink macules which become haemorrhagic. Survival depends on the degree of involvement of the heart or brain and on how early treatment of typhus with oral tetracycline is commenced.

Control

Lice are unable to survive in regularly laundered clothing. For the isolated case, it is sufficient for the patient to take a bath and change into clothes which have been washed and carefully pressed with a hot iron. All other clothing should be laundered and ironed, or stored for a month before being worn. When this is not possible, the patient and his clothing may be treated with gamma benzene hexachloride.

Pubic lice

The insects are shorter and broader than scalp and body lice, and are usually confined to the region of the pubic hair. In hirsute individuals the abdomen and thighs may be involved, and the louse is occasionally found in other hairy areas. The infestation is generally acquired during sexual intercourse.

Early lesions are inconspicuous, and soon masked by scratching. Careful examination is likely to disclose an adult insect lying immobile against the skin at the base of a hair. The lice are not easy to find without a hand lens, and the nits are dark and more difficult to see than the lighter coloured nits of scalp lice. A few patients develop small bluish grey macules on the lower abdomen and upper thighs at the sites of previous bites.

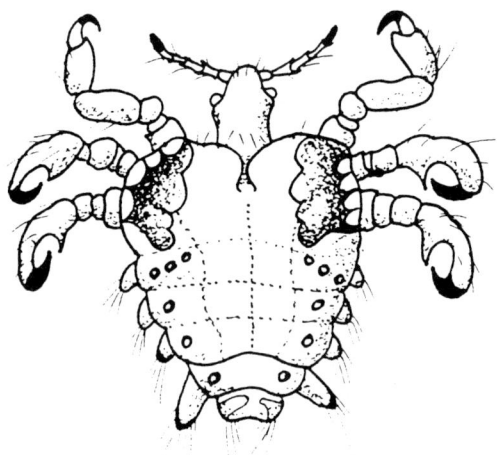

Pubic louse

Control

A lotion containing 1 per cent gamma benzene hexachloride, or 0.5 per cent malathion in an alcohol or acetone base, should be applied twice, a week apart.

Bedbugs

Bedbugs are flat, reddish-brown, wingless insects, about half a centimetre long. They live in crevices of furniture, walls and bedding, particularly in older, poorer districts. Bedbugs are nocturnal feeders and, like fleas, often sample two or three sites in a small area. There may be little or no discomfort while the insect is feeding and the patient often sleeps undisturbed. Sites most often bitten are the face, neck, wrists, back, buttocks and ankles—areas in contact with the bed.

The lesions produced vary with the degree of sensitivity. Previously unexposed patients develop a small red macule which surrounds a haemorrhagic punctum. The typical lesion in sensitised patients is a firm, itchy weal, up to 2 cm across, with a central punctum. Lesions may be vesicular and are occasionally bullous. In some patients, weals develop not only at the site of recent bites, but in previously affected areas as well.

Control

Treatment of breeding places with gamma benzene hexachloride is usually adequate, but heavy infestation may require fumigation with dichlorvos.

Papular urticaria

Papular urticaria is a common discorder, which is characterised by the formation of persistent itching papules in response to insect bites. It may be regarded as an arrest at the normally transient phase between sensitisation and development of the weal reaction. Instead of passing quickly into the phase of immediate wealing, the patient continues with the papular response for an abnormally long period. Any biting insect may cause papular urticaria, but fleas, mosquitoes, sandflies, grass mites and bedbugs are the most common.

The disease is generally one of young children. Adults may be affected when, having moved to a new district, they encounter a particular insect for the first time. It is a distressing condition which troubles many newly arrived migrants.

Clinical features

■ *Lesions* begin as small weals and evolve in a few hours to firm reddish papules, which persist for days and sometimes weeks. The papule may be surmounted by a small vesicle, and lesions are occasionally bullous. The papules are itchy and soon become crusted as the tops are scratched off.

■ *Distribution* varies with the insect involved. Mosquitoes and sandflies attack the face, neck, and other exposed areas. Fleabites are more often on the legs and covered areas, with a tendency for lesions to be clustered around the waist and other sites which are constricted by clothing. Bites from bedbugs are also clustered, but are concentrated at sites in contact with the bed. However, the distribution is used together with other evidence as an aid to the final identification of the causative insect rather than as a definite incriminatory sign on its own.

■ *New crops* consist of a cluster of approximately four lesions, all at the same stage of evolution, which are often arranged in a curved row.

Course

This usually follows a seasonal pattern, attacks most often occurring during spring and summer. The disease frequently recurs each summer for three or four years, before disappearing permanently. When there is no seasonal variation, bedbugs should be suspected.

Diagnosis

▶ **Consider and exclude**

■ *Scabies*, which is distinguished by the distribution of lesions, the characteristic burrow, and in children by the frequent involvement of palms and soles.

■ *Pityriasis lichenoides* is more a disease of young adults. When children are affected, lesions are generally of the acute, vesicular type.

■ *Bindii* is a very common weed, which infests lawns and grassland in many coastal districts of the country. During the spring and early summer months, the bindii develops spicules which penetrate the skin to form inflammatory papules, pustules and, occasionally, a somewhat psoriasiform dermatitis. Common sites of involvement include the hands, forearms, elbows, knees and soles.

■ *Recurrent impetigo* does not occur without an underlying cause. It is a common presentation of papular urticaria in children.

Treatment

Every effort should be made to protect the patient from the relevant insects. Mosquito nets during sleep, attention to flea-infested houses, cats and dogs, control of bedbug infestation, and the use of insect repellents are the measures most likely to prevent recurrences. Topical corticosteroids give some relief from the pruritus of established lesions, and the administration of systemic antibiotics is often necessary for secondary infection.

Mites and ticks

The ectoparasite of humans that completes its life cycle on the skin is the scabies mite. Other mites may cause cutaneous disease by puncturing or burrowing into the skin, but are unable to reproduce there and the infestation is self-limited. Lesions vary with host sensitivity and in previously unexposed people may cause little discomfort. In sensitised individuals, lesions are itchy weals, papules or vesicles. They are multiple and often very numerous. Distribution depends upon the mode of infestation.

Mites may be acquired by those in close contact with animals suffering from animal scabies and other mite infestations. The eruption is normally of brief duration, but repeated contact allows reinfestation, with chronic disease. Scabetic dogs and cats infested with cheyletiella are a common source in urban areas. In rural districts, the infestation may come from pigs, goats, sheep and other animals.

The starling mite is most troublesome late in the spring, when the birds leave their nests. The starling mites may enter houses through windows or ventilators close to the nests. Mites from pigeons or fowls may attack those who handle infested birds or work in poultry sheds.

Infestation of lawns with the grass-itch mite is common in south-eastern Australia during the summer months, and several mite species are responsible for the scrub itch of Queensland. Biting mites may also infest straw, hay, copra, barley and other grain.

Scabies

Scabies is a chronic infestation with the host-specific mite, *Sarcoptes scabiei var. hominis.*

Aetiology

The parasite is a slow mover until stimulated by warmth; transmission is therefore generally by skin contact, usually in bed. The adult female is less than half a millimetre long and barely visible to the naked eye. The male is smaller. The female is fertilised on the skin surface and then burrows tangentially into the stratum corneum, depositing eggs as she goes. The eggs hatch in four days, the larvae maturing on the surface 10 days later. As the life cycle is completed on the skin, untreated scabies may persist indefinitely.

The lesions of scabies are mostly a manifestation of allergy to the mite or its products. With a primary infestation, the patient remains asymptomatic for weeks after contracting the disease. Previously affected patients may develop inflammatory lesions and pruritus only hours after the female commences to burrow.

Clinical features *(Colour plates 55, 56)*

■ *The primary lesion* is the burrow—a narrow, skin-coloured or greyish ridge, 3 mm to 10 mm long. It is slightly curved or S-shaped, sometimes with a vesicle or pearly elevation at one end. Although pathognomonic, burrows are not easy to see, and are not found in every patient. There are only 10 or 11 living adult females on the skin of most patients, and only the gravid female burrows. They are most often found between the fingers, or on the ulnar border of the hand or forearm, the front of the wrist, the penis, the areola of women, and on the palms and soles of children.

■ *Secondary lesions* account for much of what is seen with scabies. They vary in number and severity, depending at least in part of the degree of allergic sensitivity of the patient.

Excoriations are common and are often infected. Frequently seen are very small urticarial papules that seem perifollicular. The surface of these is sometimes abraded. There may also be weals, pustules, crusted patches or areas of lichenification.

These non-specific secondary lesions are most commonly seen on the ulnar borders of the forearms, the anterior axillary folds, the buttocks and waist and the peri-areolar regions in females. Except in babies, the scalp and face are rarely involved and there is relative sparing of the upper back.

Reddish-brown indurated papules and nodules are a much more specific secondary sign. These are seen around the axillae and inguinal region and on the penis and scrotum. They may persist for weeks to months after eradication of the mite. They are composed of a dense dermal infiltrate rich in eosinophils.

■ *Pruritus* usually begins two to four weeks after contracting the infestation. The itch is severe and widespread, with pronounced nocturnal aggravation. The face and scalp are spared, except in infants. With the rare Norwegian scabies, pruritus may be slight or absent.

■ *Norwegian scabies* is a variant in which host responses to the parasite are in some way impaired. The mites multiply freely, forming enormous colonies which honeycomb the stratum corneum. Originally observed in lepers, Norwegian scabies occurs in patients with Down's syndrome, in mental defectives, the chronically ill, the immunodeficient and, very rarely, in apparently normal people.

The skin is scaly and thickened, especially over the hands and feet. The palms and soles are oozing, crusted and fissured. The nails are thick and lifted by subungual keratosis. Crusted and scaling plaques develop on the trunk, face and scalp. These patients are teeming with mites and provide a reservoir from which other patients and staff members are easily infested.

Diagnosis

▶ **Suspect** the diagnosis in the patient with generalised itch affecting all the body except for the face and scalp, which is worse with heat and especially in bed at night.

▶ **Consider and exclude**

■ *Body lice*, which is diagnosed by finding the lice in clothing.

■ *Papular urticaria*, which is not accompanied by burrows.

■ *Leukaemia* or *lymphoma*, particularly Hodgkin's disease, which may cause generalised pruritus with papules and nodules. There is no special sparing of the head and neck and other features are likely to be present.

■ *Dermatitis herpetiformis*, which is intensely itchy and often involves the elbows, shoulders, buttocks, belt line, and genital area. However, the scalp is frequently affected and there is mirror-image symmetry and clustering of lesions.

■ *Parasitophobia*. Patients with this disorder may claim to have scabies. These people often have a bizarre demeanour, and the objective changes are either frank excoriations or those of an associated disorder, such as senile xeroderma.

▶ **Confirm** the diagnosis

■ Microscopic identification is required of the mite, its eggs, or faecal pellets, in superficial scrapings from a burrow. The scrapings are treated with 10 per cent potassium hydroxide solution and examined with the low-power objective. It is sometimes possible to carefully lift the roof of a burrow and extract the mite with a needle point. The parasite is only a tiny speck at one end of the burrow and is difficult to remove unless a hand lens is used.

Complications

■ *Secondary infection* is very common and scabies may masquerade as impetigo or furunculosis.

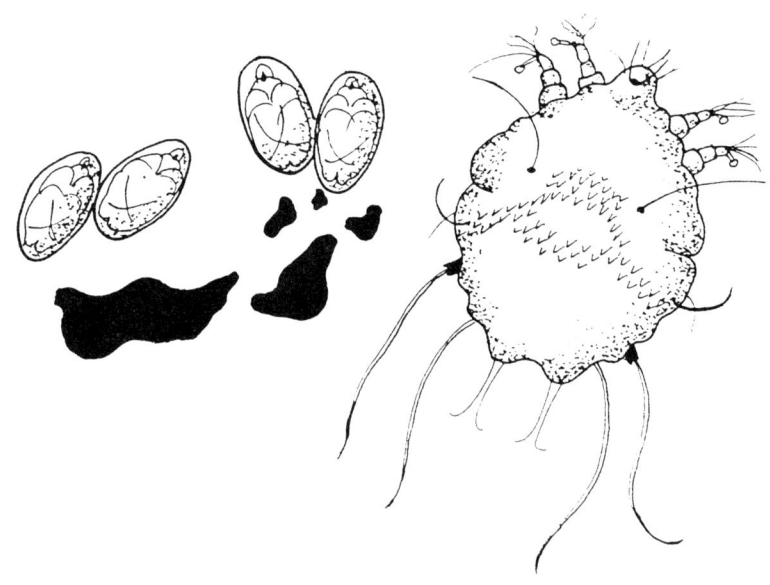

Human scabies – adult mite, eggs and faecal material

■ *Allergic contact dermatitis* may be caused by unsuitable applications.

■ *Irritant dermatitis* caused by the correct treatment is particularly common in those with atopic eczema.

Treatment

Despite a considerable potential for toxicity, gamma benzene hexachloride remains the most acceptable treatment for scabies. A 1 per cent solution is applied to all the body except for the face and scalp. After twelve hours the residue is removed by thorough washing. The sexual partner should be treated concurrently even if there are no symptoms or signs.

The neurotoxic and haematological complications due to absorption of gamma benzene hexachloride can be avoided if the skin is thoroughly dried prior to application. Alternative treatments are used in the neonate and those with widespread dermatitis or badly excoriated skin.

Alternative treatments include benzyl benzoate 25 per cent emulsion which, in many patients, is quite irritating, and 10 per cent sulphur ointment which, in addition to its irritant properties, is quite messy to use.

The mite does not survive for long off the human body and normal laundering is sufficient to destroy any parasites or larvae which might be present in bed linen or soiled clothing.

The treatment should only be repeated if there are signs of continuing active infection and the presence of mites can be demonstrated.

Ticks

Ticks are large mites, which survive as blood-sucking ectoparasites of animals. The scrub tick of Australia is retricted to bushland within a few miles of the coastline. Usually a parasite of dogs, cats, bandicoots, and other mammals, the scrub tick or its larvae may attach to the skin of people who walk through coastal bush areas.

The bite is initially painless and unnoticed. Pruritus may develop in a matter of hours, but the parasite is generally first noticed because of its size. As the tick withdraws blood its body swells to several times its previous size and within a day may form a dark, grape-like swelling, a centimetre or so in diameter, firmly anchored to the skin by its buried hypostome. If the tick drops off, a firm red infiltrated area remains for a week or two. If the tick is roughly pulled off, leaving mouth parts in the skin, a foreign body reaction follows, and may form an itchy nodule which persists for months.

Systemic symptoms may complicate attachment of multiple larvae or a single adult female, but the disturbance is usually mild. In children particularly, headache may be followed by muscle weakness, which is often confined to the limbs. In badly affected children, the paresis may extend to the trunk or lead to blurred vision and pharyngeal palsy. Deaths have occurred due to respiratory failure.

Treatment

Alcohol or ether is applied on and around the tick, which is then withdrawn by steady traction using non-toothed forceps.

Lyme disease

Aetiology

Certain varieties of Ixodes tick carry the causative spirochete *Borrelia burgdorferi*. Cases have been reported from the Hunter valley and southern coastal New South Wales.

Clinical features

■ *Skin*. Erythema chronicum migrans appears at the site of the tick bite about seven days later as a small macule that becomes a gradually enlarging warm red area with a tendency to target lesion formation. Untreated cases may reach 30 cm by three weeks then gradually resolve.

Similar but smaller and slower evolving lesions may develop widespread and distant to the bite.

Months later, in untreated patients, atrophic sclerotic plaques unrelated to previous lesions may develop on the extensor aspects of the distal portions of the limbs (acrodermatitis chronica atrophicans).

■ *Systemic*. Fluctuating lethargy, fever and headache are relatively common. Neurologic, cardiac and joint changes may appear later but serious meningo-encephalitis, myocarditis or arthritis occur in less than 10 per cent of untreated patients.

262

Diagnosis

Biopsy of skin can occasionally reveal the spirochete but demonstrating the specific circulating antibody is more reliable.

Treatment

Tetracycline one gram per day for two weeks is the preferred treatment. In children penicillin is used, and erythromycin for those allergic to penicillin. However both of those treatments, although clearing the skin changes, are less reliable than tetracycline in preventing the late systemic manifestations.

Parasitic worms

Creeping eruption (larva migrans)

Aetiology

The larvae of cat and dog hookworms hatch from eggs which are deposited in sandy soil. The parasite is able to penetrate human skin at any site in contact with infested soil, most often the feet or buttocks and posterior thighs.

Although Loeffler's syndrome is a frequently reported association, because human skin is not an appropriate breeding site, the parasite cannot survive for long periods and therefore the infestation is confined to the skin.

Somewhat similar cutaenous lesions may follow penetration of the skin by larvae of the human intestinal worm *Strongyloides stercoralis*, and by larvae of the horse botfly.

Clinical features *(Colour plate 54)*

After a variable latent period, an itchy, cord-like elevation appears in the skin. Skin-coloured or reddish, and a few millimetres wide, the lesion wanders in a tortuous fashion, following the movements of the larva. The parasite is always ahead of the lesion, which trails about a centimetre behind. The elevation may be several centimetres long and advances up to 3 cm per day. The direction is unpredictable and constantly changing, leaving a linear, arcuate or serpiginous tunnel. When more than one larva is present, there may be a maze of tangled tracks.

Treatment

The simplest approach is to freeze an area one centimetre ahead of the lesion, using liquid nitrogen. Topical applications of thiabendazole suspension, 2 per cent gamma benzene hexachloride cream, and 25 per cent piperazine ointment have all been reported effective in small numbers of patients. Systemic thiabendazole is also effective but, although a very safe drug, frequently causes unpleasant cutaneous and gastro-intestinal side effects.

Swimmer's itch

Aetiology

The disease is caused by penetration of the skin by cercarial larvae of avian schistosomes. The larvae are released into shallow lakes from species of snails which constitute the intermediate host.

The cercariae are attracted toward the surface and may enter the skin of swimmers or fishermen standing in shallow water. The larvae are unable to survive for long in human skin, but the lesions they produce may last for weeks. Individuals vary a great deal in their reaction to the parasite, depending largely on the number of larvae which enter the skin and the degree of allergic reaction which follows. As a rule, sensitivity increases with succeeding attacks, but some people remain unaffected by repeated exposure to the larvae.

The parasites infest salt water lakes at Narrabeen and Tuggerah in New South Wales, coastal lagoons and fresh water lakes in Queensland and Western Australia, and swamps and billabongs along the Murray river.

Clinical features

Lesions are often scattered over a broad band across the lower legs or thighs, depending on the depth of water in which the patient wades.

Areas protected by clothing or swimwear are unaffected. At the time of penetration there may be mild pruritus, which is follwed by the formation of reddish macules or small weals at sites of entry. Hours or days later, the lesions thicken to intensely itchy papules, often surmounted by small vesicles. The papules may become crusted or pustular but, unless perpetuated by scratching, resolve gradually over one to two weeks.

Treatment

For the first two or three days of the eruption, cold wet packs give best relief. A corticosteroid cream is more helpful later.

Intestinal parasites

Cutaneous signs produced by the intestinal parasites present in this country are non-specific. Urticaria is a rare manifestation. Threadworm infestation commonly produces perianal pruritus, which is caused by movement of the female parasite outside the anus to deposit eggs. The itch is worse at night and may extend to the vulva and even the groins. The itchy skin is red, often excoriated, and sometimes infected.

Treatment of threadworm is with a single oral dose of mebendazole.

18

The skin in systemic disease

1. Endocrine disorders
   (a) diabetes mellitus
   (b) disorders of the anterior
       pituitary and adrenal cortex
   (c) thyroid disease
   (d) hypoparathyroidism
   (e) pregnancy

2. Gastro-intestinal disorders
   (a) bowel disease
   (b) liver disease
   (c) pancreatic disease

3. Renal disease

4. Arthritis
   (a) rheumatoid arthritis
   (b) rheumatic fever
   (c) gout

5. Internal malignancy
   (a) specific deposits
   (b) non-specific signs
   (c) genetic associations
   (d) lymphoma and leukaemia

6. Histocytic disorders
   (a) histocytosis X
   (b) sarcoidosis

7. Biochemical disorders
   (a) porphyrias
   (b) hyperlipidaemias
   (c) amyloidosis

8. Nutritional deficiencies
   (a) pellagra
   (b) scurvy
   (c) kwashiorkor
   (d) zinc deficiency

One of the aspects of medicine that is most satisfying to the mind is to deduce correctly that the presenting signs in the skin are part of a systemic disease process or an indicator of disease in another organ system. Although it is not surprising that a metabolically active organ like the skin shares in the malfunctions which result from altered body metabolism, this does not mean that cutaneous disease in general merely reflects systemic disturbance. The method used to detect visceral disease is to recognise which skin signs may be an indicator of a more serious inner disorder rather than the inefficient approach of arranging for complicated laboratory investigations as part of the management of everyday dermatoses.

Elsewhere in this book, skin changes are presented and the causes discussed. In this chapter the skin signs of systemic disease are listed using the organ system and disease processes responsible for their appearance.

Endocrine disorders

1. Diabetes mellitus
2. Disorders of the anterior pituitary and adrenal cortex
3. Thyroid disease
4. Hypoparathyroidism
5. Pregnancy

Diabetes mellitus

■ *Vascular disease* produces the more serious complications of diabetes. Atherosclerosis and an altered microcirculation easily lead to ischaemic and neuropathic ulceration, or to gangrene. On the legs and feet particularly, wound healing is delayed and frequently complicated by secondary infection.

■ *Infection* in general is more common among diabetics. Bacterial infections are more severe and may be more frequent in the poorly controlled diabetic. Candida of the genital area, candida paronychia and candida intertrigo in those with diabetes is often recurrent and refractory to treatment. An uncommon variety of candida intertrigo, localised to the web space between the ring and middle fingers, is sometimes seen in those with diabetes and in virtually no other patients.

■ *Pruritus* of the genital area may be the presenting feature of unsuspected diabetes, and, even in the absence of candidiasis, unexplained pruritus vulvae or pruritus ani warrant exclusion of diabetes.

■ *Necrobiosis lipoidica (diabeticorum).* More than 80 per cent of those with necrobiosis lipoidica are clinically or chemically diabetic, but less than 1 per cent of diabetics develop the disease. The majority of patients are women. Lesions may be single or multiple and begin as firm, reddish pink nodules or plaques, usually over the shin or side of the leg. Slow peripheral extension leaves a yellowish atrophic central area. In old lesions, vessels can be seen coursing below the very thin epidermis. There is neither itch nor pain, but the severe atrophy predisposes to ulceration.

Necrobiosis lipoidica is clinically characteristic; biopsy is not often necessary for diagnosis and, with atrophic lesions, carries a real risk of persistent ulceration. *(Colour plate 57)*

■ *Diabetic dermopathy* refers to distinctive lesions that occur over the fronts of the lower legs. They begin as reddish-brown papules and evolve to small, well circumscribed areas of atrophy, which may be hyperpigmented. About two-thirds of adult male diabetics and at least 10 per cent of diabetic women develop this change. Diabetic dermopathy is seen most commonly in those who have had diabetes for many years. The cause is not known but is thought to relate to microvascular disease.

■ *Thick skin* that is waxy and tightly bound down is commonly seen on the dorsum of the hands and fingers. Insulin-dependent children and young adults with this manifestation also frequently have interphalyngeal joints that show reduced mobility. This disorder should be differentiated from scleredema which is also more prevalent among those with diabetes.

In that disorder, mucin is deposited in the dermis and sites of predilection include the neck and upper back.

- *Signs of poor control* include eruptive xanthomas and, in addition to infections and pruritus vulvae, idiopathic bullae that arise spontaneously on the dorsum of the hands and feet. The blisters are most commonly subepidermal, but can occasionally be intra-epidermal. The cause is not understood.

- *Treatment-induced changes* include urticaria and other drug eruptions. Insulin-induced lipo-atrophy at the site of injection is seen more commonly in women and children but its incidence has fallen since the introduction of more purified insulin preparations. Localised hypertrophy of fat is seen more commonly in males and is not related to purity of insulin. The raised mounds are relatively anaesthetic and therefore the patient will preferentially use this area to inject insulin. The lipohypertrophy will resolve if the sites of insulin administration are rotated.

Disorders of the anterior pituitary and adrenal cortex

- *Cushing's syndrome*. The face, trunk and buttocks are rounded by fat, while the limbs remain thin. The face and chest are oily and plethoric, and acneiform lesions are present in about 50 per cent of patients. The abdomen is protuberant and develops purplish striae. The skin is fragile, easily bruised and may be hyperpigmented. There is a high incidence of pityriasis versicolor, and tinea due to *Trichophyton rubrum*. There may be hirsutism and recession of the frontal hairline and, in women, other signs of mild virilisation.

- *Acromegaly*. Advanced acromegaly presents a striking appearance. The face is lengthened by enlarged jaws and broadened by prominent cheek bones. The brows protrude, and there is enlargement of the ears, nose, lips and tongue. The skin is thick, oily and sweats freely. There may be folds and furrows, especially over the scalp. The hands are large and fleshy, and the nails thick. Follicular pores are broad and prominent, and the hair coarse. Hyperpigmentation is common. Most of the skin changes will resolve when treatment reduces the levels of growth hormone and somatomedin, but the bone changes do not.

- *Hypopituitarism*. The skin is pale, dry, thin and sometimes finely wrinkled, but may be altered by secondary hypothryoidism. The axillary and pubic hair is scanty or absent.

- *Addison's disease*. Hyperpigmentation is an early and almost invariable sign. The whole skin darkens, but melanosis is more pronounced on sun-exposed areas and over bony prominences. Hair becomes darker, and moles more deeply pigmented. The oral mucosa is spotted with brown or bluish macules. Pigmentation is frequently marked in body folds, palmar creases, over the nipples, genitalia and in recent scars. Vitiligo is present in 15 per cent of patients.

Thyroid disease

■ *Hypothyroidism*. The skin feels thickened, cool and dry. There is generalised pallor, sometimes yellowish, which contrasts with the flushed cheeks of many of these patients. The skin is rough, somewhat scaly and may be itchy—changes which are easily mistaken for senile xeroderma. The eyelids are puffy and the eyebrows sparse. Scalp hair is coarse and brittle, often with diffuse alopecia. Axillary and pubic hair is frequently scanty.

■ *Hyperthyroidism*. Cutaneous blood flow is increased and the threshold for sweating lowered. The skin is warm and moist, and there may be palmar erythema. Scalp hair is fine, soft and may be diffusely thinned. During exacerbations, hair loss is increased and the nails are occasionally shed. Although uncommon, onycholysis confined to the ring fingers is a sign rarely seen in anything other than hyperthyroidism. Generalised pigmentation and clubbing of the digits are uncommon, late sequelae.

Pretibial myxoedema is an unusual but distinctive complication of Graves' disease, which may develop before, during, or long after effective treatment of thyrotoxicosis. Pink or purplish nodules or plaques form on the lateral or anterior surface of the lower legs. The thickening may slowly extend backwards or down to the feet. The surface is usually smooth, but prominent hair follicles may impart a pitted appearance. Microscopically, the skin shows infiltration of mucin in the lower dermis.

Pretibial myxoedema is induced via the auto-immune mechanisms that take place in Graves' disease and therefore is not seen induced by other causes.

Hypoparathyroidism

When parathyroid insufficiency results from inadvertent removal or damage to parathyroid tissue during thyroid surgery, hair loss and nail dystrophy may occur, but revert to normal after correction of the hypocalcaemia. With idiopathic hypoparathyroidism, more than 25 per cent of patients have associated cutaneous changes which persist despite treatment of the endocrine disease. The skin is coarse and dry, the hair sparse, and the nails brittle. There is a susceptibility to chronic mucocutaneous candidiasis characterised by exophytic vegetations, which most often involve the mouth, vagina and nails. These features are often merely the initial manifestation of a syndrome in which there is multiple endocrine failure.

Pregnancy

■ *Vascular changes*. The circulation is hyperdynamic, with increased cutaneous blood flow. Palmar erythema is common, and at least a few spider naevi develop in most women. There is recognisable oedema in many, and varicose veins may appear or become worse.

■ *Pigmentation*. There is generalised deepening of colour, most marked over the areolae, linea alba, and areas such as the genitalia which are normally more pigmented. Chloasma generally develops during the second trimester, and is more pronounced in those of darker complexion. Existing moles become more deeply pigmented and new ones may appear.

■ *Hair*. Increased growth of facial hair is not uncommon, and may persist after parturition. During pregnancy the percentage of scalp follicles in anagen increases, so that hair fall is decreased. After delivery there is a compensatory increase of telogen follicles, which causes a precipitate loss of hair. The rapid shedding of telogen hairs may be sufficient to cause objective alopecia, often maximal 90 days after delivery (telogen effluvium). Full recovery follows within a few months in most cases.

■ *Pruritus*. Generalised pruritus is fairly common during pregnancy. The pruritus may be a manifestation of cholestasis, but is usually unassociated with any detectable disease.

A few patients with pruritus of pregnancy develop intensely itchy papules and nodules, which often begin in the region of abdominal striae. This condition is termed 'pruritic urticarial papules and plaques of pregnancy' (PUPPP) and is seen most commonly in primagravida during the third trimester. PUPPP resolves within a few weeks of delivery, is not associated with any foetal morbidity and does not recur during subsequent pregnancies.

■ *Herpes gestationis* is a very rare itchy, polymorphous eruption of pregnancy, which evolves to a vesiculobullous rash with many of the clinical and histological features of bullous pemphigoid. A specific antibody present in the blood causes deposition of complement along the basement membrane of skin but routine immunofluorescence may not detect the very low titres of antibody present. The disorder tends to flare with parturition and sometimes with menstrual periods for some months later. There is a slightly increased risk of foetal morbidity. With subsequent pregnancies, the disease tends to occur earlier and to be more severe.

■ *Impetigo herpetiformis* resembles pustular psoriasis. Red pustular plaques are located on the trunk, axillae and groins. Pustulation is most intense around the periphery of the plaques. There is a high foetal and maternal morbidity. The rash clears with delivery. Episodes appear with every subsequent pregnancy and tend to occur earlier and be more severe. However, both herpes gestationis and impetigo herpetiformis are rare complications of pregnancy, and pruritus during pregnancy is more likely to be a result of dermatoses unrelated to the pregnancy than to its rare, specific complications. An itchy rash over the groins and perineum is more often intertrigo or candidiasis than impetigo herpetiformis.

Gastro-intestinal disease

Bowel disease

Malabsorption syndrome

The most common cutaneous signs of intestinal disease are the non-specific changes that occur in about 20 per cent of those who present with malabsorption. Children with coeliac disease often have dermatitis, sometimes for years, before intestinal features become apparent. The skin may be pale, dry and scaly, sometimes resembling ichthyosis. Follicular hyperkeratosis may result from vitamin A deficiency, and purpura or ecchymoses from hypoprothrombinaemia. With severe longstanding malabsorption, there may be digital clubbing, loss of body hair, and hyperpigmentation.

Inflammatory bowel disease

■ *Ulcerative colitis* is frequently associated with non-specific signs that follow the course of the primary disease. These include aphthous ulcers, vegetating pustular eruptions around the mouth and within the major flexures, erythema multiforme, erythema nodosum and vasculitis.

Pyoderma gangrenosum, the characteristic pattern of ulceration seen most commonly in association with inflammatory bowel disease (although usually seen during exacerbations) can occur when the ulcerative colitis is quiescent or even before it is realised the disease is present. *(Colour plate 58)*

■ *Crohn's disease* can also produce the non-specific skin signs seen with ulcerative colitis but does so less frequently. However, cutaneous involvement with the disease process of Crohn's disease is also a feature. Involvement of the mouth can produce granulomatous lesions within the lip, tongue, buccal mucosa of the cheeks and a cobblestone appearance on the palate. Perianal involvement can cause ischiorectal abscess, perianal fissures and ulceration. Similar changes can occur around ileostomy sites. Fistula formation is a characteristic feature. Persistent fistulae may form around the anus, sometimes tracking into the vagina, bladder or rectum; other fistulae erode to the surface through laparotomy scars.

Malformation syndromes

■ *Peutz-Jeghers syndrome.* The benign hamartomatous intestinal polyps of this syndrome are associated with pigmented macules on the buccal mucosa, on the face (with accentuation around the lips), and on the palms. With time, the palmar and facial pigmentation may fade after puberty, but the intra-oral pigmentation persists. Polyps arising above the ligament of Trietz may be malignant.

■ *Gardner's syndrome.* Premalignant polyps of the colon are associated with numerous epidermoid cysts that appear during late childhood. Other skin signs that may or may not be present in this autosomal dominant syndrome include fibromas (desmoids) and lipomas. Osteomas of the facial and skull bones are also common.

■ *Osler's disease* and other vascular malformation syndromes may be associated with intestinal bleeding that is often silent, detected only because the cutaneous vascular lesions are recognised.

■ *Neurofibromatosis.* Intestinal haemorrhage can also be due to neurofibromas of the bowel, as can bowel obstruction.

Skin and bowel syndromes

■ *Dermatitis herpetiformis.* By means of a multiple biopsy technique, it can be shown that almost all patients with dermatitis herpetiformis have an enteropathy. The mucosal changes resemble those of coeliac disease, but frank malabsorption is very uncommon in dermatitis herpetiformis. The enteropathy responds to a gluten-free diet and, at least in some patients, the diet also improves the course of the cutaneous disease.

■ *Acrodermatitis enteropathica.* This rare syndrome results from the malabsorption of zinc, and responds dramatically to treatment with zinc salts. Onset is usually in the first two years of life, with diarrhoea, an erosive dermatitis around body orifices, a bullous eruption of the hands and feet, and secondary candidiasis. Other features include alopecia, photophobia and personality changes.

■ *Cronkhite–Canada syndrome* is a rare disorder in which gastro-intestinal polyposis is associated with severe diarrhoea that produces hypo-albuminaemia and profound fluid and electrolyte imbalance. The skin signs are of pigmentation of the face, neck and hands, nail dystrophy and alopecia.

■ *Other diseases* frequently involve the skin and gut together. Examples are the connective tissue diseases, vasculitic diseases such as Henoch-Schoenlein purpura, thyrotoxic disease, carcinoid syndrome and mastocytosis. Extensive erythroderma can also cause dermatogenic enteropathy.

Hepatic disease

■ *Hepatocellular disorders.* Cutaneous signs very often accompany the other features of liver disease, but are by no means specific. Palmar erythema is common, but also occurs in thyrotoxicosis, pregnancy, connective tissue diseases, and in many normal people. Spider naevi are an unreliable indicator unless present in large numbers. Linear telangiectases are a frequent finding ('paper money skin') but are not confined to patients with hepatic disease.

As liver failure progresses, there may be jaundice, purpura, hyper-pigmentation of exposed skin, digital clubbing, oedema, and the enlarged abdominal veins of collateral shunts. Sparse body hair may be accompanied by gynaecomastia in men. The nails are often opaque white, except for a narrow band of erythema near the free edge. With chronic hypoalbuminaemia there may be paired white bands, parallel to the lunula.

Hyperpigmentation is a regular and usually early sign of haemochromatosis. Pigmentation is most marked on exposed skin and in the flexures. The skin is dry and thin, and may show the cutaneous signs of liver failure.

■ *Cholestatic disorders.* Generalised pruritus is a constant feature of diseases which produce elevated levels of unconjugated bile acids, and may be an early manifestation of biliary cirrhosis or drug-induced cholestasis. The pruritus of biliary cirrhosis is later accompanied by jaundice, pigmentation and xanthomas.

■ **Chronic active hepatitis.** Some patients develop distinctive crusted red papules on the trunk and legs, which heal leaving pale scars. Less characteristic lesions may be erythematous, acneiform, or purpuric. Erythema nodosum, pyoderma gangrenosum and lichen planus are also seen more frequently among patients with this disorder.

■ **Viral hepatitis.** During the prodromal phase of hepatitis B infection, immune complexes containing the surface antigen of this DNA virus and its antibody produce a transient syndrome resembling *serum-sickness*. Arthritis and mild glomerulonephritis are associated with a series of consecutive skin changes. The usual sequence is—first urticaria, then palpable purpura, followed by erythema multiforme, which is succeeded by a toxic erythema and, occasionally, a final lichen planus-like transient rash. High levels of the antibody may be associated with mixed cryoglobulinaemia which produces palpable purpuric lesions on the legs. Persistence of the surface antigen is associated with the hepatitis B-induced polyarteritis nodosa that manifests as livedo with deep inflammatory nodules arranged in a retiform pattern along the course of the artery. Occasionally these nodules may ulcerate.

In children, a particular subtype of hepatitis B, characterised by the ayw surface antigen, produces a papular dermatitis on the buttocks, face and limbs. This papular acrodermatitis of childhood (**Gianotti–Crosti syndrome**) is associated with lymphadenopathy and a mild anicteric acute hepatitis. All the signs and symptoms resolve with no treatment over a period of a few months. Similar acrolocated papulovesicular syndromes, without the hepatitis, may occur with other viruses.

Pancreatic disease

Nodular panniculitis involving particularly the trunk and lower limbs may complicate acute or chronic pancreatitis, and may be an early manifestation of pancreatic carcinoma. Patients with unsuspected carcinoma of the pancreas may present also with migratory thrombophlebitis. Glucagon-secreting tumours of the pancreas, usually carcinomatous, are associated with a distinctive syndrome in which an erosive dermatitis, involving especially the perianal region, lower trunk, buttocks, groins and thighs, is associated with a range of extracutaneous features including glossitis, diabetes, anaemia and weight loss. Purpura around the umbilicus or flanks is a well recognised sign of pancreatitis; and hyperlipidaemia may produce pancreatitis and xanthomas.

Renal disease

■ **Renal failure.** The pallor of anaemia may be partly masked by a sallow or brownish-grey discolouration. The skin is dry and scaly, and subject to recurrent bacterial infections. The distal part of the nail bed may be coloured dark brown or reddish, often with contrasting pallor of the proximal part ('half and half nail'). Pruritus, and purpura due to platelet dysfunction, are late complications. However, palpable purpura may be part of vasculitis involving both the skin and kidney. Cutaneous calcification may occur if phosphate levels are not kept low with low phosphate diet and oral administration of aluminium hydroxide.

Altered clearance of porphyrins in renal failure may induce blisters of the type seen in the porphyrias. A nodular type of follicular keratosis (Kyrle's disease) most commonly found on the legs, is seen more commonly in those with renal failure.

■ **Skin and kidney syndromes** include those with cutaneous vascular lesions such as allergic vasculitis, Wegener's granulomatosis and polyarteritis nodosa, and the defect in ceramide metabolism (Fabry's disease) that produces angiokeratomas centred around the upper thighs; the collagen diseases scleroderma and lupus erythematosus; and the malformation syndromes such as tuberous sclerosis and pseudoxanthoma elasticum.

Arthritis

There are many diseases in which cutaneous lesions are associated with arthropathy. Most of these are discussed in other chapters.

Rheumatoid arthritis

Subcutaneous nodules are present in 20 per cent of patients, mostly the more severely affected. Tests for rheumatoid factor are positive, and there is often a significant titre of antinuclear antibodies. The nodules are firm, lobulated, mobile, and painless. They are found around joints, or in areas subject to pressure and trauma. Typical sites are the elbows, hands and knees. The duration is variable, but they may persist for months. Occasionally, a nodule becomes necrotic in the centre and ulcerates through to the surface.

In patients with longstanding rheumatoid arthritis, the skin becomes shiny and atrophic, especially over the fingers. There may be linear telangiectases similar to those of lupus erythematosus, and small infarcts in the nail folds or pads of the fingers. Vasculitis may add purpuric, bullous, and ulcerative lesions, or gangrene of the fingers or toes. Leg ulcers are common in badly affected patients, and may have the features of pyoderma gangrenosum.

An eruption of small pink macules or papules sometimes accompanies the evening temperature spike, particularly in children.

Rheumatic fever

Subcutaneous nodules are smaller, and less persistent than in rheumatoid arthritis. They occur over the elbows, occiput, other bony prominences, or close to tendons. The nodules are present in 30 per cent of patients and are usually associated with rheumatic carditis. Urticaria or urticaria-like lesions are present in more than 10 per cent of patients. Crops of erythematous papules or small plaques may erupt, mainly over the trunk and proximal parts of the limbs, and enlarge peripherally with central clearing before fading completely within hours or days (erythema marginatum).

Gout

Tophi are visible accumulations of uric acid in skin or periarticular tissue. They range from a few millimetres to several centimetres in size and, if sufficiently superficial, impart a creamy white or yellowish colour to the skin. Trauma to the nodules may allow the discharge of thick chalky material. Common sites include the helix, antihelix, olecranon and prepatellar areas, and about the fingers and toes, especially the region of the first metatarsophalangeal joint.

The skin and internal malignancy

1. Specific
   (a) cutaneous metastases
   (b) Paget's disease of the nipple
   (c) extramammary Paget's disease
2. Non-specific
   (a) humoral syndromes
   (b) inflammatory dermatoses
   (c) proliferative dermatoses
   (d) arsenical keratoses and Bowen's disease
3. Genetic associations
4. Lymphoma and leukaemia

Cutaneous metastases

About 3 per cent of visceral cancers metastasise to the skin. Cutaneous metastases are usually late events, with little bearing on the prognosis. Less often, a cutaneous tumour may be the first evidence of recurrence and, rarely, a metastasis to skin may be the earliest manifestation of disease. Most cutaneous metastases are painless, rapidly growing dermal nodules. They are usually mobile, but may be fixed to the epidermis or form infiltrated plaques. They may be firm, stony hard, or relatively soft, vascular and even pulsatile. Ulceration may occur, but is uncommon.

By far the most frequent primary carcinoma metastasising to skin is cancer of the breast. More than half of all cutaneous metastases originate in the breast. The most common presentation is an inflammatory infiltration of the skin which overlies the tumour. Pink, purple or black nodules may appear, or sheets of cancer cells may slowly harden the chest wall. One-third of breast metastases occur on the scalp, as do one-fifth of metastases from cancer of other organs.

After the breast, the organs primarily involved are lung, stomach, uterus, colon, prostate and kidney. With hypernephroma, the nodule may occur long after nephrectomy, and be mistaken for granuloma telangiectaticum, squamous cell carcinoma, or amelanotic melanoma. Although the histology often shows only anaplastic carcinoma, the tissue of origin may be identifiable. The most frequent sites for cutaneous metastases are the front of the chest, scalp, and abdominal wall, but any area may be involved. *(Colour plate 65)*

Paget's disease of the nipple

A weeping or crusted lesion, which clinically resembles dermatitis, persists despite topical therapy, and slowly extends onto the areola. The disease is unilateral and, unlike atopic or seborrhoeic dermatitis, does not respond to corticosteroids. Biopsy reveals characteristic large round cells with abundant cytoplasm, which stains with the special periodic acid-Schiff (PAS) technique. There is always carcinoma of the underlying breast.

Extramammary Paget's disease

A very uncommon lesion, histologically indistinguishable from Paget's disease of the nipple, may develop in the anogenital region (and rarely, at other sites) as a sharply demarcated, itchy plaque with an oozing, crusted or scaling surface. In one-half of the patients with extra-mammary Paget's disease, there is a discoverable carcinoma, which is usually nearby but may be as distant as the breast.

Humoral syndromes

■ *Cushing's syndrome* with hyperpigmentation is the most common of unusual endocrines syndromes where tumours of non-endocrine origin secrete substances with effects similar to normal hormones.

The endocrine features parallel the course of the tumour, disappearing with its successful removal and recurring with regrowth. Anaplastic carcinoma of the lung is the most frequent primary tumour, but many others are described. Other effects of such non-endocrine tumours include gynaecomastia and precocious puberty.

■ *The carcinoid syndrome* is a striking clinical pattern associated either with hepatic metastases from a gastro-intestinal carcinoid tumour, or with carcinoid arising in bile ducts, pancreas, bronchi or ovaries. The patient suffers episodes of flushing; which are usually accompanied by bronchospasm and diarrhoea. During these attacks a vivid erythema develops on the face, neck and chest, which lasts about 15 minutes and becomes dusky before fading from the centre. With repeated attacks, permanent facial erythema and telangiectasia may develop. Although carcinoid is a serotin-secreting tumour, its cutaneous manifestations are thought to be mediated by vasoactive peptides, particularly the kinins.

■ *The glucagonoma syndrome* is the association of an alpha cell tumour of the pancreas with elevated plasma levels of glucagon, hyperglycaemia, anaemia, glossitis and a cutaneous eruption somewhat similar to pustular psoriasis. Cutaneous lesions begin as fragile vesicles or flaccid bullae, but the blisters are so superficial and easily ruptured that the patient frequently presents with polycyclic erosions fringed with a shaggy band of desquamation.

Inflammatory dermatoses

■ *Generalised pruritus.* Widespread, unexplained itching, especially in the elderly patient, should arouse the suspicion of malignant disease.

Usually, the cause will be the xeroderma so common in old people, or a drug reaction, but a few patients will be found to have lymphoma and, less often, leukaemia, or internal cancer.

■ *Dermatomyositis.* In children, there is no association between malignant disease and dermatomyositis, but in adults with onset of dermatomyositis after forty years of age, carcinoma or lymphoma is present in 25 per cent of patients.

■ *Migratory thrombophlebitis,* or *deep vein thrombosis* which cannot be attributed to the usual causes, is suggestive of carcinoma, particularly of the pancreas. Most cancers reported in association with thrombophlebitis have been inoperable.

■ *Vesiculobullous eruptions.* Atypical bullous eruptions which do not conform well to any particular pattern of bullous disease warrant a search for visceral malignant tumours.

■ *Erythema multiforme* is an infrequent manifestation of cancer, but a fairly common sequel to radiotherapy of cancer.

■ *Urticaria* has been described as a manifestation of internal carcinoma but the association, if valid, must be very uncommon indeed.

■ *Erythema gyratum repens* is a striking pattern of annular erythema with a peculiar wood-grain appearance. Its association with malignant disease is convincing.

■ *Erythroderma (exfoliative dermatitis)* is a common association of malignancy. Lymphoma and leukaemia may present this way.

Proliferative dermatoses

■ *Acanthosis nigricans* which begins in adult life is so regularly associated with visceral carcinoma that thorough investigation should be undertaken in every case. Although obese adults occasionally develop similar changes in the large flexures, the onset of itchy, progressive acanthosis nigricans in adult life is almost always associated with frank or occult malignant disease, especially if the acathosis nigricans extends to non-flexural locations. In 80 per cent of patients the tumour is an intra-abdominal adenocarcinoma.

■ *Clubbing* of the fingers and toes is a well-known association of lung cancer. The clubbing tends to be accompanied by discomfort and hypertrophic osteoarthropathy.

■ *Ichthyosis* usually begins in childhood. Onset of ichthyosis in adult life is uncommon and warrants a search for a neoplastic process, especially Hodgkin's disease.

Arsenical keratoses and Bowen's disease

The presence of arsenical keratoses and areas of arsenic-induced Bowen's disease necessitates regular examination to detect the development of carcinoma of internal organs, particularly the lung.

Genetic associations

■ *Diffuse hyperkeratosis of palms and soles* has been described in two families in which more than a quarter of those with the skin marker developed carcinoma of the oesophagus by the age of 60 years. No member of either family without the cutaneous marker developed the carcinoma.

■ *Gardner's syndrome* is the association of polyposis coli (which has a high incidence of carcinoma) with multiple benign cutaneous tumours, including epidermoid cysts, lipomas, fibromas and desmoid tumours.

■ *Peutz–Jeghers syndrome* is the association of pigmented macules around the mouth and over the digits with polyposis of the small intestine. Polyposis of the stomach and colon, which may result in carcinoma, occurs less frequently.

Cutaneous manifestations of lymphoma

One-half of all patients with lymphoma develop cutaneous changes. These changes may be the non-specific sequelae of altered function and are particularly common in patients with Hodgkin's disease. Specific lymphomatous infiltration of the skin is very uncommon in patients with either Hodgkin's disease or B-cell lymphoma, but is the cardinal feature of cutaneous T-cell lymphoma.

■ *Specific lymphomatous infiltration* may produce papules, nodules, tumours and ulcers. The colour of the lesions is very variable, but is often a striking pink, reddish brown or purple. Distribution may be widespread with a haphazard growth of papules or nodules, or lesions may be clustered or may develop peculiar arched, circular or horseshoe shapes. The texture is firm but not hard. Size may fluctuate even without treatment, and lesions may disappear spontaneously. Specific skin lesions may precede other manifestations by a long period, particularly with the small cell types of B-cell lymphoma.

■ *Non-specific skin lesions* occur more frequently in Hodgkin's disease, but the mechanisms of production are not clear. Pruritus is a common accompaniment of Hodgkin's disease, and may persist for long periods before the underlying disease becomes apparent. Scratching produces excoriations and, especially on the legs, papules may develop—Hodgkin's prurigo. The itchy skin is frequently dry and somewhat scaly, and may become frankly ichthyotic, sometimes with diffuse hyperkeratosis of the palms and soles. Acquired ichthyosis always warrants exclusion of lymphoma. The dry, scaling skin may progress to generalised exfoliative dermatitis, or erythroderma may begin as a diffuse infiltrated erythema. The hair may be lost and the nails thickened and lifted by subungual hyperkeratosis.

Lymphoma should be excluded when hair loss produced by mucin within the hair follicle lining (follicular mucinosis) manifests as widespread small boggy papules. Follicular mucinosis localised to the head and neck region is not usually associated with lymphoma.

About 25 per cent of patients with lymphoma develop hyper-pigmentation, which may be diffuse, Addisonian in distribution, or confined to areas altered by scratching. Acanthosis nigricans is not usually a feature of the lymphomas. Pallor, jaundice, purpura and ecchymoses are frequent and predictable manifestations. Urticaria and erythema multiforme are uncommon features, as is vasculitis.

Herpes zoster is a common complication of malignant disease, especially lymphoma. The infection is very frequently atypical, with a tendency to spread beyond adjoining dermatomes. It may generalise or become haemorrhagic or necrotic, and the pain is usually severe and persistent.

Cutaneous manifestations of leukaemia

As with lymphomas, cutaneous lesions of patients with leukaemia may be specific or non-specific. Specific lesions due to leukaemic infiltrates occur in about 25 per cent of patients with monocytic leukaemia, but are otherwise uncommon and tend to develop rather late in the course of leukaemia. Specific lesions of monocytic leukaemia may involve much of the cutaneous surface and frequently affect the mouth. The gums are often swollen, bright red and bleed easily with minor trauma. The trunk is the more common site of specific infiltration by granulocytic leukaemias, while specific lesions of lymphocytic leukaemias have a predilection for the face and limbs. The lesions themselves are clinically indistinguishable from those of the lymphomas.

Non-specific manifestations include pruritus, herpes zoster, purpura and erythroderma. Acquired ichthyosis and pruritus are more a feature of lymphocytic than myelocytic leukaemia.

Mycosis fungoides (Colour plate 59)

It is likely that cutaneous T-cell lymphomas constitute a small group of closely related diseases produced by malignant proliferation of helper T-cells. The more differentiated form is, at least initially, strongly epidermotropic and presents clinically as mycosis fungoides.

Mycosis fungoides is a unique lymphoma which first manifests in the skin as widespread non-indurated erythematous patches that are often misdiagnosed as eczema. This stage often persists for years before the diagnosis is made. The early histology shows a band-like upper dermal chronic inflammatory infiltrate with a number of cells showing extremely clefted and convoluted nuclei. The infiltrate gradually thickens and impinges on the epidermis. Small collections of the atypical cells appear within the epidermis. Eventually the infiltrate becomes frankly lymphomatous, with increasing numbers of atypical cells, and spreads deeper into the dermis and subcutis.

Infiltrated plaques slowly develop, often with striking arcuate, circular or horseshoe patterns, and a red or purplish colour. Pruritus is severe and difficult to relieve. Tumours evolve and tend to ulcerate. Uncommonly, the course is telescoped into a matter of months and presentation with erythroderma is not rare. Mycosis fungoides begins in and is usually confined to the skin, but, with time, lymph nodes, spleen, and other organs may be involved.

Sézary syndrome

The rare Sézary syndrome is a malignant proliferation of helper T-cells in which the malignant cells appear to have less affinity for the epidermis than in mycosis fungoides. Systemic involvement is a regular feature, with malignant cells present in blood, lymph nodes and viscera, as well as in cutaneous lesions.

Severe generalised pruritus, thick infiltrated skin, erythroderma and lymphadenopathy are invariably present. Diffuse hyperkeratosis of the palms and soles, nail dystrophy, alopecia and hyperpigmentation are less constant features.

Treatment of either mycosis fungoides or Sézary syndrome should be undertaken only by those with special knowledge of these diseases.

Histiocytic disorders

Histiocytosis-X

Histiocytosis-X may be regarded as a spectrum of disseminated granulomatous disease, in which the histiocyte dominates the microscopic picture. Although there is considerable overlap, the spectrum separates into three distinct syndromes on the basis of age at onset, degree of granulomatous reaction, severity, and prognosis.

Letterer–Siwe disease usually begins in the first two years of life as a generalised histiocytic proliferation which involves the viscera and skin, with little tendency to granuloma formation. *Hand–Schüller–Christian disease* occurs in older children. There are abundant histiocytes, but the onset is less acute, and the prognosis better than in Letterer-Siwe disease. Lesions of *eosinophilic granuloma* are often confined to bone. The onset is in older children and adults, and the prognosis is excellent.

Cutaneous manifestations

The skin lesions of Letterer-Siwe disease may precede systemic features and provide a means of early diagnosis. The earliest changes are frequently on the scalp, with redness and scaling which resemble seborrhoeic dermatitis. The characteristic lesions are discrete, yellow-brown scaling papules, a few millimetres in diameter, on the scalp, face, neck and trunk. Some lesions are vesicular, and tiny pustules may form close to the hairline. Coalescence of papules produces scaly or weeping plaques which are sometimes crusted, and often purpuric. In fulminating cases, purpura may be the only cutaneous manifestation. Persistent ulceration of the mouth or perineum is common.

The onset of Hand–Schüller–Christian disease is insidious, and more often marked by osseous than cutaneous involvement. Bony lesions may be discovered because of cyst-like swellings on the scalp, chronic ear discharge, or loss of teeth. Cutaneous lesions are present in about one-third of patients. Yellowish-brown papules are characteristic, but dark scaly patches and multiple xanthomas may occur. Proptosis is a classic, but relatively uncommon, sign. Diabetes insipidus is present in 50 per cent of patients.

Sarcoidosis

Cutaneous sarcoidal granulomas are present in 10 to 35 per cent of patients with systemic sarcoidosis. However, similar lesions frequently occur in the skin without other evidence of systemic disease. Whether or not these cutaneous granulomas should be considered as valid lesions of sarcoidosis is debatable. For the present it may be better to reserve the diagnosis of sarcoidosis for patients in whom visceral involvement is demonstrable, accepting the presence of cutaneous sarcoidal granulomas only as indicating the need for adequate assessment and follow-up to detect the possible development of ocular and visceral sarcoidosis.

Histology

An outstanding feature of sarcoidosis is the histological uniformity of lesions in all affected organs. The characteristic microscopic lesion is a granuloma with insignificant central necrosis. Circumscribed clusters of epithelioid cells with few, if any, giant cells are surrounded by a light infiltrate of lymphocytes. As the granuloma matures, fibroblasts appear at the periphery and fibrosis follows.

Clinical features

The most common cutaneous manifestation of sarcoidosis is erythema nodosum, which develops in about one-third of cases, occurs early in the course, and is accompanied by hilar lymphadenopathy.

Specific lesions range in colour from purplish-red to yellow or brown, often beginning as violaceous papules or nodules which later fade to brown. Plaques may form by coalescence of discrete foci or as a more diffuse granulomatous infiltration. Expanding nodules or plaques with central clearing may form annular lesions with some resemblance to granuloma annulare.

Papular lesions can occur at any site, but favour the face, limbs, old scars, and sites of recent trauma. Nodules and plaques are more common on the trunk, buttocks, limbs and face. Involvement of the nose, earlobes, fingers and toes produces a striking clinical picture (lupus pernio), which is frequently accompanied by digital bone cysts and pulmonary sarcoidosis.

Diagnosis

Granulomatous infiltrates may also occur with chronic infections, vasculitis, Hodgkin's disease, and in response to exogenous irritants such as talc, silica or beryllium. Sarcoid-like granulomas in a skin biopsy support the suspicion of sarcoidosis, but the diagnosis is insecure when it is based on cutaneous features alone.

Gallium-67 accumulates in active lesions of sarcoidosis, but the accumulation is not specific and is more useful in repeat scanning for progress than for diagnosis. Angiotensin-converting enzyme activity is usually raised in active sarcoidosis, but the test is not specific, and is not reliably positive in patients with active disease.

The Kveim test is not longer performed because of the high rate of false-positive results.

Treatment

Cutaneous sarcoidosis is rarely an indication for systemic therapy. With oral corticosteroids improvement occurs, but generally lasts only for as long as the steroid is continued. Minor lesions are better left untreated. A fluorinated steroid applied under plasic occlusion, or injected intralesionally, may accelerate resolution of troublesome lesions.

Biochemical disorders

Porphyrias

Porphyrins are produced throughout the body, and function as components of haemoglobin and some enzymes. Small amounts are normally excreted in the urine as coproporphyrin and uroporphyrin, and in the faeces as coproporphyrin and protoporphyrin. The porphyrias are primary disturbances in the metabolism of porphyrins or their precursors as a result of enzyme defects.

Photosensitivity is an outstanding feature of all porphyrias affecting the skin, and is a result of photo-excitation of 'resonant' porphyrin molecules. The activating wave-lengths approximate 400 nm and are not filtered off by window glass nor by the usual UV-B sunscreens. The various porphyrins differ in lipid solubility, and localise at different levels in the skin, which accounts for clinical characteristics peculiar to one or another of the porphyrias. Of the porphyrias which affect the skin, only the three more frequently encountered ones are discussed here.

Porphyria cutanea tarda

Predisposition to porphyria cutanea tarda is associated with defective function of uroporphyrinogen decarboxylase and in some families is inherited as an autosomal dominant characteristic. In other individuals, the enzyme is localised to the liver and manifests as a result of exposure to specific toxins. In either case, expression of the clinical disease usually follows chemical injury to the liver, most often by alcohol.

Clinical features *(Colour plate 60)*

Blisters, sometimes haemorrhagic, develop on light-exposed areas, often leaving milia as they heal. The skin is fragile, minor knocks producing blisters or small erosions which heal slowly. Exposed skin develops an aged, weather-beaten appearance, with hyperpigmentation. There may be pale, scarred areas which resemble plaques of scleroderma. Facial hypertrichosis is common, particularly around the eyes and upper parts of the cheeks. Associated diseases include cirrhosis of the liver and diabetes.

Pathology

The bullae are subepidermal, with minimal inflammatory infiltrate. The pattern of excretion of urinary prophyrins is diagnostic. There is a marked increase in uroporphyrin (8-carboxyl-porphyrin) and 7-carboxyl-porphyrin, with lesser increases of 6- and 5-carboxyl-porphyrins. There is a moderate increase of coproporphyrin excretion in both urine and faeces. The serum iron level is frequently elevated and liver function tests usually provide evidence of hepatocellular disease. Only a few laboratories are currently able to measure the enzyme.

Treatment

The patient should be urged to abstain from alcohol, and should be advised of the adverse effects of sunlight. Most patients can be successfully treated by phlebotomy. At each venesection 400 to 500 ml of blood are removed, and the venesections are repeated at intervals of two to four weeks. Five or six phlebotomies are sufficient to achieve remission in most cases, but the haemoglobin, serum iron and iron-binding capacity need to be monitored.

For patients in whom even mild anaemia might prove dangerous, chloroquine therapy is an effective alternative. However, the rapid flushing of porphyrin from the liver by chloroquine may be accompanied by fever, malaise, abdominal pain, and biochemical evidence of acute hepatic toxicity. The risk is considerably reduced by a low-dose schedule in which only 125 mg of chloroquine is administered twice a week. Safety of the low-dose regimen is further enhanced if the patient is treated by one to four phlebotomies before commencing the chloroquine.

Porphyria variegata

Although inherited as an autosomal dominant trait, predisposition to porphyria variegata may remain unsuspected until unmasked by pregnancy or administration of a drug, particularly a barbiturate.

Clinical features

Cutaneous changes similar to porphyria cutanea tarda are combined with the systemic features of acute intermittent porphyria—abdominal pain, vomiting, mental disturbances, neuropathy, epilepsy, and even bulbar palsy. Systemic features are more prominent in women, while cutaneous lesions frequently dominate the clinical picture in men.

Pathology

The defective enzyme is protoporphyrinogen oxidase. During an acute attack, there are elevated levels of urinary coproporphyrin as well as the porphyrin precursors δ-aminolaevulinic acid and porphobilinogen. However, the total urinary porphyrins are generally much lower than in patients with porphyria cutanea tarda. Moreover, the ratio of uroporphyrin to coproporphyrin is less than 1:1, whereas in porphyria cutanea tarda the ratio usually exceeds 5:1. During remission, faecal coproporphyrin and protoporphyrin are increased.

Treatment

There is no specific treatment for porphyria variegata, but the systemic component of acute episodes needs careful management. Glucose infusion and haematin infusions have been reported successful.

The patient should be protected from trauma and sunlight, and should be warned of the drugs likely to precipitate an acute attack. These include barbiturates, sulphonamides, alcohol, oestrogens, griseofulvin, methyldopa and chloroquine.

Erythropoietic protoporphyria

The disease is inherited in autosomal dominant fashion. The onset is in childhood, with burning and tingling of the skin after exposure to sunlight. The discomfort begins within minutes of exposure, at first with no objective changes. Over a period of time, the backs of the hands develop a cobblestone thickening, the nose becomes scarred, and the lips pursed. Rarely, there is redness and swelling similar to sunburn, and blistering or purpura that is restricted to light-exposed areas.

There is an increased incidence of cholelithiasis and structural changes in the liver. The prevalence of serious liver disease is unknown but rapidly progressive hepatic failure is an occasional complication of protoporphyria which can result in death.

Pathology

The levels of urinary porphyrins remain normal. Faecal excretion of protoporphyrin is increased, but the diagnosis is established by estimation of the red-cell protoporphyrin concentration, which is grossly elevated. The defective enzyme is ferrochelatase, which is normally used to chelate protoporphyrin with iron to form haem.

Treatment

As with other porphyrias, the activating wavelengths are in the UV-A band, which makes protection difficult, short of using an opaque sunscreen such as zinc cream or titanium dioxide. Good symptomatic relief for most of these children is provided by β-carotene taken by mouth, but the long-term effect, if any, on the hepatic changes is unknown.

It would seem prudent for patients to avoid known hepatotoxins, particularly alcohol, and in view of the rapid deterioration of liver function which may occur in patients with protoporphyria, even subtle changes in liver function should be carefully assessed. As cholestyramine has been found to remove protoporphyrin from the liver, minor alterations of liver function may indicate the need for liver biopsy as a prelude to cholestyramine therapy.

Hyperlipidaemias

Histiocytes within the dermis phagocytose lipids. When lipid-laden foamy histiocytes form aggregates that are visible as pinkish-yellow nodules or plaques, the collections are termed xanthomas and the levels of plasma lipids are almost always elevated. The raised levels occur either as a primary disorder or secondary to biliary cirrhosis, nephrotic syndrome, myxoedema, severe uncontrolled diabetes or, occasionally, myelomatosis or leukaemia.

The recognition of xanthomas associated with hyperlipidaemia usually initiates treatment that can reverse potentially serious atheromatous cardiovascular disease.

Clinical features *(Colour plate 61)*

■ **Xanthelasma** Small yellow or brown papules form on the upper lid, close to the inner canthus. The papules coalesce, and extend laterally as a soft band across the eyelid. Xanthelasma generally affects both upper lids and sometimes the lower lids as well.

■ *Tuberous xanthomas* are yellow to orange-brown papules or nodules. They develop in the dermis and subcutaneous layer over bony prominences, particularly the elbows, knuckles, knees, heels and buttocks. Larger nodules may be lobulated and reach several centimetres in diameter. Tuberous xanthomas are generally asymptomatic, but may be tender to pressure.

■ *Tendinous xanthomas* are firm subcutaneous nodules attached to tendons or the ligaments around joints. They are formed by a diffuse infiltration of lipid within the tendon, and are found mostly on the Achilles tendons, the tendons of the hands and feet, knees and elbows.

■ *Eruptive xanthomas* tend to appear suddenly, in crops. They are extremely itchy, brownish-yellow papules, often surrounded by an erythematous halo. Buttocks, thighs and trunk are the common sites.

■ *Plane xanthomas* are soft, yellowish or tan streaks or plaques, most frequently found on the face, neck, upper trunk and palms. Plane xanthomas are very uncommon. They may occur alone or with other xanthomas.

Xanthoma-lipid associations

No xanthomatous lesion is specific for any particular abnormality of lipid metabolism. A complete physical examination and assessment of plasma lipids is necessary in every case. However, some clinical patterns are at least suggestive of the type of lipoprotein involved.

■ *Xanthelasma* is more often an isolated abnormality in patients with normal lipoprotein levels, but if the patient is a child or young adult, plasma lipids are commonly elevated and the rise is usually due to low density lipoprotein (LDL) cholesterol.

■ *Tuberous xanthomas* are found in familial hypercholesterolaemia or familial combined hyperlipidaemia.

■ *Tendinous xanthomas* are usually typical of familial hypercholesterolaemia but may be seen in any patient with raised LDL cholesterol.

■ *Eruptive xanthomas* are associated with very high triglyceride levels and are therefore a feature of the elevated VLDL levels seen with familial hypertriglyceridaemia. However, they may be associated with any lipid disorder except familial hypercholesterolaemia. Uncontrolled diabetes is still the most common cause. *(Colour plate 61)*

■ *Plane xanthomas* may be associated with normal lipid levels, especially in patients with myelomatosis. When hyperlipidaemia is present, the biochemical abnormality is usually impaired conversion of the chylomicron remnant particle to low density lipoprotein.

■ *Juvenile xanthogranuloma* is a benign, self-limiting lesion with no associated disturbance of plasma lipids. Lesions may be solitary or multiple, and generally appear in the first year of life as well-defined, yellowish-red nodules, most frequently on the scalp, face or trunk. After an early increase in size, the nodules gradually resolve within a few years.

Most patients with xanthogranuloma suffer no more than a mildly disfiguring dermatosis of limited duration. However, xanthomatous deposits occasionally form in the uveal tract and cornea, and minor visceral involvement may occur. There is a very inconstant association with neurofibromatosis and, less frequently, myeloproliferative disease.

Amyloidosis

Amyloid may be deposited in the skin of patients with myeloma, or with primary systemic amyloidosis. It is doubtful if cutaneous lesions ever result from amyloidosis that is secondary to prolonged inflammation or infection. Amyloid may, however, occur in the skin alone, in the absence of detectable visceral involvement.

■ *Cutaneous lesions of systemic amyloidosis.* In both primary systemic and myeloma-associated amyloidosis, the mucocutaneous surfaces are involved in about one-third of the cases. Clinically, the lesions of either type are indistinguishable from those of the other, most often forming waxy yellow papules or nodules on the eyelids, face, scalp, upper trunk, and major flexures. Occasionally, the amyloid is deposited as firm waxy plaques or, more diffusely, as a sclerodermoid thickening of the face and hands. Small infiltrated vessels are easily ruptured by trauma, and rubbing or squeezing frequently produces petechiae or ecchymoses in affected and, sometimes, in apparently unaffected skin.

The gingivae may be thick, spongy and bleed easily after minor trauma, and the tongue may be thickened in a diffuse or spotty fashion. Macroglossia is present in about 15 per cent of patients.

■ *Localised cutaneous amyloidosis.* When amyloid is limited to the skin, without systemic involvement, the deposits are usually small and restricted to the dermal papillae. Clinically, there may be a persistent, intensely itchy eruption of grey or yellowish brown hyperkeratotic papules, usually on the legs (lichen amyloidosis), or the patient may present with poorly demarcated, rippled areas of pigmentation, generally on the legs or back (macular amyloidosis). Rare nodular and tumefactive variants occur.

Nutritional deficiencies

In practice, nutritional deficiencies are almost always multiple and more often the result of malabsorption than of dietary insufficiency.

The patient, though often pale, may be hyperpigmented, usually in an Addisonian pattern. Terminal hair may be fine, sparse and show premature greying, and the nails brittle and easily cracked along their free edges. The skin tends to be dry, sometimes with follicular hyperkeratosis, and there may be an erythematous, scaly dermatitis. The tongue and buccal mucosa are frequently red and sore, and the lips tender, fissured and crusted. Oedema is common and there may be a haemorrhagic diathesis.

Pellagra

Produced by deficiency of nicotinic acid, pellagra is most commonly seen in the alcoholic but may occasionally be produced by drugs such as isoniazid and, rarely, occurs in the carcinoid syndrome.

The tongue is swollen, sore and bright red. There is dermatitis of light-exposed areas and usually also at sites of friction, particularly the groins and perineum. The dermatitis resembles sunburn and is followed either by hyperpigmentation or scaling with hypopigmentation.

Scurvy

This is still occasionally seen in infants or adults who have a low intake of fruit. Perifollicular haemorrhages or painful deep haematomas are usually the most prominent signs. Closer inspection will reveal friable gums and coiled 'corkscrew' hairs.

Kwashiorkor

This may occur in the neglected child in whom severe protein depletion is almost invariably accompanied by oedema. The skin takes on a reddish brown or purplish discolouration and may crack in a crazy-paving pattern. Patchy desquamation is followed by hypopigmentation.

Zinc deficiency

Acrodermatitis enteropathica is indicative of zinc deficiency, which is usually seen in those who have had severe muscle loss following injury and have had prolonged intravenous alimentation.

19

Connective tissue diseases

1. Lupus erythematosus
2. Scleroderma
3. Eosinophilic fasciitis
4. Dermatomyositis
5. Mixed connective tissue disease
6. Sjögren's syndrome

Lupus erythematosus (LE)

This is an uncommon disorder with a wide range of expression which varies from mild chronic disease of a single organ to a severe multisystem illness that may be rapidly fatal, especially if there is serious renal or central nervous system involvement.

Although systemic disease may be present in lupus erythematosus with no skin signs, and the presence or absence of systemic involvement cannot be determined with certainty on the basis of skin changes, the various patterns of cutaneous lupus erythematosus tend to indicate subsets of patients with a relatively predictable risk of developing a certain degree of systemic severity. The skin signs therefore play a large part in indicating how intensively the patient with lupus erythematosus needs to be followed.

Aetiology

The disease occurs in all races, at all ages, and in both sexes, but has its highest incidence among young to middle-aged women, and is possibly endocrine dependent. There appears to be a genetic predisposition to the development of LE, with a pronounced clustering of cases in particular races and families. Certain subsets of lupus erythematosus have very strong associations with particular HLA antigens.

Whatever the level of predisposition, the history often suggests that LE is precipitated by agents external to the patient. Sunlight causes aggravation of skin lesions in one-third of patients, and systemic disease in a smaller proportion. Cutaneous lesions may develop at the site of burns, trauma or exposure to cold. In up to 10 per cent of patients with systemic LE, the disease is drug-induced.

Pathogenesis

There is clearly a disturbance of immunological function. There are reduced numbers of circulating lymphocytes, especially T lymphocytes. The function of supressor T lymphocytes is impaired. It is thought that, secondary to these changes, there is hyper-reactivity of B lymphocytes, with increased synthesis of immunoglobulin and enhanced production of a wide range of auto-antibodies. The increased gamma globulin production results in increased ESR in vitro.

The more serious manifestations of LE relate to the production of the antibody most characteristic of lupus erythematosus, which is antibody directed against double-stranded DNA. This antigen–antibody combination is very potent at forming immune complexes that cause small vessel damage, especially to those of renal glomeruli.

Antibodies may be directed against specific tissue antigens and cause damage in that way. The haemolytic anaemia of LE and thrombo-cytopenia are examples of that type of reaction. Antiphospholipid antibodies, by reacting against phospholipid in the test reagent antigens in vitro, produce a false positive reaction for syphilis and prolong phospholipid-dependent coagulation tests. In the patient, however, antiphospholipid antibody, by reacting against vascular endothelial cells, produces thromboses in deep veins, livedo and leg ulcers due to thromboses in superficial vessels, and miscarriages due to placental vessel thromboses.

In the skin, antibodies are deposited in the basement membrane zone at the junction of the dermis and epidermis. This can be demonstrated by direct immunofluorescence of skin biopsy in 90 per cent of cutaneous lesions. In more than 60 per cent of those with systemic disease this can also be demonstrated in clinically uninvolved skin. How this relates to production of skin lesions is uncertain, as is the exact mechanism of many other manifestations of this disease.

Histology

Despite the many and varied clinical appearances of skin changes in this disease, histology is relatively uniform when the skin is directly involved in LE.

The basal cells of the epidermis show intracellular oedema of a type known as hydropic degeneration. A patchy infiltrate of lymphocytes appears around blood vessels and hair follicles. There is hyperkeratosis which extends into the hair follicle producing follicular plugs. Some basal cells undergo eosinophilic condensation of the cytoplasm, become smaller, lose the nucleus and 'drop' into the papillary dermis. These are termed 'apoptotic bodies' or 'Civatte bodies'. Secondary to the epidermal basal cell damage, melanin may be deposited into the dermis ('pigmentary incontinence') and engulfed by macrophages.

Clinical patterns

The division of LE into clinically based subsets with the aim of predicting systemic severity is effective because, although activity of disease may fluctuate, disease pattern is usually constant for that patient.

The subsets are grouped according to risk and severity of systemic involvement.

1. Chronic cutaneous disease

In this subset there is negligible risk of systemic symptoms and when these occur, they are of minimal severity, such as mild lymphopenia.

■ *Discoid lupus erythematosus* begins as a well circumscribed pink or red plaque, frequently on the face, scalp, ear or neck. The nose and cheeks may be more or less symmetrically involved to produce the classic butterfly distribution. Scaling becomes more pronounced, tending to bulge down into dilated hair follicles so that small keratinous plugs are seen on the undersurface of lifted scale (*carpet tacking*). Telangiectasia becomes more prominent and the centre of the plaque becomes depressed and scarred. If the scalp is involved, the scarring destroys the hair matrix and scarring alopecia results.

■ *Oedematous pink plaques*, generally few in number, often solitary, may develop on the face or neck and resemble lesions of urticaria. Unlike urticaria the plaques persist and frequently develop a purplish tinge. Scarring is not a feature.

2. Low risk of mild extracutaneous disease

The following clinical subgroups feature only a low risk of extracutaneous disease, the severity of which is not great. Arthralgia and haemolytic anaemia are typical of the systemic involvement in this category.

■ *Disseminated discoid lupus erythematosus* shows classic plaques identical to localised discoid LE but there are large numbers of lesions found in places other than the head and neck region. Typically the back, chest and dorsal aspect of the distal forearms are involved but, in some patients, the limbs may be just as heavily covered.

■ *Lupus erythematosus profundus* is a rare manifestation in which the fat beneath the dermis (the panniculus) is primarily involved in a lobular pattern. Persistent, well-defined subcutaneous nodules become tethered to the overlying skin, which is not always affected by LE. Considerable scarring follows and produces depressed areas. Sites most often involved are the cheeks, upper arms and buttocks.

■ *Chilblain lupus erythematosus* presents as vascular looking red plaques on the fingers. The proximal nail fold capillaries are usually thrombosed, tortuous and dilated in a much more prominent manner than is generally seen with other manifestations of LE or any of the various collagen diseases.

3. Frequent, moderately severe extracutaneous disease

The next three subsets are characterised by frequent and moderately severe extracutaneous disease; but severe renal and central nervous system disease is only seen in the rare patients within these clinical groups who have DNA antibodies.

■ **Subacute lupus erythematosus** is characterised by papulosquamous or annular lesions. Photosensitivity is often very pronounced but the typical lesions are also found in non sun-exposed parts of the trunk. Unlike disseminated discoid LE, scarring is not a feature. Patients have antibodies against extractable antigens Ro and less commonly La. These are detected by precipitating antibody techniques and are therefore either absent or present, unlike other lupus antibodies which are reported as a titre. These auto-antibodies are also found in two other varieties of lupus erythematosus which are characterised by annular lesions, neonatal LE and that caused by congenital deficiency of complement components.

■ **Drug-induced lupus erythematosus** has a low rate of skin changes, but when present usually manifests as extensive discoid LE or very similar to acute systemic LE. However, although there is a low rate of central nervous system or renal involvement, there is a very high prevalence rate of arthralgia, and pulmonary disease. Antinuclear factor is usually directed against histone which produces the homogeneous pattern, antinuclear factor test result.

■ **Lupus anticoagulant syndrome** is (as previously explained) probably better considered as an antiphospholipid antibody syndrome. Skin changes are those of livedo and also leg ulcers. The thromboses that characterise this disorder are responsible for the high risk of miscarriage during pregnancy, but although thrombosis of spinal cord vessels may produce a transverse myelitis, central nervous system involvement is not usually a feature of this disorder.

4. *High risk of severe manifestations* (Colour plate 62)

Lupus erythematosus that has anti-DNA antibodies present in high titre carries a high risk of severe manifestations of extracutaneous disease. In this subset, variation in disease activity is common and therefore patients must be monitored closely.

■ *Acute lupus erythematosus* typically presents as recent onset of symmetrical redness, plaques, telangiectasia or coalesced papules distributed over the cheeks and nose. This pattern is usually worsened by sun exposure and may present as acute photosensitivity involving exposed areas away from the face and neck.

■ *Immune-complex induced vascular changes* include nail fold telangiectasia, necrosis of nail folds and fingertips, and cutaneous vasculitis presenting as either palpable purpura or a fixed urticaria that, unlike ordinary urticaria, takes longer than 48 hours to fade.

The return of these signs or their appearance for the first time in a patient with LE previously well controlled, suggests a return of disease activity.

■ *Other signs of active disease may be:*

━ *Mucous membrance lesions* which commence as reddish-purpuric areas progressing to painful ulceration that heals with scarring.

━ *Hair loss* at the frontal margin of the scalp caused by hairs which snap and break. Telogen effluvium may also be induced by acute worsening of LE. However, neither of these patterns of alopecia are associated with scarring of the scalp which characterises discoid LE.

— *Vesicular lesions* similar to dermatitis herpetiformis appear as grouped vesicles on an erythematous base, distributed on the trunk and hips. As with dermatitis herpetiformis, the vesicles are subepidermal and have collections of neutrophils at the tips of the dermal papillae. To complete the confusion, the vesicles respond well to dapsone and have IgA deposited in the basement membrane zone. However, the immunoreactants are in a linear band rather than just at the tips of the papillae.

Other organs

With severe systemic disease, low-grade fever and weight loss are common, but the outstanding complaint is fatigue. Fatigue is present in almost all untreated patients, and is often the presenting complaint. Joint symptoms are present in 90 per cent of patients, a striking feature being the degree of discomfort in relation to objective changes. Muscle pain, weakness and tenderness are frequently associated, but severe muscle weakness is unusual.

Renal involvement is a serious complication and an important cause of death from LE. Lupus nephritis may present as nephrotic syndrome, which develops in 10 per cent of patients with systemic disease, and is frequently complicated by hypertension. Pyelonephritis may occur, particularly in those treated with corticosteroids. Immunosuppressive therapy may be complicated by infective episodes, sometimes with organisms normally of low pathogenicity.

Pericarditis is very common, and there may be cardiomyopathy and endocarditis. Pleural effusion, mottled pulmonary infiltration, disordered oesophageal motility and episodes of colicky abdominal pain are all frequent manifestations. Neuropsychiatric features are common, while epilepsy and evidence of 'organic brain disease' occur in about 15 per cent of cases. There is often hepatosplenomegaly and lymphadenopathy, but virtually any organ may be affected.

Diagnosis

▶   **Suspect** lupus erythematosus in the patient with erythema and scaling on the face especially if there is associated photosensitivity or systemic symptoms.

▶   **Consider and exclude**

■ *Rosacea.* Scaling and atrophy are not features of rosacea and pustules are not an expression of LE. The marked fluctuation of rosacea is not seen in LE.

■ *Seborrhoeic eczema.* The scale is yellowish, soft and greasy, and does not resemble more adherent white or grey scale of LE.

■ *Psoriasis.* Atrophy does not occur. Scratching produces the typical silvery opaque scale whereas with LE scratching often removes the scale.

■ *Pemphigus foliaceous.* Biopsy may be the only means of distinguishing doubtful lesions.

■ *Photosensitivity* due to other causes is confined to light-exposed areas, is itchy, lacks the characteristic scale of LE and has an eczematous histology.

▶ **Confirm** the diagnosis of cutaneous LE by biopsy, as many forms may have negative antinuclear factor testing.

▶ **Assess** the extent of systemic disease and determine the likelihood of future severity by looking for anti-DNA antibodies and recognising the subset of LE.

Treatment of lupus erythematosus

■ *Acute systemic LE* should be managed only by those with a special knowledge of the disease and with access to adequate laboratory facilities. The outlook for affected patients is now considerably better than in the past because exacerbations and remissions are now recognised earlier and due to the use of oral steroids, immunosupressives, antimalarials, and techniques such as plasmaphoresis.

■ *Discoid LE* usually responds to the use of fluorinated topical corticosteroids and the avoidance of sun exposure by protective clothing and sunscreens. Resistant areas may require the intralesional injection of steroid. When widespread and unresponsive to topical corticosteroid, antimalarial therapy is often helpful but if used, eye toxicity should be watched for by an opthalmologist. The persistent hyper- and hypopigmentation and scarring that result when discoid lesions resolve can be covered with cosmetics, and the scarring alopecia with a wig.

■ *Lupus panniculitis and subacute LE* usually respond well to antimalarials and these agents are sometimes also helpful in controlling extremely photosensitive LE. Oral prednisolone is sometimes necessary for these varieties of LE.

Scleroderma

Scleroderma is an uncommon disease of skin and viscera which is characterised by local vascular changes and altered connective tissue.

Aetiology

The cause is unknown but, because there is a variety of immunological abnormalities found in a variable proportion of patients, an auto-immune pathogenesis is proposed. The commonest type of antinuclear antibody staining is of a speckled pattern but the most characteristic ANF pattern, rarely seen in any disorder other than scleroderma, is the nucleolar pattern which correlates well with antibody against topoisomerase (scleroderma 70 antigen). It is uncertain if and how these antigens or antibodies are involved in pathogenesis.

Histology

The microscopic appearance of the skin changes is remarkably consistent, no matter what the clinical pattern of involvement. Early on, a mild lymphohistiocytic infiltrate is present around vessels and at the dermo-epidermal junction. Later on collagen bundles are thickened, more closely packed, and stain more eosinophilic. There is a reduction in the number of hairs, and fat is lost from around eccrine sweat glands. Dermal vessels become thickened and hyalinised.

Clinical features

The skin is almost always involved, but involvement of other organs is variable. Patterns of skin involvement provide a reasonable guide to extent and severity of systemic involvement.

Morphoea *(Colour plate 63)*

A form of scleroderma confined to the skin and sometimes called 'localised scleroderma', morphoea may occur at any age, but is predominantly a disease of children and young adults, with a female-to-male ratio of three to one.

■ *The typical lesion* begins as a skin-coloured or purplish oedematous plaque, anywhere on the body. Over weeks or months, the colour changes to yellowish-white, except at the periphery, where a violaceous zone persists. The shape is usually round or oval, and the surface smooth and waxy. The lesion gradually evolves to a depressed sclerotic plaque, which is free of hair, and incapable of sweating. The plaque persists for years, but may eventually resolve completely, sometimes leaving a residual patch of hyperpigmentation. Lesions may be solitary or multiple, and range in size up to 20 cm.

■ *Guttate morphoea* is characterised by multiple superficial lesions, less than a centimetre in diameter and usually on the trunk. Unlike lichen sclerosus et atrophicus, which may look similar, there is no overlying epidermal atrophy.

■ *Linear morphoea* occurs mostly in children, usually as a single linear band of sclerosis on one limb. The lesion may be very extensive and penetrate to underlying muscle and bone. Involvement of the forehead and scalp is frequently associated with atrophy of bone, producing considerable disfigurement.

■ *Generalised morphoea* is a rare variant in which broad plaques extend to involve large areas, particularly on the trunk. Sclerosis over the chest and abdomen is occasionally sufficient to cause respiratory difficulty.

Diffuse scleroderma (progressive systemic sclerosis)

This pattern has a high incidence of internal organ involvement, although the rate of progression is variable. There are three distinct modes of onset.

■ *Acral onset.* Most patients present with a long history of Raynaud's phenomenon, to which the changes of acrosclerosis are gradually added.

Typically, sclerosis is preceded by oedematous thickening of the digits, often with arthralgia. The thickened skin gradually hardens, becomes bound down and shiny. In some patients there is no tumid phase, and the digits insidiously develop a smooth tapered appearance with atrophy of the tips of fingers and toes. The digits may be shortened by resorption of bone from the distal phalanges, and flexed by contractures. Small ulcers are common on the fingertips and over the interphalangeal joints, sometimes extruding a chalky material. The sclerosis extends proximally on the limbs, and may involve the face and trunk.

The face becomes taut and expressionless, with a smooth forehead, pinched nose and puckered mouth. Telangiectases appear on the lips, face and hands, often with a distinctive angular or rhomboidal shape. There may be generalised hyperpigmentation and areas of hypopigmentation, particularly on the trunk.

■ *Onset without Raynaud's syndrome* occurs in about 5 per cent of patients. Ivory or yellowish plaques begin on the trunk and gradually extend peripherally onto the face and limbs. Visceral involvement may occur, but is probably no more frequent than in patients with the more usual acral presentation. Whereas the acral onset is three times as common in females, the onset without Raynaud's syndrome occurs in both sexes with equal frequency.

■ *CRST syndrome* is a mild form of acral onset, in which cutaneous deposits of calcium (calcinosis) are combined with Raynaud's syndrome, sclerosis of fingers and toes (sclerodactyly), and macular telangiectases. Skin changes other than the calcification tend to remain confined to the distal limbs. However, apart from a low prevalence of renal disease, systemic involvement is common. Oesophageal dysmotility is almost universal, pulmonary involvement may be severe, intestinal scleroderma may occur, and about 5 to 10 per cent of patients with primary biliary cirrhosis have CRST syndrome. The disorder is more frequent in females and is associated with the presence of an antibody that reacts with centromeric chromatin.

Internal involvement

Variable combinations of fibrosis, vascular change and neurological dysfunction may occur in organs other than the skin.

Oesophageal motility disorders are frequent and produce dysphagia. Involvement of the lower portion is most common and may result in oesophageal reflux which, if severe, can produce strictures. Similar problems of motility can occur throughout the intestinal tract, producing abdominal pain, bowel diverticulae and the problems of the blind loop syndrome such as diarrhoea or malabsorption. Impaction of faeces due to poor bowel motility is not uncommon.

Pulmonary involvement may be predominantly fibrosis, which will produce restrictive defects, diffusion defects, ventilation–perfusion mismatch, or cor pulmonare. However, primary pulmonary hypertension with no involvement of lung parenchyma is not uncommon, even with seemingly mild cutaneous disease. In addition to right heart disease secondary to pulmonary disease, cardiac conduction pathways may become fibrosed, resulting in conduction defects and arrhythmias.

Renal involvement is, typically, secondary to constriction of the arcuate interlobular arteries. This change, which is signalled by the onset of microscopic haematuria, used to be a non-treatable terminal event.

However, the prompt use of drugs that inhibit the angiotensin-converting enzyme is now able to reverse this previously fatal disorder.

Course

The course for individual patients is unpredictable, but tends to be worse for males and for older age groups. The pulmonary changes are permanent and do not respond to therapy. Renal involvement generally indicates a poorer prognosis but is not incompatible with a prolonged and relatively benign course. For many patients, scleroderma follows a protracted course with long periods in which the disease remains stationary.

Diagnosis

▶ **Suspect** scleroderma in the patient with thickened, bound-down skin.

▶ **Consider and exclude**

■ *Scleredema*, which can usually be suspected clinically by its sudden onset and distribution over neck and face, and can be confirmed histologically by preservation of appendages in affected skin and deposition of mucin.

■ *Diabetic thick skin*, although acral in distribution, is not associated with Raynaud's phenomenon and has none of the vascular signs of scleroderma.

■ *Lichen sclerosus et atrophicus* may mimic guttate morphoea but is papular, has epidermal atrophy, and lacks the purplish edge.

■ *Porphyria cutanea tarda.* Sclerodermatous change may be difficult to distinguish, especially if there is associated cutaneous calcification. Distribution is mainly on the sun-exposed areas of the face, scalp, chest and hands. Porphyrin testing confirms the diagnosis.

■ *Eosinophilic fasciitis* is clinically distinctive, and is characterised by an elevated sedimentation rate, hypergammaglobulinaemia, and eosinophilia. However, progression to scleroderma has been reported.

■ *Occupational* exposure to vinyl chloride, epoxy resin, certain organic solvents and some pesticides, may lead to cutaneous changes clinically and histologically indistinguishable from scleroderma. Particularly with vinyl chloride disease, the cutaneous sclerosis may be accompanied by systemic illness, but the visceral changes differ from those of scleroderma.

■ *Addison's disease* and *haemochromatosis* may be suggested in patients with hyperpigmentation, but the diseases are otherwise dissimilar.

■ *Sclerodactyly* is not pathognomonic of scleroderma. It may occur in other connective tissue diseases, or be associated with Raynaud's syndrome without any evidence of systemic disease.

▶ **Confirmation** of the diagnosis using special tests is not usually necessary, as clinical appearances are sufficiently characteristic. However, anticentromere antibody is required if the CRST syndrome is suspected, and skin biopsy is helpful in cases of morphoea.

▶ **Assess** the extent and severity of systemic involvement on the basis of history and the appropriate tests.

Treatment of scleroderma

There is no specific treatment. Physiotherapy helps to prevent contractures, and protection from cold reduces vasospastic episodes. Vasodilator drugs are of doubtful value, with the calcium channel blockers the most frequently reported as helpful. Improvement after sympathectomy is inconsistent and transient. Penicillamine is sometimes of benefit in linear scleroderma. The administration of corticosteroids may be necessary when simpler measures fail to relieve the arthritis of scleroderma, but are not otherwise useful.

Eosinophilic fasciitis
(diffuse fasciitis with eosinophilia)

Eosinophilic fasciitis is a very uncommon syndrome in which cutaneous changes, rather like those of scleroderma, are combined with peripheral blood eosinophilia and elevated serum levels of IgG. An inflammatory infiltrate, predominantly of lymphocytes, histiocytes and plasma cells, invades deep fascia in the affected areas and may involve the fibrous trabeculae of subcutaneous fat and the deeper zone of the reticular dermis. Fibrosis may be added.

The disease has a fairly rapid onset, sometimes noted to follow an episode of unusually strenuous physical exertion. After a brief prodromal period in which muscle pain and tenderness may be accompanied by a low-grade fever, subcutaneous thickening develops, generally over the limbs and, less frequently, the trunk. There may be frank oedema in affected areas, the course of veins may be apparent as prominent linear depressions or gutters, and reduction in joint mobility may be a feature.

Whether oesinophilic fasciitis is a distinct entity or merely a variant of scleroderma is not yet clear. Deep biopsy of typical scleroderma may show thickening and inflammation of the fascia, and some patients with oesinophilic fasciitis evolve to true scleroderma. However, the very persistence of scleroderma contrasts with the regular response of eosinophilic fasciitis to systemic corticosteroid therapy.

Dermatomyositis

Dermatomyositis is a rare syndrome which combines necrotising myositis of voluntary muscle with a range of cutaneous lesions.

Aetiology

The disease occurs at all ages, with a peak incidence in the fifth and sixth decades. In 25 per cent of patients over the age of 40, there is an associated malignant tumour; the neoplasm is most often an adenocarcinoma, but all types of malignancy have been reported in association with dermatomyositis, including melanoma, sarcoma, lymphoma and leukaemia. There is no association with malignant disease in children.

Histology

Histological change may be very similar to that of lupus erythematosus, with hydropic degeneration of the basal cells of the epidermis and a perivascular and periappendageal lymphohistiocytic infiltrate. However, deposition of mucin within the dermis is often evident with the use of special stains. Biopsy of affected muscle is sometimes more helpful in diagnosis.

Clinical features

■ *Cutaneous.* Skin lesions may precede, accompany or follow the myositis, or the presenting symptoms may be fever and malaise. Areas of oedema and purplish erythema develop on the face, trunk or limbs, and are at first transient. The centrofacial area is often involved, usually with some degree of scaling. The erythema is not as sharply demarcated as with LE and affects the eyelids, which are puffy and have a lilac tinge.

Red or purplish plaques are frequently present on the back of the hands, affecting particularly the skin over knuckles. Vascular proliferation is often conspicuous, especially over the elbows, knees, and other bony prominences. The nail folds are swollen and red, and there may be telangiectases or mottled erythema over the thenar and hypothenar eminences, as in lupus erythematosus. Flattened red or purplish papules over the knuckles are particularly characteristic, but are not an early feature. With time, the plaques tend to become atrophic, sometimes with poikiloderma. In adults there may be sclerodermoid changes, often with severe episodes of Raynaud's syndrome.

An unusual presentation is of rapidly spreading erythema and telangiectasia, which affects mainly light-exposed areas. Oedema is marked and may progress to bulla formation. Diffuse thinning of scalp hair is a frequent association.

■ *Other organs.* The myositis is bilateral, with a predilection for muscles of the shoulder and pelvic girdles, and variable involvement of other muscle groups. Affected muscles are tender, painful and weak, sometimes with oedema of overlying skin. The patient may complain of difficulty in climbing stairs, brushing her hair or rising from a chair. There may be dysphagia, dysarthria and weakness of eye movements. The muscles of respiration may be affected, with hypoventilation. Fibrosis follows the inflammatory phase and, especially in children, may lead to severe contractures, with calcification of muscle and subcutaneous tissue. Children also frequently develop a vasculitis that involves skin, subcutaneous fat and gastro-intestinal tract.

Course

Quite apart from its association with malignancy, dermatomyositis is a very serious disease with a significant mortality and considerable morbidity among survivors. Respiratory failure and aspiration pneumonia are common terminal events. The prognosis of dermatomyositis is much improved by aggressive systemic therapy, despite the risks associated with doses of corticosteroid adequate to control the disease.

More than 10 per cent of patients suffer a severe progressive disease which is fatal within a year or two. Permanent remission may occur spontaneously or with therapy, particularly in children, but the majority of patients follow a chronic fluctuating course with serious disability.

Laboratory findings

Serum levels of creatine phosphokinase, aldolase and lactic dehydrogenase are raised during the inflammatory phase of the myositis, and may parallel the activity of the disease. Urinary creatine excretion is usually the best guide to disease activity. Although many different antinuclear antibodies may be found, none are specific for the disease, they are often not present, and none are clinically useful in defining subsets.

Diagnosis

▶ **Suspect** the disease in a patient with symmetrical proximal myopathy who has a rash in the hands, face and eyelids.

▶ **Consider and exclude**

■ *Lupus erythematosus.* This is frequently accompanied by a degree of myositis, and the cutaneous lesions may be similar. However, the distribution of plaques on the back of the hands is different, and skin over the larger joints is rarely affected by LE. Laboratory findings may allow diagnosis of borderline cases, but a sharp distinction is not always possible.

■ *Mixed connective tissue disease.* Raynaud's phenomenon is usually prominent. Antibody to ribonucleoprotein is present in high titre.

■ *Giant cell arteritis* is suggested by the history and confirmed by biopsy of an affected vessel.

■ *Myopathy* other than that due to connective tissue diseases is not accompanied by the cutaneous features of dermatomyositis.

▶ **Confirm the diagnosis** by electromyography, elevated muscle enzyme levels, and biopsy from an affected muscle.

▶ **Assess** the possibility of underlying malignancy in patients over 40 years of age. Assessment is initially on the basis of history, examination and simple tests such as chest X-ray, liver function tests and full blood examination. Any suspicious changes are then taken further.

Treatment of dermatomyositis

Corticosteroids are usually used. 60 mg to 100 mg of prednisone daily is usually sufficient to achieve initial control of the disease. The dose is then tapered to the smallest amount that is adequate to maintain suppression, often between 5 mg and 15 mg daily. Maintenance therapy usually needs to be continued for at least a year or two. About 20 per cent of patients, mainly those with the acute form of the disease, either respond poorly to corticosteroids or are unable to tolerate the dose required to maintain suppression. Addition of a cytotoxic drug, usually azathioprine or methotrexate, will generally be necessary to control the disease in such cases. Myositis may sometimes be controlled without the rash fading. In that situation, use of antimalarial tablets will often improve the rash without necessarily influencing the myositis.

Mixed connective tissue syndrome

It is not too uncommon for patients to have features of more than one connective tissue disease. In some cases the range of symptoms and signs is so wide as to defy a more precise diagnosis than 'a connective tissue disease'. In most of these patients, however, the overlap is most pronounced in the initial stages, and a more definite pattern gradually emerges. Rarely, there is a true overlap syndrome in which, for example, a patient with lupus erythematosus later develops dermatomyositis.

There is another small group of patients with a distinctive mixture of features to which the term 'mixed connective tissue disease' has been applied. Among these patients, arthralgia or arthritis is almost universal, and there is a high incidence of myositis and Raynaud's syndrome. There may be cutaneous changes resembling early scleroderma, particularly a sausage-like thickening of the fingers; less often there are lesions identical to those of lupus erythematosus or dermatomyositis.

The serum of these patients contains a high titre of antibodies to a saline-extractable nuclear antigen sensitive to ribonuclease (ribonucleoprotein). The use of oral corticosteroids in these patients produces a prompt resolution of the inflammatory manifestations such as myositis and arthritis, but the non-inflammatory changes (such as Raynaud's phenomenon, sclerodermatous change or pulmonary hypertension) do not respond. Therefore the long-term outcome for these patients is a scleroderma-like syndrome.

Sjögren's syndrome

Sjögren's syndrome is a characteristic type of lymphocyte-mediated destruction of glandular tissue. Most commonly the lacrimal and salivary glands are affected, but the process may also involve glandular structures in the upper and lower respiratory tract, the gastro-intestinal tract, the vagina and also the eccrine and sebaceous glands of the skin.

Aetiology

The disorder is usually associated with a connective tissue disease, most commonly rheumatoid arthritis, but a primary form also exists. Antibodies to extractable antigens Ro and La are found in most of those with primary Sjögren's syndrome but are not found in the secondary variety.

Clinical features

Dryness of mucous membranes and the skin give rise to the presenting symptoms. The mouth and throat may be smooth, red, and dry, with hoarseness and difficulty in mastication. Dysphagia and atrophic gastritis may reflect further gastro-intestinal involvement. The eyes feel gritty and inflamed, and are unable to produce tears. Affected skin is dry, scaly and itchy. Most patients are females and pruritus vulvae is a common complaint.

The primary form is also associated with extraglandular manifestations in about one-quarter of those affected. The changes include renal tubular atrophy and fibrosis, muscle atrophy, and pulmonary fibrosis. The skin of the legs may also develop purpura due to hyperglobulinaemia and vasculitis.

Diagnosis

In the appropriate clinical setting the diagnosis is rapidly confirmed by demonstrating reduced tear production with Schirmer's test and, in the primary form, by also finding the characteristic antibody.

Treatment

Lubricant eyedrops relieve the ocular discomfort. Simple emollients are helpful for the pruritus. The purpura and prefibrotic stage of the extraglandular manifestations of the primary form may be controlled by oral steroids or immunosupressives, if treated prior to the fibrosis developing.

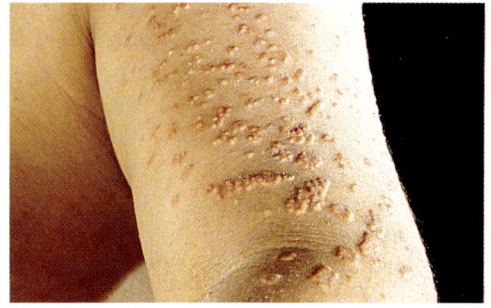

61. Eruptive xanthomas

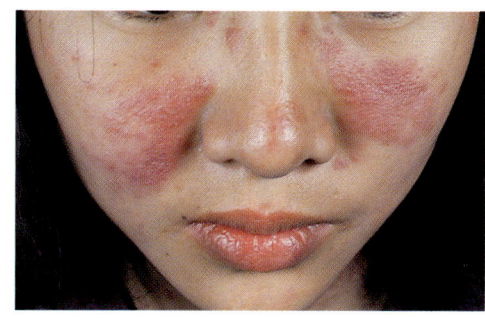

62. Lupus erythematosus

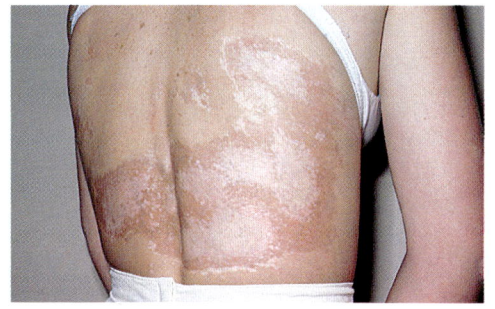

63. Morphoea

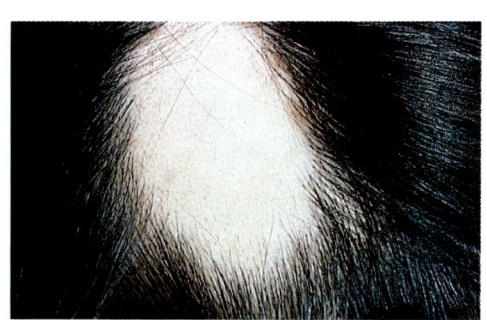

64. Alopecia areata

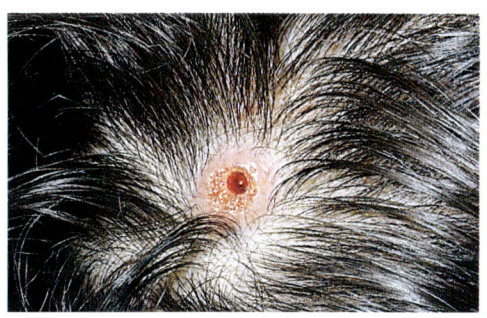

65. Alopecia due to metastasis

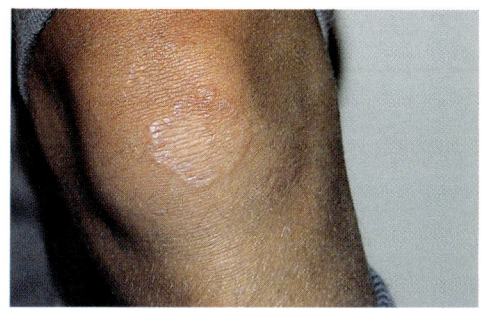

66. Granuloma annulare

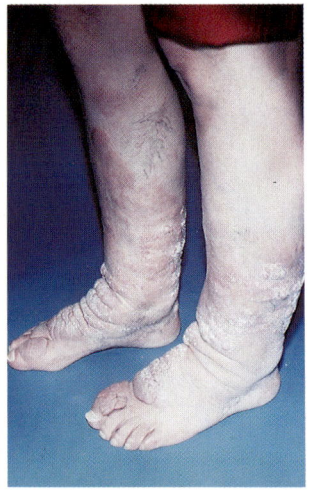

67. Pretibial myxoedema

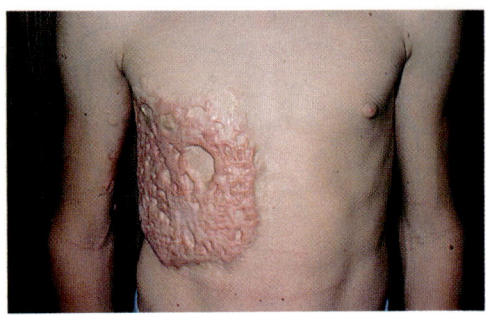

68. 'Cheloid following burn

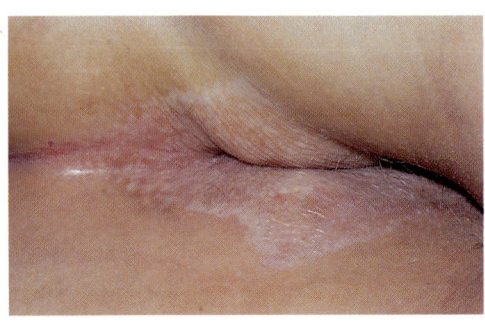

69. Lichen sclerosus et atrophicus

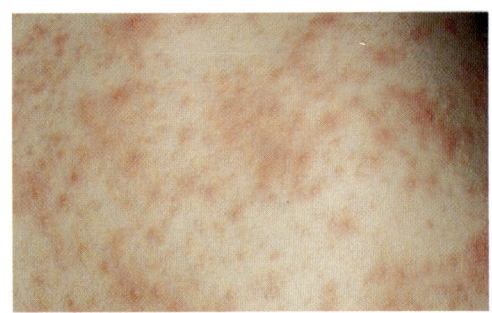

70. Miliaria rubra

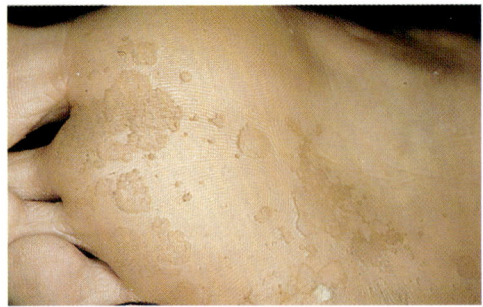

71. Pitted keratolysis

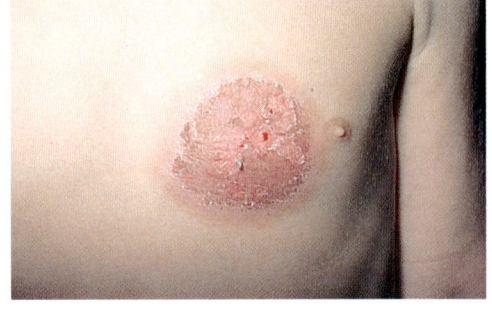

72. Fixed drug eruption

20

Diseases of hair

1. Alopecia
   (a) physiological
   (b) androgenetic
   (c) telogen effluvium
   (d) diffuse
   (e) alopecia areata
   (f) tinea
   (g) traumatic
   (h) cicatricial
2. Hypertrichosis and hirsutism

3. Hair shaft abnormalities
   (a) monilethrix
   (b) pili torti
   (c) pili annulati
   (d) trichothiodystrophy
   (e) trichorrhexis nodosa
   (f) peripilar casts
4. Dandruff
5. Hair colour
6. Permanent waving

Alopecia

Alopecia can be caused by disorders directly involving the hair shaft so causing the hairs to break; alterations in the hair cycle so that a larger proportion of hairs are in the falling out phase; disorders primarily involving the skin so that hairs in that region are secondarily involved; and by biochemical changes to which the actively growing hairs are sensitive.

To distinguish between these it is helpful to conduct the history and examination so that the following questions can be answered. Is the hair loss localised, generalised or patchy? Are the hairs breaking or are they coming out by the roots? Is the number of hairs lost more or less than the physiologically normal one hundred per day? Does the scalp look abnormal? Has the patient taken drugs or had health problems that could produce biochemical changes influencing hair growth?

This results in a small list of possible diagnoses relevant for that patient which can then be differentiated by appropriate tests.

Physiological alopecia

At birth the scalp hairs of humans are all at the same stage of the hair growth cycle and quickly enter the regressing phase (*catagen*) in a wave progressing from the frontal to the occipital region. Although the hairs then enter the telogen phase in another wave, they re-enter the actively growing phase (*anagen*) at different rates to achieve the randomly distributed hair cycle pattern characteristic of adult human scalp hair. The loss and replacement are usually gradual and hardly noticed. When shedding is more abrupt, the infant may have temporary diffuse alopecia, beginning at the frontal hairline and resembling the baldness of men. In some babies, the alopecia is noticeable only over the occipital region, where the head rubs on the pillow.

During puberty most boys and some girls lose the curved frontal hairline of childhood and develop triangles of permanent hair loss, in the fronto-parietal region on each side. This appears to be dependent upon circulating androgen levels and does not require the genetic predisposition to male pattern alopecia.

Androgenetic alopecia

The onset and progression of male pattern baldness are androgen-dependent. Minor degrees occur in normal women but the typical pattern is almost entirely confined to men. It is likely that the predisposition is genetically inherited as a polygenic autosomal dominant trait with clinical expression requiring the presence of androgen levels that are normally only found in men.

Pathophysiology

Under the influence of androgens, affected follicles become progressively smaller in successive hair cycles and are eventually reduced to diminutive vellus hair remnants with a shortened anagen phase and lengthened telogen phase. The enzyme 5 alpha reductase that converts testosterone to dihydrotestosterone in tissues is necessary for this to occur. Androgenetic alopecia will only occur if the increased conversion to dihydrotestosterone takes place in genetically predisposed follicles.

Clinical features

■ *In men* the earliest change is generally a progressive frontoparietal recession of the hairline. The rate of recession varies a great deal. There may be only gradual progression over many years or there may be a rapid extension within a year or two. Simultaneously, a round or oval area of thinning develops on the crown and may progress to a definite patch of baldness. Enlargement of the area and coalescence with the receding hairline eventually leaves only a horseshoe of hair around the scalp margins.

This too may be lost, producing total baldness. Incidence and severity increase with age. By the age of fifty, about 50 per cent of men have some degree of baldness. Because hairs are present but not seen because they are small, the patient notices apparent reduction in hair density without any obvious increase in hair fall.

■ *In women* the process begins as a fairly uniform thinning of hair over the crown, which produces an oval area with a reduced density of hairs around which there remains a broad circular band in which the number of hairs is unaltered. The distribution resembles a minor degree of male-pattern alopecia except for the persistence of an unaffected frontal fringe. With increasing age, reduction of hairs in the central

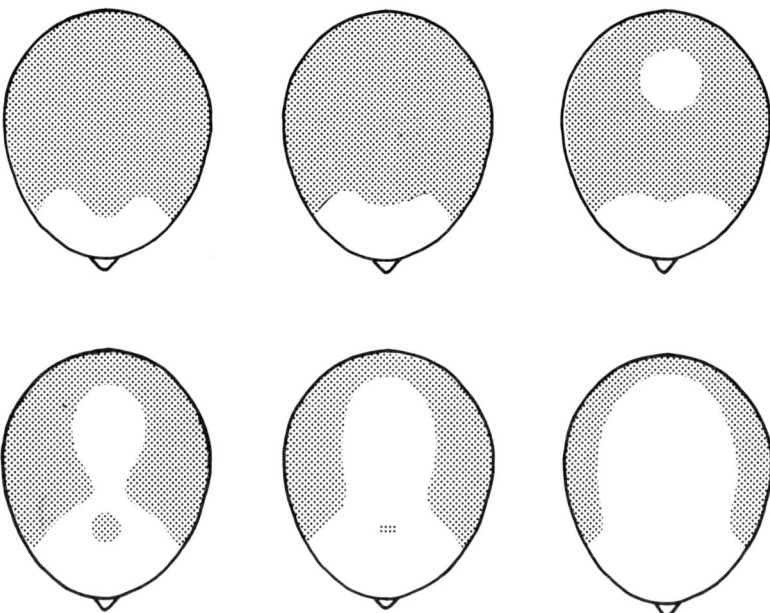

Male-pattern alopecia

area becomes more severe, but the pattern remains unchanged. A distribution and course resembling androgenic alopecia of men is exceptional in women and indicates the need for careful assessment of endocrine function.

Diagnosis

▶ **Suspect** the diagnosis of androgenetic alopecia when there is
- typical pattern
- history of reduction in hair density without obvious increase in hair fall
- family history in males on either side of family
- normal looking scalp

▶ **Consider and exclude**
- severe telogen effluvium, which may unmask a mild genetic tendency to male pattern baldness
- diffuse alopecia in a female which is due to endocrine or other systemic disturbance

Treatment

Philosophical acceptance is often best counsel, but a well made wig should be suggested for those unduly embarrassed by baldness. Grafting of follicles from the occipital and parietal regions resistant to the involutional effects of androgens gives satisfactory results when performed on selected patients by those experienced in the technique. Minoxidil solution applied to the vertex of the scalp may induce vellus hairs in this region to return to adult type terminal hairs in about 30 per cent of selected patients. Frontal and fronto-parietal hairs do not respond.

Clinical improvement is slow to begin and then progresses gradually. However, if treatment is ceased the hairs once again rapidly regress to vellus follicles.

Telogen effluvium

Following a severe disturbance such as completion of pregnancy, major illness or injury, rapid weight loss, surgical procedure or emotional upset, an abnormally large number of hairs may spontaneously prematurely complete the anagen phase and move to the catagen phase which they quickly complete and move into the telogen phase. Weeks later this large number of telogen hairs are pushed from the follicle by the newly emerging anagen hairs beneath them in the same follicle or are released by minor traction.

Clinical features

About 25 per cent of scalp hairs must be lost before diffuse alopecia becomes apparent. This does not often occur with telogen effluvium, so the patient is likely to complain of increased hair fall rather than alopecia. However, shedding may be severe enough to cause diffuse thinning or to reveal latent male-pattern baldness. Even in severe cases, alopecia due to telogen effluvium is temporary and is almost always followed by a return to normal within a few months as the proportions of hairs in each phase return to normal.

Diagnosis

▶ **Suspect** telogen effluvium when there has been
- preceding event approximately 6 weeks prior to onset
- hairs shed in large numbers
- diffuse, even involvement of scalp
- normal-looking scalp

▶ **Consider and exclude**
- *diffuse alopecia areata*, in which there are still signs to indicate hair is falling out from coin-shaped patches. Exclamation mark hairs usually are present.
- *anagen effluvium* due to cytotoxic drugs, in which hairs break off rather than fall out by the roots.
- *chemical trauma* to hairs which has caused them to break.

▶ **Confirm by**

- *microscopic examination* of hairs which should reveal a telogen count greater than 25 per cent. Telogen hair roots contain no pigment and are club-shaped, rather like a small cotton bud.

- *pull test*—if when plucking hairs for microscopy, tugging gently on a clump of hairs picked up between thumb and index finger releases 10–20 hairs (compared with normal 3–5 hairs per tug), microscopy is sometimes considered unnecessary.

Diffuse alopecia

Hair loss in myxoedema and hypopituitarism involves not only the scalp, but also the eyebrows, axillae and pubic region. Hormone replacement therapy is followed by regrowth in all areas. Hair loss may follow starvation and malnutrition, severe debilitating illness, and deficiency of iron or zinc. Diffuse alopecia is a feature of hypoparathyroidism and may occur with secondary syphilis, lupus erythematosus and dermatomyositis.

The rapidly dividing cells of the hair matrix are especially sensitive to antimitotic drugs. Suppression of mitoses in the anagen follicle by such drugs as colchicine, methotrexate, 6-mercaptopurine and cyclophosphamide may cause reversible diffuse alopecia. Excessive intake of vitamin A, or treatment of thyrotoxicosis with carbimazole or thiouracil, may also produce diffuse thinning. Dose-related hair loss is a sequel to anticoagulant therapy and with high doses there is frank alopecia. Thallium and other poisons are rare causes.

However, there are many patients with diffuse non-cicatricial alopecia in whom careful history, examination and investigation reveal no specific cause.

Alopecia areata

Alopecia areata is a common disease, characterised by one or more circumscribed areas of hair loss, which develop without apparent cause on otherwise normal skin.

Aetiology

Alopecia areata is most common in children and young adults, but can occur at any age. A family history of the disease in more than 10 per cent of patients suggests a genetic predisposition. There is an increased association with several diseases regarded as auto-immune and a significant incidence of thyroid and gastric parietal cell antibodies. In active lesions there is an infiltrate of predominantly helper T lymphocytes around the dilated vessels beneath the hair matrix. Active lesions grafted on to athymic mice regrow hair, which suggests that T lymphocytes mediate the induction of hair loss in this disorder. In approximately 20 per cent of patients, significant psychological events seem to trigger the onset of the disorder.

Histology

In early active lesions there is an infiltrate of lymphocytes around the vessels beneath the hair matrix with an increase in the proportion of hairs in catagen and telogen phase. Later, as the hairs become arrested in early anagen, and are smaller, small numbers of lymphocytes remain in clumps beneath the follicles around the sites of the former papillae.

Clinical features (Colour plate 64)

One or more discrete areas of hair loss appear suddenly, generally on the scalp. There is no discomfort and the lesion is often first noticed by a relative. The affected area is well-defined and usually completely devoid of hair. Vellus hairs are sometimes spared and in older patients grey hairs may remain. A very occasional pigmented hair may also persist in the lesion. Characteristically deformed 'exclamation mark' hairs are generally recognisable at the edges of recent or expanding lesions. The exclamation mark hair is a short broken hair, a centimetre or so long, with a frayed tip and a shaft which tapers towards the scalp.

Although most common on the scalp, alopecia areata can begin on the chin, eyebrow, a limb, or at any other hair-bearing site. Lesions may rapidly reach a maximum size or may enlarge slowly and coalesce with other affected areas. Nail changes are associated in 10 per cent of cases, but develop more frequently in patients with extensive alopecia. Brittleness, superficial pitting, ridging and, rarely, onycholysis may occur. There is a markedly increased incidence of alopecia areata among atopic individuals, and a less pronounced association with thyrotoxicosis, vitiligo, pernicious anaemia, Down's syndrome and juvenile-onset diabetes.

Course

There is a tendency for some regrowth of hair within a few months, but the course is otherwise unpredictable. Quick permanent resolution may occur, or the initial lesion may be followed by others. Regression in one area may proceed simultaneously with extension in another, or all areas may return to normal, only to be followed by the appearance of new lesions in the same or other areas. Recurrences are very commn, occurring sooner or later in most patients. In a few, relentless progression leads to involvement of the whole scalp (alopecia totalis) or the whole body (alopecia universalis).

The prospects for satisfactory regrowth are less favourable in patients with asthma or atopic dermatitis, and are decidedly unfavourable in those with steady progression of lesions, with alopecia totalis or universalis, and when the eyebrows, eyelashes and nails are affected.

Diagnosis

▶   **Suspect** alopecia areata when there is
- patchy hair loss
- normal scalp
- exclamation mark hairs at periphery
- sparing of grey hairs

▶   **Consider and exclude**

- *tinea capitis*, which is accompanied by some degree of erythema and scaling. Hairs are broken rather than shed and there are no exclamation mark hairs.

- *traumatic alopecia*, which is patchy, poorly defined and never causes complete baldness.

- *secondary syphilis* and *lupus erythematosus*, which both may cause patchy alopecia but have other features of the disease present.

▶   **Confirmatory tests** are often not required.

- *Biopsy* may be necessary to confirm the diffuse form and to distinguish trichotillomania which shows intrafollicular damage to hair shaft and dumping of pigment into the follicle.

- *Exclusion tests* for tinea, syphilis and lupus erythematosus are occasionally needed.

Treatment

While the disease remains confined to one or two small areas, a measure of reassurance is justified. When larger areas are affected or the alopecia is progressive, undue optimism is neither prudent nor kind. It is better to explain the position honestly to the patient or parent. At the same time, the value of a placebo is not to be despised in diseases for which there is no specific treatment. Sedatives and tranquillisers are useful only to lessen the upset caused by the disease.

Minor lesions with evidence of regrowth are better left untreated. When improvement is delayed, or for larger lesions, applications of a fluorinated steroid ointment combined with plastic occlusion sometimes accelerate resolution. Intralesional injections of a corticosteroid frequently promote regrowth, but the benefit is often transitory. The administration of systemic corticosteroids is rarely justifiable for the treatment of alopecia areata. There is no real evidence of long-term benefit, and in most cases the hair continues to grow only while the dosage is maintained at a level which is unacceptable over long periods for a disease posing no threat to life.

Gentle irritation of the scalp will frequently induce regrowth, for reasons that are not well understood. This can often successfully be achieved using the irritant properties of dithranol cream.

Induction and maintenance of an allergic contact dermatitis on the scalp will produce regrowth of hair in nearly two-thirds of those with alopecia areata. Most experience has been obtained using di-nitrochlorobenzene-induced allergy, but because this substance, which is absorbed, is mutagenic to bacteria and therefore possibly carcinogenic, diphencyprone or squaric acid dibutyl ester are sometimes chosen as the allergen.

Alopecia areata has an unpredictable high spontaneous recovery rate, which makes the efficacy of newer treatments such as PUVA and topical Minoxidil difficult to assess.

Tinea capitis

Although in Australia there are four fungi that account for almost all cases, by far the commonest is *Microsporum canis*. This is predominantly an infection of children and, in addition to patchy hair loss, produces associated scaling and redness of the involved scalp. The hairs break off rather than being shed, and under Wood's light hairs infected with *M. canis* fluoresce a bright green.

Treatment with topical antifungal agents is ineffectual because they cannot penetrate into the involved hairs. Treatment with oral griseofulvin is required until the hairs no longer fluoresce. This is usually about 10 to 12 weeks. Although oral ketoconazole is effective, its use should be reserved for specifically indicated situations because the long term use makes hepatotoxicity a definite risk to consider.

Traumatic alopecia

Hair plucking (trichotillomania) is a relatively common cause of alopecia in children. The hairs may be simply pulled from the scalp, but are often extracted by winding hair around a finger or broken by rubbing the scalp. Usually only a single area is affected, with an irregular, poorly defined outline. Short regrowing hairs cannot be grasped by the child, so that the area is not completely bald. There is a stubble of hairs of various lengths, and the scalp itself is usually normal, although there may be a little scaling. In a child, trichotillomania is generally no more than an undesirable habit comparable to thumbsucking and confined to times of preoccupation or fatigue. In adults, trichotillomania is a more serious disturbance and is frequently associated with significant psychological problems.

Considerable tension may be imparted to hair by tight plaiting, by tightly winding hair around rollers or curlers, and by upswept hair styles. The tension may be sufficient to drag hair from follicles, particularly at the scalp margins (traction alopecia). Vigorous massage or brushing, especially with stiff nylon brushes, may cause hair loss in normal people, but significant alopecia is more likely when hairs are fragile, either because of structural abnormalities or from previous chemical trauma.

Cicatricial alopecia

Irreversible alopecia follows any process which destroys follicles. Thermal and chemical burns, deep folliculitis and large doses of radiation cause permanent hair loss. Alopecia due to tinea is not usually cicatricial, although some permanent damage may be caused by a kerion. Such scarring diseases as lupus vulgaris, morphoea, scleroderma, lupus erythematosus, necrobiosis lipoidica, and primary or metastasising tumours all produce irreversible alopecia. *(Colour plate 65)*

Hypertrichosis and hirsutism

Hirsutisim is excessive hair growth in women or children of a distribution which would be normal for men. Hypertrichosis is excessive hair growth which is either localised or distributed more widely, in a pattern not corresponding to that of normal men.

Hypertrichosis

There are very rare families in which affected individuals fail to shed the longer, silky lanugo hair of foetal life. Instead of being replaced by vellus, the lanugo persists and continues to grow throughout life. There is also a rare acquired form of the disease, which is generally encountered as an association of visceral carcinoma or other serious debilitating disease.

A circumscribed area of hypertrichosis in the lumbosacral region ('faun tail') is frequently the surface marker of a spinal anomaly, while excessive hair growth is a common feature of melanocytic naevi and other developmental defects. Acquired localised hypertrichosis may develop in plaques of pretibial myxoedema or over the cheeks and lateral parts of the forehead in patients with porphyria variegata and porphyria cutanea tarda. More extensive hypertrichosis may be a feature of acromegaly, juvenile myxoedema, and Hurler's syndrome.

Iatrogenic hypertrichosis may follow therapy with dipheylhydantoin, corticosteroids, minoxidil, diazoxide, psoralens, cyclosporin and, perhaps, streptomycin. Drug-induced hypertrichosis is more frequent in children and generally disappears after withdrawal of the drug.

Hirsutism

The presence of a vellus fuzz over the upper lip and chin is very common in women of all races and has no sinister significance. Some women, particularly those of southern or eastern European extraction, develop coarser, longer hair on the face, without any clinical evidence of endocrine dysfunction. Standard methods of investigation have been largely unrewarding and such cases have been regarded as 'idiopathic', and attributed to an unusual sensitivity to normal levels of circulating androgens. More sophisticated methods of investigation have demonstrated subtle endocrine abnormalities in many of these women.

Virilising tumours and other causes of frank masculinisation are more likely to be accompanied by menstrual irregularities, deepening of the voice, acne, increased muscle mass, clitoral hypertrophy, increased growth of hair in other areas and recession of the frontal hairline. Coarse hair over the chest, shoulders and back, a masculine physique and decreasing breast size are suggestive signs. Pelvic examination may disclose ovarian enlargement. Investigation and treatment of such patients is the province of the endocrinologist.

However, in the absence of frank virilisation, major menstrual disturbance, acromegaly or Cushing's syndrome, the finding of normal levels of serum testosterone and dihydro-epiandrostenedione sulphate (which is a reliable indicator of adrenal androgen production) indicates that the patient can be assumed to have idiopathic hirsutism.

Symptomatic treatment of hirsutism

It is important that the various adrenal, ovarian and hepatic causes of hirsutism be excluded. However, even when a remediable cause is discovered, symptomatic treatment is needed for the majority of those women in whom the hirsutism tends to persist after correction of the cause.

Mild cases can be satisfactorily masked simply by bleaching dark hair with hydrogen peroxide. Shaving is effective, but strongly resisted by most women, often because of the rough feel of emerging hair. The mistaken belief that shaving encourages more rapid growth of coarser hair is also a common deterrent. Abrasive pads are less suitable for the face than for other areas.

■ *Waxes.* Cosmetic waxes melt at a relatively low temperature and are applied as a liquid. The wax sets on the skin and plucks embedded hairs as it is peeled off. The method is somewhat painful, but has the advantage that the hair regrows with a naturally pointed tip, and the bristly feel of hairs truncated by shaving or depilatory creams is avoided.

■ *Depilatory creams.* Most depilatory creams now contain thioglycolates which do not have the unpleasant smell of older sulphide preparations. They are reasonably effective, but are powerful primary irritants which are poorly tolerated by sensitive skins. Allergic contact dermatitis to thioglycolate may also occur, but is rare.

■ *Electrolysis.* The aim is to permanently destroy the hair matrix without scarring. When there are many hairs, the method is tedious, painful and expensive. Too brief or too weak a current leaves the hair attached, while too strong a current is followed by scarring. Even in expert hands, minor inflammation may occur in the follicle, leaving a small pit. Electrolysis should never be used on patients who are known to form cheloid.

■ *Spironolactone.* In high doses this is a functional anti-androgen in peripheral tissues. A period of at least four months is required before results can be seen and about one year before the cosmetically desired result of apparent reduction in hirsutism due to paler shorter thinner hairs is achieved. Blood levels of sodium and potassium need to be monitored and the drug should not be taken during pregnancy, because of its feminising effects on the foetus.

Hair shaft abnormalities

Temporary defects of the hair shaft may result from malnutrition, severe illness, or the effect of drugs. The calibre and growth of hair is altered by endocrine disorders, and abnormalities may occur in rare genetic syndromes either as part of a generalised ectodermal defect or, for example, associated with gross aminoaciduria. Occasionally, malformations occur as a distinctive isolated defect. Many of these variations of structure cause no trouble, but a few result in alterations of cosmetic significance.

Monilethrix (beaded hair)

Thickened nodes or spindle-shaped swellings, about a millimetre apart, are separated by abnormal constrictions of the hair shaft. The beaded hairs emerge from small follicular papules and break before reaching two centimetres in length. Monilethrix may affect part or all of the scalp, the eyebrows, eyelashes, axillary and pubic hair. Affected areas are covered by a short, dull stubble.

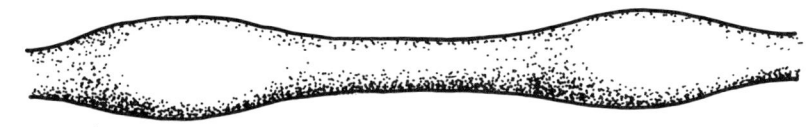

Monilethrix

The disorder is inherited in an autosomal dominant manner with a high degree of penetrance but with variability in expression. X-ray diffraction reveals that an abnormal keratin is present. Except in very young hairs, cuticle cells are lost from the nodes yet the hairs break between the nodes.

Pseudomonilethrix is due to trauma from overlapping hairs in normal individuals. It is seen only in scalp hair and the cuticle is intact. Normal hair shape occurs quickly once the cause is removed.

Pili torti (twisted hair)

The hair is twisted up to 180° on its axis at several points along the shaft. Affected hairs are brittle and may break at points of twisting to leave a stubble which resembles, but is longer than, that of monilethrix. The hairs are flattened as well as twisted, and may coexist with monilethrix. When pili torti is the only abnormality present, hairs generally reach 5 cm or so in length before breaking. The disorder may affect only part of the scalp, or abnormal hairs may be scattered over the scalp with normal hairs between. In reflected light, hair altered by pili torti has a characteristic spangled sheen. Although originally described as an autosomal dominantly inherited disorder occurring in people who were otherwise normal, pili torti is more commonly found as a minor component of other more complex neurectodermal developmental disorders.

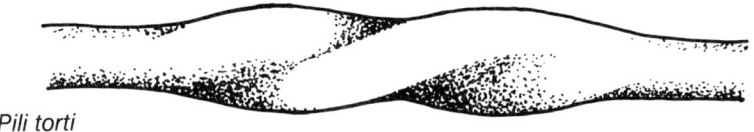

Pili torti

Trichothiodystrophy

Sulphur deficient hair, produced either as a part of a variety of congenital neurectodermal disorders or by severe protein malnutrition as in kwashiorkor, has a very weakened cuticle that is often lost. The weakened hairs break with a clean transverse split. The hairs are dry and slightly coarse tending to break off as they emerge near the surface. Hair loss is aggravated by the trauma of brushing. Patients may show alopecia of the scalp, eyebrows and eyelashes.

Microscopy reveals a very characteristic clean transverse break, but under polarised light the diagnostic feature of alternating light and dark transverse bands can be seen.

Pili annulati (ringed hair)

The cortex contains air-filled cavities along the length of the hair, together with a distinctive abnormality of cuticle cells. In reflected light the defects appear as light bands alternating with the darker areas of normal cortex seen with the naked eye and confirmed under the microscope. As a rule, affected hairs are not unduly fragile, and the alternating bands may add quite an attractive sheen to the hair.

Trichorrhexis nodosa

Nodular swellings develop on the hair in response to mechanical or chemical trauma in predisposed individuals. Microscopically, the nodes have an appearance like two interlocking brushes, a change produced by longitudinal splitting of fibres without complete fracture. Although affected hairs are fragile at the nodes, the swelling usually occurs towards the tip of the hair where fracture causes little cosmetic disturbance. There is a variant of trichorrhexis nodosa, more common in black races, in which the nodes form proximally and predispose to more serious hair loss.

Peripilar casts

Abnormal adherence of the external root sheath causes the formation of short, whitish cylindrical bands of keratin, which are usually widely spaced at intervals along the hair. They resemble nits, but are larger and slide freely towards the tip of the hair, unlike nits which are firmly attached. They can be destroyed by the application of retinoic acid liquid.

Dandruff

Dandruff is the normal desquamation of loosely adherent parakeratotic scale diffusely from a non-inflamed scalp. The shed scale is 'trapped' in hair, and visible; conversely, dandruff is not visible on bald areas.

Increased epidermal turnover is occurring but the cause is not known. The incidence and severity are generally greatest during the second decade, when 50 per cent of the population is affected, which suggests that androgenic stimulation of sebaceous glands possibly plays some role. Topical agents effective against pityrosporum yeasts frequently help control dandruff but it is possible to abolish all microflora from the scalp without reducing dandruff. Zinc pyridinethione and selenium sulphide present in antidandruff shampoos are locally cytotoxic and reduce epidermal turnover.

However, dandruff is physiological and treatment is necessary only for cosmetic reasons. Most patients can achieve satisfactory control with overnight application of a cream containing 4 per cent liquor picis carbonis and 2 per cent salicylic acid once or twice a week.

Should there be persistant or heavy scaling, consider the diagnosis of psoriasis or seborrhoeic dermatitis.

Hair colour

■ *Greying*. Reduced activity of follicular melanocytes may dilute the colour of individual hairs to grey, but loss of melanin in a single hair is eventually complete. Diffuse greying results from a mixture of white and pigmented hairs, and usually begins on the temples, which spread to the rest of the scalp and, later, to the beard and moustache. Hair on the chest, axillae and pubic region is affected last or not at all. Age of onset is genetically programmed and is generally between 30 and 50 years. Premature greying is almost always an isolated abnormality, but is more frequent among patients with hyperthyroidism and pernicious anaemia, and may be a manifestation of dystrophia myotonica or such rare hereditary syndromes as progeria and the Rothmund–Thomson syndrome.

■ *Rapid whitening*. Once formed, hair cannot be depigmented except by exogenous agents. Areas of depigmentation may, however, develop rapidly with vitiligo, and the hair may appear to become white in a patient with extensive alopecia areata when only pigmented hairs are shed. Severe malnutrition and protein depletion are rare causes of hypopigmented hair. Chloroquine may produce irregular bleaching of fair hair, an effect not seen in dark-haired individuals.

■ **Accidental discolouration**. Hair may be discoloured by contact with salts of copper or cobalt in industry, resulting in spectacular shades of green or blue. Greenish discolouration has also been reported from contact with copper-containing algicide in the water of swimming pools, and from excessive amounts of copper in household tap water. Yellow or brownish tints may be caused by contact with picric acid, resorcin and dithranol. The tars of cigarette smoke may stain the moustache or frontal hair of grey-haired smokers.

■ **Hair dyes and bleaches**. When properly used on normal hair, dyes cause few problems. Most adverse reactions come from the oxidative ('permanent') dyes. Paraphenylenediamine and paratoluylenediamine both have considerable sensitising potential. Rinses and semi-permanent dyes rarely give trouble, and henna, the only vegetable dye used with any frequency, is a very rare sensitiser.

Hydrogen peroxide is contained in many bleaches and, if used too frequently or applied for too long, produces structural changes in the hair shaft. The hair becomes dull, dry and fragile, often with trichorrhexis nodosa. The weakened hair is susceptible to breakage and is particularly vulnerable to the chemicals used in permanent waving.

Permanent waving

A reducing compound, usually a thioglycolate, is applied to break disulphide bonds between the peptide chains of keratin. The pliable hair is then straightened, waved or curled by moulding over rollers or other devices. Oxidants are used to restore the disulphide bridges, 'setting' the hair into its altered shape.

Waving lotions are powerful primary irritants. Careless application may cause chemical burns of the scalp and prolonged application leaves hair dull, fragile and prone to breakage. Elastic bands are sometimes used to hold hair on rollers and may cut through the softened hair if applied too tightly. Waving lotions easily damage hair which is naturally fragile or which has been made so by hydrogen peroxide or other chemicals.

21

Diseases of nails

1. The normal nail
2. The abnormal nail
3. The nail folds
4. Tumours about the nail

The nail changes associated with many cutaneous and metabolic diseases have been described in other chapters.

Therefore, rather than describing the changes caused in nails by each disease, discussion in this chapter is confined to the topics listed.

The normal nail

The normal pink colour of nails is produced by the rich blood supply of the bed which is seen through the translucent, adherent nail plate. At the lunule, where the nail is separated from the vessels by cells of the matrix, the colour is obscured. The nail plate is normally 0.5 mm to 1.0 mm thick and is firmly attached to the epidermis of the nail bed. The dermo-epidermal junction of the bed differs from other areas in forming a pattern of parallel longitudinal ridges. Fine dermal capillaries pass beneath the ridges and, when ruptured, form the characteristic linear 'splinter haemorrhages'.

The rate of nail growth varies considerably between individuals, and is slower on toes than fingers. Fingernails grow about one millimetre per week, whereas toenails grow approximately one-third this rate. With increasing age, nail growth is slower, even when the circulation and general health are normal. Nails of elderly people are frequently dull and opaque, and may show longitudinal ridging. Particularly on the toes, they are often thick and brittle, sometimes with superficial flaking or splitting.

The abnormal nail

Nails are the product of a rapidly dividing matrix. The proximal matrix forms the dorsal (superficial) portion of the nail plate and the distal matrix is responsible for the ventral (deep) portion of the nail plate.

Surface abnormalities of the nail plate therefore reflect changes in the proximal zone of the matrix whereas pathology of the distal matrix induces alteration of the deep portion of the nail plate. The metabolically active matrix cells are vulnerable to nutritional and systemic changes, and to cytotoxic drugs. Depression of mitoses is reflected later by an altered nail plate. Deformed or discoloured nails may provide evidence of systemic disease, but the abnormalities are often non-specific and may be reproduced by local factors, or occur without apparent cause. Pathology in the nail bed usually induces local nail plate detachment (onycholysis).

Resilience

The limited flexibility of nails is decreased by a fall in their water content. Resilience is impaired by repeated contact with lipid solvents, detergents and alkaline compounds. Excessive manicuring and the frequent use of solvents to remove nail polish may leave nails which are more easily split and broken. The dry, easily chapped skin of xeroderma and ichthyosis is frequently accompanied by nails which are dry and brittle. Nails altered by psoriasis and tinea are often brittle and crumbly, while nails thinned by lichen planus or hypochromic anaemia are fragile and easily broken. Many people, however, have brittle nails for which no cause can be found.

Compared to skin and hair, the keratin of nails is harder because the keratin matrix protein has a higher sulphur content, which is mainly present as cystine. Koilonychia is produced when nails with a low cystine content are remoulded by mechanical trauma. In addition to iron deficiency anaemia, this appearance may be caused by exposure to oils and organic solvents.

Thickness

Nail hypertrophy may follow a single injury or repeated minor trauma. Poorly fitting shoes or a weight dropped onto a toe are typical causes. Thickened nails may occur as an isolated genetic defect and are a characteristic feature of hidrotic ectodermal dysplasia. True thickening may be a manifestation of psoriasis and Darier's disease, but is less common than apparent thickening due to subungual hyperkeratosis, with which it may coexist.

Surface

■ *Sheen*. The normal lustre of the nail surface is dulled by age, and by diseases which alter the thickness of texture of the nail. The sheen is enhanced in nails which are used for habitual scratching, and is often combined with bevelling of the free edge.

■ *Pitting*. A few pits are faily common in normal nails and are of no significance. Pitting is a frequent finding in psoriasis, and may follow dermatitis which involves the proximal nail fold. Shallow pits are an uncommon association of alopecia areata.

■ *Longitudinal furrow or split.* A split or depression along the length of a nail can be the permanent sequel to an injury involving the matrix. A mucous cyst just proximal to the cuticle often causes longitudinal furrowing. Some patients produce a depression along the nail by constantly scratching the surface as a habit tic. The depression is crossed by irregular ridges, which results in a characteristic deformity.

'Median dystrophy' is a very uncommon abnormality, which is characterised by a longitudinal canal or split in the nail plate close to the midline. The split begins at the cuticle and extends distally, often with short lateral branches. The aetiology is unknown, but some patients give a history of preceding injury.

■ *Transverse furrow.* A depression across the nail plate may follow any temporary cause of reduced mitoses in the matrix. When systemic in origin, all nails are affected, and the furrows are known as Beau's lines. Measles in children or any severe illness in adults may be sufficient to produce the depression some weeks later. The deformity appears first just beyond the cuticle, passing distally as the nail grows. Occasionally, the furrow penetrates the full thickness of the nail, with shedding of the distal portion.

Cold injury or severe attacks of Raynaud's syndrome may produce transverse furrows confined to one or a few nails. Multiple irregular depressions may follow dermatitis of the proximal nail folds.

■ *Ridging.* Some degree of longitudinal ridging is not uncommon in normal nails and may be exaggerated in the elderly or in those with peripheral ischaemia. The ridging is often interrupted, giving the appearance of longitudinal beaded lines. Children occasionally develop quite severe ridging of all twenty nails with the loss of normal nail lustre. In most of these children the cause is not apparent, and the nails revert to normal after approximately two years. Identical changes may be produced by lichen planus, psoriasis, eczema, and alopecia areata.

Transverse ridges are often the result of using a nail file to push the cuticle back from the nail plate. When the injury is repeated, the nail may develop a suggestive pattern of regular parallel ridges. Irregular transverse ridging may complicate dermatitis involving the nail folds.

■ *Pterygium* is a distinctive pattern of scarring that produces destruction of the nail plate and fusion of the nail bed with an expanded proximal nail fold. The central portion of the cuticle grows over the nail and becomes attached to it. The nail is slowly split into two parts which become smaller as the pterygium enlarges. Eventually, the nail may be completely destroyed.

The deformity may complicate vasospastic or other causes of digital ischaemia, and is an uncommon sequel to lichen planus. In some patients, no cause is apparent.

Colour

Separation of a nail from its bed alters the normal pink colour to white or yellowish. Tinea occasionally begins as a chalky white crumbling spot on the surface of a toenail, but small white spots and transverse streaks are usually due to trauma to the proximal nail fold. Arsenical poisoning is a rare cause of transverse white stripes. Like those due to trauma, arsenical streaks are in the nail plate and grow distally with the nail. This contrasts with the paired white bands of hypoalbuminaemia, which reflect changes in the nail bed. A milky white opacity of the nail beds may develop in hepatic failure, or occur as a rare genetic abnormality.

Psoriatic nails may be yellow or brownish, and a round yellow area in the centre of a nail is particularly suggestive of psoriasis. Yellow or brown discolouration can be produced by tinea, candidal paronychia, pityriasis rubra pilaris, ionising radiation, and occasionally, by prolonged tetracycline therapy. Exogenous dyes produce discoloration in which the proximal end is the same shape as the cuticle, whereas systemic causes of discoloration have a proximal end shaped like the lunule. Subungual haematoma involving the proximal end of the nail plate grows out with a transverse proximal margin. Pseudomonas infection complicating paronychia or distal onycholysis may stain the adjoining nail bright green or bluish black. A rare but characteristic greenish yellow discolouration of all twenty nails occurs in the yellow nail syndrome.

Azure blue lunulae are a marker of Wilson's disease and should not be confused with the deeper blue of lunulae discoloured by phenolphthalein. Dark discolouration of the nail bed is an uncommon reaction to phenolphthalein in proprietary laxatives, or to chloroquine and other antimalarial drugs. Longitudinal brown or black bands are quite common in black-skinned people, but, in whites, may be the only evidence of a melanocytic naevus or melanoma of the matrix. Systemic administration of cytotoxic drugs may produce transverse black lines.

Red lunulae are a recognised sign of cardiac failure, chronic airways disease or carbon monoxide poisoning, but may also be seen with collagen diseases and severe psoriasis. A red distal half of the nail bed can occur with renal failure.

Separation (onycholysis)

A single injury may detach the proximal part of the nail from its bed, usually with an associated subungual haematoma. Distal separation can follow a single injury or repeated minor trauma, as from the wearing of tight shoes. Distal separation may also follow chemical injury by primary irritants, especially formaldehyde in nail hardeners. Onycholysis can also result from allergic contact dermatitis to acrylic resin, which is used to make sculptured artificial nails and is found in glues used to attach substances to the nail plate.

Psoriasis, dermatitis, tinea and erythroderma are frequent causes of 'spontaneous' separation, and the nails may be partially or completely detached in thyrotoxicosis, hypothyroidism, peripheral vascular disease and, rarely, severe hyperhidrosis. Onycholysis may occur as part of a phototoxic drug eruption, most often due to psoralens or tetracyclines, particularly demethylchlortetracycline.

Separated nails should be carefully trimmed back to the line of attachment, to avoid accumulation of foreign matter between nail and bed. Debris is gently removed with a soft brush, not the point of a nail file. Any application which is used should be bland and non-irritating, effective against both yeasts and bacteria, and cause evaporation of water. Thymol 3 per cent in alcohol is suitable.

Splitting into layers

Repeated wetting and drying of nails may lead to separation of small surface flakes toward the free edge. The condition is largely confined to women and the use of nail lacquer has been suggested as a contributing factor.

Subungual haemorrhage

Haemorrhage beneath the nail is a common and painful sequel to injuries which involve the distal phalanx. Early release of the blood by boring a hole through the nail plate not only relieves discomfort but usually prevents shedding of the nail later.

Although a classic sign of bacterial endocarditis, splinter haemorrhages are present in many patients with chronic diseases of the heart and lungs. They are a frequent finding in healthy manual workers, in patients with connective tissue diseases, and in those with psoriasis or tinea of the nails.

Digital clubbing

Clubbing begins with a filling-in of the angle between the proximal nail fold and the nail plate. There is an increase of fibrovascular tissue beneath the proximal fold and lunule, producing abnormal motility on pressure. The nail becomes thick and more curved than normal. Enlargement of the distal phalanx follows. Most patients have cyanotic heart disease, chronic lung disease or bronchial carcinoma. Other associations include ulcerative colitis, cirrhosis and thyroid disease. There is also a familial form.

The nail folds

Acute paronychia

Acute bacterial infection of a nail fold is usually preceded by some simple injury. A needle prick, picking at the nail fold, and similar forms of minor trauma, are common causes. The organisms most often involved are *Staphylococcus aureus*, *Streptococcus pyogenes* and *Pseudomonas aeruginosa*.

Clinical features

The nail fold is swollen, red, painful and tender. Suppuration often develops and gentle pressure on the fold may force a bead of pus onto the nail plate. The infection sometimes extends deeply, forming a small lake of pus which lifts the adjoining nail from the bed.

Treatment

An appropriate antibiotic should be administered systemically. Cool soaks using an aqueous solution of aluminium acetate (1:40) are helpful, but it may be necessary to promote drainage by carefully puncturing the fold close to the nail with the tip of a scalpel.

Chronic paronychia

Chronic inflammation of the nail fold is a very common disorder, which is mostly confined to those whose hands are frequently immersed in water. It is particularly common among housewives, barmen and cleaners. Other predisposing causes include diabetes, and thumb-sucking in children.

Clinical features

The nail fold is swollen, rounded and sometimes red. The normal close contact between fold and nail plate is lost, leaving a space in which water may accumulate. Chronic paronychia is not usually painful, but acute episodes punctuate the course, with pain, tenderness and sometimes suppuration. There may be secondary candidal or chronic bacterial infection, especially with pseudomonas.

The nail gradually becomes irregularly ridged, furrowed and discoloured. The nail adjoining infected folds may be yellowish brown or, with pseudomonas infection, bright green to black. With time, the size of the nail may be decreased. Generally, several fingers are affected and there is often an associated chronic dermatitis of the hand.

Treatment

Attention to the aetiological factors is essential if a prolonged course is to be avoided. The patient should minimise contact with water, soap, detergents, lipid solvents and other irritant compounds—a formidable undertaking for the housewife with young children. Cleaners and barmen may require a period of dry work to allow healing, which should not be considered complete until the cuticle has reformed.

After washing up or working in the laundry, the patient should thoroughly rinse and dry the hands. Loose rubber gloves with cotton inner gloves have theoretical advantages when wet work is unavoidable, but, in practice, the maceration produced by sweating often outweighs the protection which is provided. If gloves are used, they should not be worn for more than 10 minutes at a time. Cultures will often demonstrate *Candida albicans*, in which case clotrimazole, miconazole or amphotericin B may be applied with benefit. Applications of 10 per cent sulphacetamide in alcohol, or 2 per cent thymol in alcohol, to the nail fold, four times daily, are helpful. For a few patients who are unresponsive to an adequate trial of conservative management, surgical marsupialisation of the nail fold may be necessary.

Ingrown toenail

Overcurvature of the nail plate and minor orthopaedic deformities predispose to penetration of the nail fold by the lateral edge of the nail. Clipping the nail too short and picking or cutting away the corners of the free edge frequently initiate penetration. Tight shoes and high heels are contributing factors.

Clinical features

A lateral nail fold, almost always of the first toe, becomes swollen, red and painful. Secondary infection is common and adds to the swelling. Granulation tissue forms around the buried nail edge and pus may ooze from the groove beneath the nail fold.

Treatment

A period of rest, avoidance of further nail-clipping, the administration of systemic antibiotics, and attention to footwear may be sufficient to allow the nail to grow out. The affected nail should then be trimmed only in a straight line and no shorter than the tip of the toe. Persistent inflammation may necessitate avulsion of the nail. If recurrences follow regrowth, removal of the nail and matrix may be necessary to achieve permanent relief. However, such procedures are inappropriate for the elderly patient, or for others with a compromised peripheral circulation.

Tumours about the nail

Warts

Viral warts involving the distal portion of the lateral nail folds commonly grow under the nail plate. The resultant onycholysis and hyperkeratosis is often mistakenly diagnosed as tinea. Warts growing on the proximal nail fold, if treated with diathermy or by surgical methods, will produce scarring of the nail matrix and subsequent nail dystrophy.

Mucous cyst (myxoid cyst)

The mucous cyst is a poorly defined dermal swelling which develops insidiously and may reach a centimetre or so in diameter. The fingers, particularly the nail folds, are a common site. When the cyst forms in the proximal fold, pressure on the matrix may lead to the formation of a longitudinal depression in the nail. There may be fluctuations in the size of the cyst, but inflammatory episodes are not a feature. Surgical excision is frequently followed by recurrence, but injection of triamcinolone into the cyst gives a good cure rate.

Subungual exostosis

The bony outgrowth forms a hard swelling beneath the nail, usually towards the free edge on one side. The first toe is the digit most often affected. The tumour gradually displaces the overlying nail, with considerable pain from the pressure of a shoe. The subungual surface of the nodule occasionally becomes eroded and secondarily infected. There may be a superficial resemblance to ingrown toenail, but the nail is lifted by a subungual exostosis, not buried in the lateral nail fold. The outgrowth is visible on X-ray and is easily excised.

Glomus tumour

The nail bed is a common site for the benign glomus tumour. The lesion is purplish red, painful and extremely tender to pressure. Excision is curative.

Granuloma telangiectaticum

In a nail fold, the red, fleshy pyogenic granuloma may be mistaken for granulation tissue around an ingrown toenail. The similar appearance of squamous cell carcinoma or amelanotic melanoma at the site necessitates microscopic examination of the excised nodule.

Melanocytic naevus

A pigmented longitudinal band in the nail plate of a white-skinned patient points to a pigmented lesion of the matrix. Although often a junctional naevus, the responsible lesion may be a melanoma. Excision and histological assessment of the affected matrix is therefore necessary.

Kerato-acanthoma

Subungual kerato-acanthoma begins with rapidly increasing pain, together with swelling and redness of the distal phalanx. Subungual swelling lifts the nail from its bed and causes pressure necrosis of underlying bone. Local excision is curative.

Bowen's disease

Bowen's disease of the nail bed usually begins in a lateral nail fold, later spreading to the bed. In its early stages, the appearance is quite nondescript and the lesion is generally treated as dermatitis or tinea. Later, keratin gradually accumulates over the entire nail bed, with separation and eventual slow destruction of the nail. The variable appearance, even of advanced lesions, makes diagnosis very difficult without biopsy. Adequate excision with or without grafting is acceptable treatment, but microscopically monitored excision (Mohs' technique) combines total removal with maximal preservation of normal tissue.

Squamous cell carcinoma

Nail bed carcinoma may form an expanding nodule, which resembles granulation tissue growing around the free edge of a nail. The carcinoma may masquerade as chronic paronychia, but only one digit is affected, and the usual accompaniments of paronychia are lacking. Carcinoma of the nail bed is rare and unlikely to be diagnosed without biopsy. The tumour is removed either by amputation of the distal phalanx, or by Mohs' excision.

Melanoma

Although rare, melanoma should be considered in the differential diagnosis of atypical lesions of the nail fold or bed. Melanoma may masquerade as granulation tissue or chronic paronychia, as a small wart under the free edge of the nail plate or in a nail fold, or as granuloma telangiectaticum. Melanoma of the matrix may present as a dark stripe down the length of the nail plate, but any disturbance of pigmentation beneath or around the nail should arouse suspicion of melanoma.

22

Diseases of the dermis and fat

Dermis

1. Atrophy
   (a) ageing
   (b) striae
   (c) Ehlers-Danlos syndrome
   (d) localised atrophy

2. Thickening
   (a) solar damage
   (b) granuloma annulare
   (c) perforating elastoma

3. Expansion
   (a) lymphoedema
   (b) mucinoses
       scleredema
       pretibial myxoedema
       scleromyxoedema
   (c) amyloidosis
   (d) lipoid proteinosis

4. Sclerosis
   (a) hypertrophic scar
   (b) cheloid
   (c) fibromatoses
   (d) lichen sclerosis et atrophicus
   (e) scleroderma
   (f) pseudoscleroderma
       syndromes

Fat

1. Atrophy
   (a) insulin atrophy
   (b) progressive partial
       lipodystrophy
   (c) total lipoatrophy
   (d) post-inflammatory lipoatrophy

2. Inflammation
   (a) panniculitis
   (b) lobular panniculitis

When the dermis and fat are the site of primary pathology the visual impression, aided by palpation, is usually that of either atrophy or thickening. Dermal thickening may be due to altered collagen and elastin, ground substance infiltration, or dermal sclerosis. Fat involvement is usually poorly defined on palpation because of the dermis intervening between the probing fingers and the fat. Change is discerned as atrophy or inflammatory nodules.

Dermal atrophy

Ageing

Cutaneous atrophy is a regular accompaniment of ageing. The dermis is thinner and has less collagen than the skin of younger individuals. There are changes in the ground substance and in elastic fibres which are reflected clinically as fine wrinkles, reduced elastic recoil and is heightened by a concurrent reduction in fat. The epidermis shows only minimal macroscopic change, although functional alterations include poor wound healing and reduced barrier function. However, the signs of innate ageing are subtle when compared with the skin changes attributable to chronic sun damage, which is what the non-medical person normally equates with ageing skin.

Dermal atrophy is also a feature of the rare premature ageing syndromes, such as acrogeria, which is confined to the skin of the hands and feet, and the disorders with systemic involvement, such as progeria and Werner's syndrome.

Atrophic striae ('stretch marks')

The precise aetiology of striae is unknown. Mechanical stresses determine their direction, but the underlying cause is probably endocrine. They are common in pregnancy, Cushing's syndrome, and at adolescence, particularly in girls and, reputedly, in diabetics. Prolonged topical therapy with fluorinated corticosteroids may induce striae, mostly in the flexures or at sites which are treated under plastic occlusion.

Clinical features

Striae begin as smooth, weal-like, purplish elevations, up to a centimetre or more wide and many centimetres in length. As the colour fades to white, the lesions shrink to wrinkled, atrophic linear bands. During pregnancy, striae develop from the second trimester onwards, over the abdomen, buttocks, thighs and breasts. In adolescent girls the bands typically form on the buttocks and thighs, while boys tend to develop striae in a transverse pattern on the lower back.

Treatment

There is no effective method of prevention or treatment. Adolescents can be reassured that the lesions become much less conspicuous with time.

Ehlers–Danlos syndrome

There are numerous genetically determined disorders of collagen production which can manifest as this syndrome. Inheritance can be dominant or recessive.

The dermis is atrophic, slightly lax and hyperelastic. Minor wounds gape and heal with broad atrophic scars, often with underlying spongy nodules. The dermis is friable and will not hold sutures well. Easy bruising is usually a feature.

As part of a generalised disturbance of collagen production in many organs, there may be extreme flexibility of joints, multiple hernias, bladder and bowel diverticulae, arterial aneurysm and rupture, and valve prolapse.

Localised atrophy

■ *Injury* of various types will characteristically result in atrophic scarring. Examples include radiation damage, mechanical injury over bony prominences, occasional chemicals and discoid lupus erythematosus.

■ *Primary macular atrophy* (anetoderma) refers to a group of rare conditions in which small areas of dermal atrophy (one to two centimetres in diameter) occur without preceding inflammation. They may be soft bladder-like protrusions on the trunk and shoulders, or areas that are barely visible yet can be readily felt.

■ *Perifollicular elastolysis* is an uncommon complication of acne on the chest and back in which acne resolves to leave small, 1 mm to 2 mm diameter, white to yellow macules centred around hair follicles.

Thickened dermis

Solar damage

Aetiology

As with the epidermis, solar-induced change in the dermis is the net effect of incident radiation, inherent protection qualities and repair mechanisms. Experiments confirm that UV-B (290–320 nm) induces most of the effects. UV-A can also produce change but a greater quantity of radiation is required and even then the outcome is not as damaging. People of Celtic origin are more prone to cutaneous solar damage when compared with others of equal pigmentation exposed to similar radiation. This probably reflects abnormal repair mechanisms but so far no abnormality has been identified.

Histology

The papillary and upper reticular dermis is thickened by the accumulation of basophilic thickened and branched fragmented elastotic fibrous material. Special studies indicate that although there is a fourfold increase in normally functioning cross-linked elastin, this is small in comparison to the huge amount of non-functional degenerate elastotic material. Solar damage reduces the papillary capillary plexus and results in compensatory vasodilation of deeper vessels.

In addition, late changes include epidermal atrophy, mild dysplasia of keratinocytes, localised increase in melanocytes and eventually, reduction in the amount of collagen producing thinning of the dermis. In some areas overlying the basophilic elastotic change, the papillary dermis becomes thickened, homogeneous and eosinophilic (colloid degeneration).

Clinical features

The skin has a leathery texture and is sagging and wrinkled. In parts such as the nape of the neck, deep furrows are present. The vascular changes produce sallow telangiectatic skin and small venous lakes. Paradoxically, during the summer months, sun-damaged skin may look red because of an abnormal extreme prolongation of the vasodilatory response to acute sunburn. Changes within the epidermis induce blotchy pigmentation, depigmentation and surface atrophy. The elastotic dermis imparts a yellowish colour and where there is colloid degeneration, this shows as coalesced small macular yellow dots. A late change is dermal atrophy as a result of a reduction in collagen. This, combined with the atrophy of fat and dermis caused by innate ageing, reduces support for dermal vessels, causing them to rupture with minor trauma. The resultant ecchymoses typically seen over the dorsum of the distal forearms and hands persist for weeks and fade without the usual colour changes that accompany bruising. In the periorbital regions, comedones and keratinising cysts may be prominent. Solar keratoses and skin cancers are usually present.

Treatment

Repair of the dermal changes will slowly occur to a degree if there is a reduction in the amount of incident radiation. Topical retinoic acid enhances this repair and, in addition, induces angiogenesis in the papillary dermis and a return towards normal of the mild keratinocyte dysplasia and melanocytic changes.

Granuloma annulare

Granuloma annulare is a common, benign dermatosis which is characterised clinically by firm papules often grouped in an annular pattern.

Aetiology

Incidence is greatest among children and young adults. The precise cause is unknown, but lesions frequently occur at sites subject to minor trauma. Reports of an association with diabetes are conflicting, although there is firm evidence of reduced glucose tolerance in patients with multiple scattered lesions.

Histology

Beneath a normal epidermis, areas of degenerate collagen are surrounded by a palisade of histiocytes and an infiltrate of lymphocytes and fibroblasts. A few giant cells are sometimes present. This pattern of an area of altered hypocellular connective tissue surrounded by a cellular palisaded infiltrate is termed 'necrobiosis', and is also seen with rheumatoid nodules and necrobiosis lipoidica.

Clinical features (Colour plate 66)

The primary lesion is a firm, asymptomatic, pink or whitish papule or nodule. Peripheral enlargement and central clearing produce the typical raised circular border and slight central atrophy. Irregular thickening of the border gives a characteristic 'string of pearls' appearance, more pronounced when the skin is stretched. Common sites are the dorsum and sides of the fingers, back of the hands, the elbows and knees.

Unusual variants include nodules without central clearing, a generalised eruption of small but otherwise typical lesions, giant lesions many centimetres across, a widespread macular form, papules that extrude altered dermis through surface perforations, and a rare ulcerating form. However, in most patients granuloma annulare is clinically characteristic.

Diagnosis

▶ **Suspect** granuloma annulare when skin-coloured papules are present with a tendency to annulus formation.

▶ **Consider and exclude**

■ *Warts*, which are skin-coloured and share the same common sites of involvement. They are, however, an epidermal change.

■ *Sarcoid* involving the skin is frequently annular. Lesions do not show beading of the border and the histology is of cellular granulomas without connective tissue change.

■ *Leprosy* produces papules and plaques with annulus formation but lesions are commonly anaesthetic and the histology is of cellular granulomas.

■ *Syphilis* in the tertiary stage is often annular. However, surface change is prominent, the face is usually involved, and serology is positive.

■ *Lichen planus* uncommonly presents as annular lesions that are usually found in association with more typical flat topped violaceous papules elsewhere. Mucosal changes when present are a helpful feature. Biopsy is of a band-like infiltrate of lymphocytes in the papillary dermis.

■ *Necrobiosis lipoidica*, although similar histologically, rarely causes confusion clinically if lesions are established. Early lesions, although papular, are more pink-looking and tend to be present over the shin rather than on the knee or ankle.

▶ **Confirm** the diagnosis, when there is doubt, by biopsy.

Treatment

Treatment is unnecessary for most patients. Cosmetically significant lesions may be treated with corticosteroids either applied under plastic occlusion or injected intradermally into the lesion. However, enthusiasm for intralesional steroids should be tempered by awareness of the atrophy which may follow their injudicious use.

Perforating elastoma (elastosis perforans serpiginosa)

Perforating elastoma is a very uncommon lesion, probably caused by a defect of elastic tissue. More than one-third of those affected have an associated disorder of fibrous proteins, usually pseudoxanthoma elasticum, Ehlers-Danlos syndrome, or Marfan's syndrome. Penicillamine, which affects cross-linking of fibrous proteins, may induce this disorder.

Histology

There is a stream of abnormal connective tissue with a large elastic fibre component, which begins high in the dermis and winds through the epidermis to the surface, where a keratinous papule surrounds the opening of the canal.

Clinical features

Individual lesions are firm, skin-coloured or reddish papules with a horny plug in the centre. The papules are frequently arranged in a circular, arched or horseshoe shape, which surrounds an area of normal or slightly atrophic skin. The clusters are generally only a few centimetres in diameter, but may be much larger. In the majority of patients, only one region is affected, most often the back or sides of the neck, the lower face, the upper or lower limbs.

Perforating elastoma begins in children or young adults and persists for years, new papules appearing as old ones heal. Resolution ultimately occurs, but the disease may last a decade or more.

Treatment

The risk of cheloid precludes surgical excision. Even a small biopsy may trigger cheloid formation. Cosmetic improvement can be achieved by gently curetting out the centre of the papules, or by stripping the keratinous plugs with repeated application of sticky tape. Cryotherapy is often of benefit. Dermabrasion will make the condition worse.

Expansion of the dermis

Lymphoedema

Chronic lymphoedema can impart a woody feel to the thickened dermis. The epidermis is often hyperkeratotic and papillomatous over the lower legs and feet producing an appearance known as *mossy foot*. Fluid may ooze to the surface and secondary infection is a common complication.

Mucinoses

A woody thickening of the dermis is also produced by mucinoses. Biopsy and special stains reveal abundant mucin in the dermis between collagen fibres.

■ *Scleredema* has an abrupt onset and often follows a streptococcal or respiratory infection. The disease usually begins on the face or neck, and may spread to the shoulders and upper trunk. Involvement of other areas is uncommon but the tongue, pharynx, pleura, voluntary and cardiac muscles may all be affected. Resolution occurs in most patients within a year or two. The disease is more persistent in diabetics. There is no treatment.

■ *Pretibial myxoedema (Colour plate 67)* produces a 'peau d'orange' appearance, coarse hairs within the area and is associated with Graves' disease although it can occur after the hyperthyroidism has been controlled. Other features include exophthalmos and the presence of long-acting thyroid stimulator (LATS) within the blood.

■ *Scleromyxoedema* (lichen myxoedematosus) is characterised by papules that coalesce to form large plaque-like areas. The hands and forearms, and the upper trunk neck and face are the areas of predilection. A characteristic paraprotein which is a cationic IgG is found in the blood.

Melphalan is extremely helpful in causing resolution of the skin changes even though the paraprotein may still be present in the same amounts.

Amyloidosis

Localised cutaneous amyloidosis without systemic involvement most commonly presents as sheets of small hemispherical itchy papules that are a transparent grey or hyperpigmented, hyperkeratotic and localised to the shins. Asian males are especially predisposed. The amyloid probably arises from the epidermis and stains variably. A battery of stains is best used to diagnose this variety. Deep tumours within the dermis are rarely seen. A non-indurated pigmented macular form also occurs.

Primary systemic amyloidosis or myeloma associated amyloid may deposit within the dermis. Amyloidosis secondary to chronic inflammation does not involve the skin. In systemic amyloidosis, firm waxy yellow plaques occur, especially in the eyelids. Deposition of amyloid within the walls of small blood vessels prevents them constricting and therefore pinching the skin typically produces purpura both within the plaques and in normal-looking skin.

Lipoid proteinosis

This is a rare, recessively inherited condition in which hyaline material is deposited within the dermis of the oral cavity and larynx.

Histology

PAS-positive material is deposited around vessels and sweat glands and in broad bands within the reticular dermis. Unlike the lipid storage diseases, in which the abnormal material is within macrophages of histiocytes, in this disorder the hyaline material that contains lipid is lying free within the dermis.

Clinical features

The disorder is progressive during childhood but does not seem to proceed during adult life. Yellowish-brown nodules and plaques are most conspicuous on the face. The changes often appear in areas of trauma such as the palms, fingers, knees and elbows. Small papules typically appear along the eyelid margins. Laryngeal involvement is usual and produces a characteristic hoarse whispering voice. On the soft palate and tonsils, infiltrates are often visible as yellowish-white areas. Similar changes may be seen on the undersurface of the tongue, which is enlarged, firm and has a limited range of movements.

Diagnosis

▶ **Consider and exclude**

■ The *porphyrias* and, in particular, erythropoietic protoporphyria which may, in the early stages, look similar. However, although these conditions may produce PAS-positive material in a perivascular location, in lipoid proteinosis the hyaline is also around sweat glands and photosensitivity is not a feature.

■ *Lichen myxoedematosus* has the abnormal gamma globulin.

■ *Systemic myxoedema* may also present with hoarseness but thyroid function is normal in lipoid proteinosis.

Treatment

Because prognosis is good, treatment is not necessary. Skin changes can be cosmetically improved by dermabrasion. Voice changes may be returned towards normal by laryngeal surgery.

Sclerosis

Hypertrophic scar

Aetiology

Increased synthesis of collagen is an integral part of dermal repair after injury. Normally, collagen production is coordinated with the needs of repair and the end-result is a fibrous scar. If the synthesis of collagen is excessive, the scar is hypertrophic.

Histology

Normal collagen bundles are replaced by fibrillary collagen that tends to be aligned parallel to the skin surface. Elongated thin fibroblasts are increased in number. Elastin is absent. Adnexal structures are reduced in number or totally absent.

Clinical features

The hypertrophic scar does not extend beyond the area of trauma and is slowly remodelled by the dermis. It may be regarded as a temporary aberration of normal healing and usually resolves within eighteen months or so. Areas particularly prone to this pattern of healing include anterior chest, upper back, and thyroidectomy scars. Thermal injury commonly induces this type of reaction.

Treatment

Intralesional injection of steroid is useful for areas that are not too extensive. For areas not under tension, surgical revision is often effective.

Cheloid

In genetically predisposed people, hypertrophy after injury may be not merely a reversible excess of collagen, but a sustained synthesis by abnormally proliferating fibroblasts (cheloid). The proliferation bears little relation to the needs of repair, is not reversed with time, and proceeds beyond the area of injury.

Aetiology

Genetic predisposition is more frequent in oriental and black races, and in some families. Even in predisposed individuals there is a pronounced regional variation of susceptibility. Cheloids occur more often on the presternal and deltoid regions, the upper part of the trunk, the neck and the earlobes. The eyelids, forehead, palms and soles are rarely affected.

Cheloids are most prevalent in young adults and are rare at the extremes of life. The cheloid is usually a sequel to known injury, particularly burns and scalds, but some patients form cheloid at sites of injury so minor as to escape notice. Thyroidectomy and vaccination scars are common sites. Cheloid is more frequent in the presence of infection or foreign matter, and is more likely to complicate surgery when the wound is under tension.

Histology

There is a nodular accumulation of thickened homogeneous collagen fibres, arranged in a rather haphazard pattern. Plump fibroblasts lie parallel to the collagen bundles, which are separated by abundant mucin. Many capillaries and a patchy inflammatory infiltrate are present in early lesions, but decrease along with a reduction in the number of fibroblasts as the cheloid matures.

Clinical features *(Colour plate 68)*

The developing cheloid is an itchy, tender, reddish thickening, which soon grows beyond the edges of the wound. Firm, claw-like extensions spread from the margins of the swelling, which continues to enlarge for months or years. Having reached a maximum size, the lesion persists indefinitely. Cheloids are generally rounded or lobulated, but may become sessile or pedunculated. Serious contractures may complicate cheloids around joints.

Diagnosis

▶ **Consider and exclude**

■ *Hypertrophic scar*, which does not extend beyond the margins of the wound and regresses within eighteen months or so.

■ *Scar sarcoid* is neither itchy nor tender, usually arises in old scars, and can be distinguished microscopically.

■ *Dermatofibrosarcoma protuberans* and other neoplasms of connective tissue may require histological differentiation.

Treatment

Particular care is necessary with surgical procedures which involve the neck and upper chest, especially in patients known to be cheloid-prone. In predisposed patients, cheloid can be prevented by X-ray treatment of surgical wounds within two weeks of operation. Simple excision of an established cheloid is usually followed by recurrence. Excision should therefore be combined with adjuvant therapy designed to reduce postoperative fibrous hyperplasia. Various devices have been used to apply constant pressure to the site of excision and have given good results when maintained for a minimum of four to six months. X-ray therapy may also be combined with surgical excision of cheloid to prevent recurrence.

Intralesional triamcinolone is effective if used early while cheloid is forming, but old lesions are more difficult and, if not unduly disfiguring, are probably better left untreated.

Fibromatoses

There is a group of cutaneous disorders which are characterised by abnormal fibrous hyperplasia, frequently associated with a predisposition to cheloid formation. The hyperplasia may be restricted to a single syndrome, or there may be a combination of more than one type. Only the three more common forms are considered here. These are Dupuytren's contracture, knuckle pads, and Peyronie's disease.

Fibromatosis of palms and soles (Dupuytren's contracture)

The disease is inherited as an autosomal dominant characteristic. The incidence rises with increasing age and there is considerable sex-limitation to males. There is a significant association with other fibroblastic proliferative disorders, particularly knuckle pads. The increased incidence in epileptics and alcoholics is unexplained.

Clinical features

Bilateral involvement is usual and all four extremities may be affected. A firm painless nodule arises in the palm or sole, and extends slowly in the palmar or plantar fascia. On the hand, the thickened aponeurosis becomes palpable as firm bands stretching below the skin. Digital extension is progressively restricted as fibrous contracture bends affected fingers toward the palm. The fourth or fifth finger is affected first; other fingers follow, but the thumb is rarely involved. On the sole, nodular thickening is similar but seldom progresses to contracture of the toes.

Treatment

A patient who is unable to place his hand flat on a table top, palm down, has at least a 30° joint deformity and warrants assessment for surgical relief.

Knuckle pads

The knuckle pad is a well-circumscribed thickening of skin over the dorsum of an interphalangeal or metacarpophalangeal joint. The toes are rarely affected. In some families the condition is inherited as an autosomal dominant trait.

Clinical features

A callus-like thickening develops insidiously over one or more knuckles, usually the proximal interphalangeal. Onset is in early adult life and the lesions persist indefinitely, enlarging slowly, but not extending beyond the skin over the joint. Knuckle pads are painless and skin-coloured, with a flat or domed surface.

Treatment

Surgical excision is invariably followed by recurrence, sometimes cheloidal. Regression follows the intralesional injection of corticosteroids, but recurrences are the rule.

Peyronie's disease

The disease begins in middle age or later, as a tumour-like fibroblastic proliferation of penile connective tissue. A firm subcutaneous nodule or plaque forms on one side of the penis and slowly spreads. Fibrous contracture follows, with pain and deformity of the erect penis. Intralesional injection of triamcinolone is a painful, but frequently effective, treatment.

Lichen sclerosus et atrophicus

Lichen sclerosus is an uncommon disease of unknown aetiology in which striking white lesions form in the skin. The anogenital region is a particularly frequent site, especially in prepubertal girls and postmenopausal women.

Histology

In early lesions the epidermis is thick and hyperkeratotic, and overlies an upper dermal band of oedema and homogenised collagen. The band appears structureless and separates the epidermis from a mid-dermal zone of lymphocytic infiltrate. Epidermal atrophy gradually replaces acanthosis as the infiltrate becomes scattered and scanty.

Clinical features *(Colour plate 69)*

- The *characteristic lesions* are firm, ivory-white papules a few millimetres in diameter, which are closely aggregated into vivid white patches. Individual papules may become depressed and hard, while others coalesce to form solid white plaques, usually with discrete papules still visible around the margins. The induration lasts for years, but may eventually soften to an atrophic patch of leucoderma. Lesions are occasionally deep brown in colour, particularly in dark-skinned individuals.

- *Distribution* in females is most often to the anogenital region, where a characteristic figure of eight pattern forms over the vulva and around the anus. The glans or prepuce may be affected in men. Extragenital lichen sclerosus is usually bilateral, with a predilection for the upper part of the trunk and the front of the wrists. However, lesions may occur anywhere on the skin and in the mouth.

- *Course.* This varies a good deal with the age of the patient. In adult women with anogenital involvement, severe vulval pruritus is the rule, and there may be progressive atrophy with narrowing of the introitus. Although previously regarded as a precursor of leukoplakia and carcinoma, vulval lichen sclerosus is now believed to be a benign condition. However, the issue remains unsettled, with a reported incidence of squamous cell carcinoma which ranges from 0 to 10 per cent in different published series.

The prognosis is better in girls, many cases resolving at puberty. In men, genital involvement may lead to phimosis and meatal stricture. Extragenital lesions are usually asymptomatic.

Treatment

There is no satisfactory treatment. Corticosteroids do not influence the course, but may relieve the pruritus of vulval lesions. Simple emollients are also very useful in reducing discomfort. Applications of testosterone proprionate have been successfully used to induce resolution of vulval disease in some prepubertal cases. However, the prognosis is better in girls, with about two-thirds of patients spontaneously improving or resolving completely at or about puberty.

Doubtful areas of erosion or thickening should be biopsied to exclude premalignant dysplasia and carcinoma. In the absence of either, surgical measures are indicated only to relieve late cicatricial complications.

Scleroderma

■ *Localised* cutaneous involvement manifests as morphoea. Typically a purplish oedematous area evolves over months to produce a pale, slightly depressed sclerotic plaque with a violet or brown periphery. Slowly, over many years, the area of sclerosis becomes a uniform ivory or brownish colour. The plaque then apparently remains static but, several decades later, spontaneous resolution may be noted.

■ *Diffuse* scleroderma most commonly begins on the distal limbs following a period of Raynaud's phenomenon. The skin is shiny, taut and bound down. Skin lines are lost from the dorsum of the fingers and the patient is unable to completely clench the fingers to make a fist. Often small ulcers appear on the fingers in association with atrophy of the finger tip pulp. Facial involvement produces a taut expressionless appearance with a smooth forehead, pinched nose, puckered mouth and mat-like telangiectases around the lips.

Pseudoscleroderma syndromes

In many other diseases, for reasons that are often not well established, dermal fibrosis occurs unrelated to preceding local injury. The resultant change produces fibrotic bound-down skin mimicking scleroderma.

■ *Porphyria cutanea tarda* induces fibrosis predominantly in sun-exposed areas, even though porphyrins are known to stimulate fibroblasts to produce collagen without sun exposure being necessary. The porphyria has usually been active for years.

■ *Carcinoid syndrome*. The fibrosis occurs predominantly on the legs and other signs of this tumour-induced disease are present.

■ *Rheumatoid arthritis* is associated with shiny atrophic, bound-down sclerotic skin over the hands and fingers.

■ *Diabetes mellitus*. Thick skin also involves the hands.

■ *Phenylketonuria* produces widespread sclerosis which is usually seen during the first year of life and can be reversed by exclusion of phenylalamine from the diet.

■ *Bleomycin* induces fibrosis not only of the skin but also the lungs. Changes can resolve months after the drug is ceased.

■ *Occupational exposure* to organic solvents and vinyl chloride manufacture produces acrocyanosis as well as sclerosis. Characteristically, X-ray of the hands reveals osteolysis of the distal phalanges.

Atrophy of fat

■ *Insulin atrophy* is now rare, since human insulin manufactured by genetic engineering has replaced animal insulins for routine use. However, well-defined areas of subcutaneous atrophy may still develop occasionally if sites are repeatedly chosen for insulin injection. The patient is usually a young woman or child and the first lesions begin to appear, within two years of starting insulin, as depressions that are relatively insensitive. Improvement occurs when affected sites are avoided for future injections.

■ *Progressive partial lipodystrophy*. This rare disorder usually begins between five and fifteen years of age with a progressive loss of subcutaneous fat, which starts on the face and spreads downwards. Atrophy stops above the hips and the legs may, in fact, be abnormally fat. The face develops an aged, cadaverous appearance. There may be hyperglycaemia, hyperlipidaemia, and glomerulonephritis.

■ *Total lipoatrophy*. Total lipoatrophy is a rare metabolic disorder which begins early in life, with progressive loss of subcutaneous and visceral fat. The face is gaunt, the body muscular and sometimes acromegaloid. There is hepatosplenomegaly, elevation of plasma lipids and decreased glucose tolerance.

■ *Post-inflammatory lipoatrophy* is a well recognised outcome of lupus erythematosus profundus and deep granuloma annulare, which are both disorders that produce a lobular panniculitis.

Inflammation of fat

Panniculitis

Inflammation of the subcutaneous fat (the panniculus) has, in the past, had a very confusing nomenclature. Despite a wide variety of causes, most cases look very similar clinically, with tender reddish nodules involving predominantly the lower legs, and women being much more commonly affected than men. Biopsy is usually performed as an aid in directing the search for a cause rather than for confirming panniculitis, which is evident clinically.

Aetiology

Panniculitis produced by vasculitis and polyarteritis nodosa may occur secondary to infections such as hepatitis, tuberculosis and bacterial upper respiratory tract infections, or secondary to various drugs. Cessation of oral steroids may also be followed by panniculitis. Lipolytic enzymes released during acute pancreatitis or by pancreatic tumour may be responsible. Direct injury either by cold, trauma or introduced substances is identified in some cases. In many patients there is no discernible cause.

Histology

The normal panniculus is divided into large lobules by septae which are downgrowths of dermal connective tissue. Depending upon the cause, pathology is either predominantly within the septae and peripheral portions of the lobules (septal panniculitis), or primarily within the central portions of the lobules (lobular panniculitis).

■ In *septal panniculitis*, inflammatory cells and, later, histiocytes, giant cells and fibrous tissue expand the septae. Portions of the periphery of fat lobules show fat cell necrosis with phagocytosis of lipids by macrophages. This pattern is seen with erythema nodosum, a deep continuation of necrobiosis lipoidica or scleroderma, and small vessel vasculitis or polyarteritis nodosa.

■ *Lobular panniculitis* usually manifests as an intense inflammatory infiltrate where lipocyte necrosis produces lipid-laden foam cells that coalesce to form giant cells. Processes producing this variety include injury, granuloma annulare, lupus erythematosus, large vessel vasculitis and leukaemic infiltrates. Pancreatitis produces a specific lobular panniculitis, in which there is virtually no inflammation, and fat cells are destroyed to leave only cell outlines.

Clinical features

Early nodules are pink, red or purplish elevations, usually on one or both lower limbs. They are oedematous, ill-defined, and a little tender. Size ranges from one to several centimetres. Lesions may be solitary, few or numerous, and may form as a single eruption or in crops over a period. Typically, the oedema subsides and gradual resolution follows over a few weeks, leaving a slightly depressed, hyperpigmented area. Individual nodules may coalesce or expand to form a large plaque, or extend and slowly migrate over a limb. Occasionally, nodules break down and discharge a brown oily fluid. Although most common on the legs, nodular panniculitis can occur anywhere on the limbs or trunk, and may involve mesenteric or retroperitoneal fat.

The ESR is generally elevated, often with leucocytosis, fever and sometimes anaemia.

Treatment

A search for underlying disease should be made in every patient. Rest, salicylates, and firm bandaging are usually sufficient to relieve discomfort while resolution occurs. Severely affected patients may respond to prednisone, 60 mg daily for the first week, with gradual reduction over the following four weeks. Oral administration of tetracycline, potassium iodide, and fibrinolytic agents have each been reported effective in small groups of patients.

23

Disorders of sweating

1. Eccrine
   (a) hyperhidrosis
   (b) hypohidrosis
   (c) diseases associated with increased sweating
2. Apocrine
   (a) body odour
   (b) apocrine miliaria
   (c) hidradenitis suppurativa

Eccrine disorders

Hyperhidrosis

Hyperhidrosis is sweating which is excessive in relation to environmental circumstances. It may be generalised or restricted to certain areas.

Generalised hyperhidrosis

When cutaneous vasodilatation is inadequate to prevent a rise in body temperature, further cooling is provided by evaporation of sweat. Eccrine glands are stimulated by neural impulses which originate in hypothalamic cells and pass via the medulla and lateral horn cells to sympathetic fibres. Heat-induced sweating is most abundant over the trunk, where evaporation from the large flat surface is more effective in reducing body temperature.

■ *Generalised sweating* is a normal thermoregulatory response to increased environmental temperatures or strenuous exercise. Defervescence of fevers is accompanied by profuse sweating, and generalised hyperhidrosis may persist into convalescence, long after the fever has abated. In most non-febrile diseases with hyperhidrosis, the patient responds as if the hypothalamic threshold were lowered. Thyrotoxicosis, acromegaly and gout may be accompanied by sweating at normal body temperatures. Hypothalamic hyperhidrosis also occurs with lymphomas, chronic infections, alcoholism and after withdrawal of narcotics. Tumours and other lesions of the hypothalamus are rare causes.

■ *Episodic hyperhidrosis* is a feature of shock, hypoglycaemia, dumping syndrome, phaeochromocytoma, treatment with antipyretic or emetic drugs and, paradoxically, in some patients with spinal cord injuries. Episodic sweating localised to the face may be induced by eating. When gustatory sweating is physiological, it is distributed symmetrically. Pathological gustatory sweating is unilateral and is produced by autonomic dysfunction often secondary to diabetes, herpes zoster or parotid gland pathology.

■ *Apparent or compensatory hyperhidrosis* occurs in unaffected areas of skin in patients with a substantially reduced number of functioning eccrine glands after only minor exertion or small elevations of environmental temperature. Compensatory hyperhidrosis of the face may be a misleading sign in patients with incomplete anhidrotic ectodermal dysplasia, and other causes of reduced sweating.

■ *Psychological factors* are not often relevant to generalised hyperhidrosis. In many patients there is no discoverable cause, emotional or otherwise.

Localised hyperhidrosis

Although sharing the eccrine response to increased body temperature, the palms, soles and axillae are especially sensitive to emotional stimuli. Most people have clammy palms and soles at times of fright, severe anxiety, or intense concentration, and the axillae may be affected in the same way, either alone or together with the palms and soles. Some individuals experience sweating from these areas with very minor stress, and the response may be excessive and prolonged. Palmoplantar hyperhidrosis often begins in childhood but the axillae are seldom affected before puberty.

Severe palmar hyperhidrosis causes embarrassment and may interfere with the patient's occupation. Sweaty hands can be a serious handicap for typists, clothing sales assistants, those handling fine metal objects, and people in many similar occupations. Apart from being unpleasant, plantar hyperhidrosis predisposes to interdigital intertrigo, and to contact dermatitis from substances leached out of shoes. Patients with axillary hyperhidrosis are troubled by soiled, sweat-soaked clothing, but the secretion, which is predominantly derived from eccrine glands, does not cause axillary odour.

Treatment of hyperhidrosis

Most patients are children or young adults and, for these, slow improvement can be confidently predicted. When not unduly severe, hyperhidrosis is best managed with explanation and reassurance. Sedatives and tranquillisers are of very limited value. Propantheline and similar anticholinergic drugs are generally ineffective, even in doses sufficient to produce unpleasant side-effects. They are equally disappointing when applied topically. Aluminium salts, formaldehyde and glutaraldehyde act by obstructing eccrine ducts rather than by reducing secretion, and may cause contact dermatitis and axillary miliaria.

For axillary hyperhidrosis the most effective topical agent is an alcoholic solution of 20 per cent aluminium chloride hexahydrate, but irritant contact dermatitis is frequent. This agent is not effective in reducing palmoplantar hyperhidrosis. Mild plantar hyperhidrosis can be controlled with dilute formalin footbaths. The theoretical problem of contact allergy to formalin can be minimised if application is confined to the soles. Iontophoresis using tap water gives temporary relief, which is of variable duration for patients with moderate severity palmoplantar hyperhidrosis, but can be repeated.

Surgery is used in severe cases. Excision of a small block of skin and subcutaneous tissue from the vault of the axilla removes the eccrine sweat glands and effectively relieves axillary hyperhidrosis in most patients. The excision of an area about 4 cm × 2.5 cm usually suffices. However, results are best when the area of maximal sweating is first defined by the starch-iodine method. For palmar or plantar hyperhidrosis, cervicodorsal or lumbar sympathectomy is an effective but radical measure, difficult to justify except for very severely affected patients.

Hypohidrosis

Complete inability to sweat is very rare, even in patients with 'anhidrotic' ectodermal dysplasia. Extensive anhidrosis may complicate hypothalamic lesions, syringomyelia, spinal transection, peripheral neuropathy, leprosy or scleroderma, and is a temporary consequence of generalised miliaria. Significant hypohidrosis occurs with Sjögren's syndrome and hypothryroidism, and may follow intoxication with mepacrine, heavy metals, or large doses of anticholinergic drugs.

Clinical features

Very few patients complain of inability to sweat normally. Infants may be brought for advice regarding unexplained pyrexia, and older patients present because of headache, malaise, and fatigue in warm weather or with exercise. There may be dizziness, nausea, and symptoms resulting from hyperventilation. Examination is likely to reveal only tachycardia and an elevated temperature.

Hypohidrosis renders the patient vulnerable to the effects of exercise and environmental heat. Physical work in hot weather may lead to complete collapse of thermoregulation, peripheral circulatory failure, and death.

Treatment

In the absence of a remediable cause, management amounts to explanation and avoidance of the factors producing thermal stress. Badly affected patients are well advised to move to cooler regions.

Diseases associated with increased sweating

1. Miliaria
   (a) crystallina
   (b) rubra
   (c) profunda
2. Intertrigo
3. Pitted keratolysis
4. Juvenile plantar dermatosis

Miliaria

Miliaria is a papular or vesicular eruption due to sweat retention caused by occlusion of eccrine ducts.

Aetiology

The eccrine pore is easily blocked by altered keratin, which prevents the escape of sweat to the surface. The gland continues to respond to thermal stimuli until pressure within the duct exceeds the pressure of secretion, when further sweat production ceases. The keratinous obstruction is usually shed in one to two weeks so that, in the absence of further damage to the pore, the condition is self-limited.

Sweat retention occurs in sunburned skin and in patches of dermatitis, where it contributes to the pruritus. Widespread miliaria is generally the result of prolonged sweating in hot environments, particularly with high relative humidity. The macerated poral cells are altered to form a keratotic plug which obstructs the lumen—a process facilitated by the overgrowth of micrococci that accompanies hydration of the eccrine pore. In hot dry climates, miliaria is more or less confined to areas covered by clothing and to the flexures, where the immediate environment is more humid. Miliaria is common in the napkin area of infants who wear rubber or plastic pants for long periods, or on the back of bedridden patients when evaporation of sweat is impeded by rubber undersheets.

Histology

■ *Miliaria crystallina* is the most superficial form. A small surface plug overlies a vesicle in the stratum corneum, which communicates with an eccrine duct.

■ *Miliaria rubra* develops when thermal stress leads to extravasation of sweat through the damaged eccrine duct into the stratum spinosum. A tiny area of dermatitis develops in which there is spongiosis and infiltration by inflammatory cells.

■ *Miliaria profunda* complicates miliaria rubra when impaction of the eccrine duct by a secondary plug produces dilatation of the lower epidermal and dermal portions of the duct. Seepage of sweat into the superficial papillary dermis may then produce a deep vesicular lesion.

Clinical features

■ *Miliaria crystallina*. Lesions are tiny, clear, superficial vesicles, which are fragile and quickly ruptured. There is neither pruritus nor erythema and, occurring mostly in the axillae and groins, the lesions are easily overlooked. Miliaria crystallina has little clinical importance.

■ *Miliaria rubra (sweat rash, prickly heat)*. The primary lesion is a small vesicle or papule on an erythematous base. With many contiguous lesions, coalescence produces large patches of erythema dotted with papules or vesicles, which may become pustular. Only the palms and soles are never affected, although the face is generally spared, except in infants. The trunk and large flexures are common sites. *(Colour plate 70)*

Pruritus is severe, but tends to be intermittent and is aggravated by any stimulus to sweating. Extensive involvement may lead to significant hypohidrosis, with fatigue and heat intolerance. Miliaria rubra is a relatively common cause of disability among miners, pastrycooks, foundry workers, and others who work in hot surroundings.

■ *Miliaria profunda*. The deep form of miliaria is invariably preceded by prolonged or recurrent miliaria rubra. Lesions are discrete whitish papules, two or three millimetres in diameter, most numerous on the trunk, but with some involvement of the limbs. There is neither pruritus nor erythema, except from associated miliaria rubra. The clinical picture is dominated by the effects of hypohidrosis.

Treatment

The patient should be moved to a cool environment, and activity should be reduced to a minimum. Clothing should be loose, light, and made of cotton material. Alcohol intake is better avoided. Greasy and irritating applications are unsuitable. A lotion consisting of salicylic acid 3 per cent, menthol 1 per cent and chlorhexidine 0.5 per cent in alcohol will accelerate resolution by alleviating the obstruction, causing evaporation of the sweat and preventing secondary infection. When possible, the patient is treated in an air-conditioned room or ward. Too frequent bathing, and the excessive use of soap are discouraged.

Intertrigo

Intertrigo is dermatitis of apposing skin surfaces. The immediate cause is mechanical, but the effects of friction are magnified by obesity, warm weather and maceration induced by sweating. Miliaria, scratching and secondary infection tend to perpetuate the inflammation.

Clinical features

Intertrigo occurs in the groins, natal cleft, axillae, beneath pendulous breasts, in skin folds of the obese, and between the toes. Affected skin is red, itchy and a little tender. With the onset of bacterial infection, inflammation is increased and frank cellulitis or impetigo may develop and spread beyond the flexure. Fissuring deep in the fold is common and with secondary infection may produce a smelly, purulent crevice. Flaccid pustules, a shaggy, festooned border and soft, soggy scaling suggest secondary candidiasis.

Diagnosis

Persistent intertrigo unresponsive to treatment may indicate that mechanical effects are not the cause. Many rashes preferentially localise to the flexures and a biopsy may be required to achieve the correct diagnosis.

▶ **Consider and exclude**

■ *Tinea*, which has a more definite border, is not strictly confined to surfaces in close contact, and can be excluded by examination of scrapings. Topical steroid application may mask the inflamed border but actually makes the microscopic visualisation of fungi easier.

■ *Erythasma* produces a brownish pink discoloration covered with a delicate wrinkled scale. Wood's light examination will reveal a coral pink fluorescence.

- *Flexural psoriasis* retains the rich red colour of psoriasis elsewhere, although surface scaling is often minimal and instead there is a glazed look. Other sites are likely to be affected.

- *Seborrhoeic dermatitis* spreads out beyond the skin folds and is usually associated with lesions of the scalp and other seborrhoeic areas.

- *Hailey–Hailey disease*, although vesicular, often presents as crusted coalesced erosions.

- *Darier's disease* may present as greasy flexural plaques formed by the aggregation of the typical keratotic papules. Nail changes are often present.

- *Histiocytosis X* is suspected if the flexural rash looks like seborrhoeic dermatitis but has petechial haemorrhages within the area.

Treatment

The patient with acutely inflamed intertrigo is better treated by rest in bed, with the affected skin surfaces separated. Secondary infection with bacteria or candida is treated using the appropriate agents. Topical therapy is as for acute weeping dermatitis. Cool wet packs will dry out the oozing surface in two to three days. A corticosteroid lotion or cream may then be substituted until healing is complete. Greasy applications should not be used.

Attention should be directed to prevention of recurrences. Diabetes should be excluded, obesity needs to be corrected and appropriate cotton garments substituted for occlusive pantyhose or nylon underpants. The patient is reminded to rinse soap thoroughly from the flexures while showering, and to dry the skin carefully afterwards. Women with submammary intertrigo benefit from a suitable uplift bra. A simple, unscented powder is useful if applied sparingly to dry skin. Mothers should be made to understand the role of rubber or plastic pants in producing intertrigo and miliaria of the napkin area of infants.

Pitted keratolysis *(Colour plate 71)*

Being confined to plantar skin and usually asymptomatic, pitted keratolysis is probably considerably more common than is generally realised. Mostly during summer, small, superficial, circular erosions form over weight-bearing areas of the sole. With coalescence, polycyclic or irregular lesions reach a centimetre or more in size. The erosions may be tender and uncomfortable, especially with sweating.

Hyperhidrosis is frequently associated and the macerated stratum corneum provides a favourable site for bacterial overgrowth. Several organisms, most often actinomycetes or corynebacteria, have been held responsible for the condition, but large numbers of aerobic diphtheroids are regularly found.

Treatment

Control of the sweating will be effective, as will topical antibiotics, but recurrences are very common.

Juvenile plantar dermatosis

Like intertrigo, juvenile plantar dermatosis is a dermatitis of complex aetiology in which friction and sweating constitute two important features. Plastic and rubber footwear, nylon socks and a vulnerable atopic skin are other relevant factors.

The dermatitis is confined to plantar skin, particularly in its distal part. Affected skin becomes reddish, glazed and tender, and may develop painful fissures. The course is fluctuating but prolonged, although most affected children improve over the years. It is exceptional for the disease to persist into adult life.

Avoidance of occlusive footwear, the substitution of cotton for nylon socks, and the regular application of simple emollient creams provide considerable relief. Topical corticosteroids are generally no more effective than bland applications.

Apocrine disorders

Body odour

Patients with dermatoses in which there is widespread hyperkeratosis, as in pityriasis rubra pilaris or generalised erythroderma, often have an unpleasant musty odour, probably due to bacterial decomposition of keratin. A similar smell may come from patients with diffuse palmo-plantar keratoderma, particularly when there is associated hyperhidrosis. Eccrine sweat is normally odourless, except in those fond of onions and garlic. Smelly eccrine sweat is produced by the excretion of arsenic, in phenylketonuria, and in a few other rare metabolic disorders.

In the vast majority, however, unpleasant odours emanating from the skin are the result of bacterial degradation of apocrine sweat. Apocrine secretion has no smell, but its decomposition products are responsible for the characteristic body odour. Most of the so-called body odour originates from the axillae. Apocrine glands are present in other areas but in the axillae are larger and more densely distributed. Axillary hair adds to the effect by storing apocrine sweat, debris, and bacteria.

Axillary odour can be substantially reduced by the regular use of a bactericidal soap and by shaving the axillary hair. Antibiotic creams are effective, but not often necessary, and carry the risk of contact sensitisation.

Treatments effective in eccrine hyperhidrosis also reduce apocrine sweating and are therefore helpful. Young children with an abnormal odour should be investigated to exclude aminoaciduria and other metabolic causes.

Apocrine miliaria

Apocrine miliaria is a chronic papular eruption, confined to apocrine areas and caused by retention of apocrine secretion.

Aetiology

Keratinous occlusion of the apocrine duct is followed by rupture of its contents into the stratum spinosum, with secondary inflammation. The cause of the primary keratinous plug is unknown. Although occasionally seen in men, apocrine miliaria is largely confined to women of child-bearing age and appears to be endocrine dependent.

Clinical features

Small round perifollicular papules are present in areas of apocrine secretion. They are intensely itchy, particularly after stimulation of apocrine secretion by stress or excitement. The papules are numerous in the axillae and pubic region, with occasional lesions around the areolae and on the trunk.

The course is prolonged, the disease generally persisting at least until the menopause. Remission often occurs during pregnancy, and in many women an improvement takes place while they are taking the contraceptive pill. Slow regression after the menopause is common, but is not invariable.

Treatment

A cream containing 0.1 per cent tretinoin provides very useful relief but is irritating and may need to be combined or alternated with hydrocortisone cream. Severely affected women who do not respond to topical tretinoin, or to hormone therapy, may need surgical excision of affected areas.

Hidradenitis suppurativa

Hidradenitis suppurativa is a chronic inflammatory disease which occurs in the areas most densely covered with apocrine glands.

Aetiology

The precise details are not well understood. Poral occlusion may play a role, as evidenced by the frequent finding of grouped comedones in the affected region, and the common association with other follicular occlusion diseases such as severe cystic acne, pilonidal sinus and the sterile dissecting cellulitis of the scalp. Group F streptococci may play a part initially, but most bacteria that are isolated are merely secondary invaders. Shaving, use of axillary deodorants, or depilatory creams have not been confirmed as playing a role. Although more common in the obese, the condition is not uncommonly seen in those of slender build. Onset after middle age or before puberty is very rare. In women, the axillae and inframammary folds are more frequently affected, while men tend to develop the disease in the groins and perianal region. However, any sites may be affected, singly or in combination, in either sex.

Clinical features

Early lesions are usually solitary, small, tender nodules in the subcutaneous fat. The overlying skin reddens as the abscess softens and slowly breaks through to the surface. Healing is followed by fibrosis and, as new nodules evolve, the site becomes distorted by scarring. Sinuses form and intermittently discharge, while the subcutis is gradually undermined by burrowing purulent tracts. A persistent low-grade inflammation is interrupted by recurrent episodes of acute cellulitis.

Severe hidradenitis suppurativa may extend from the axillae across the chest, with scarring sufficient to restrict movements of the arm. From the groins, the disease may spread to the perineum, buttocks and scrotum, or burrow into the anal canal to form fistulae. Hidradenitis suppurativa can become a chronic intractable disease with considerable debilitation, anaemia, and even systemic amyloidosis.

Treatment

In the early stages topical clindamycin used on a regular basis is very helpful. Although the initial bacteria isolated are often streptococci, penicillin has little effect. Short term use of an orally administered corticosteroid can reduce the severity of an acute flare.

If the patient presents with a draining abscess, the pus should be cultured and an appropriate antibiotic prescribed. Metronidazole is usually the most effective oral antibiotic. It needs to be taken for several weeks but, because prolonged use can induce peripheral neuropathy, metronidazole can only be used intermittently. Orally administered retinoids have been helpful in some patients, but more needs to be known about their use before these agents can be regarded as first-line treatment.

Surgery is required for more advanced stages. Sinuses should be opened completely, and the base cauterised. Incomplete excisions do more harm than good. For longstanding cases with much scarring, it may be necessary to excise and graft the whole affected area.

24

Drug eruptions

1. Aetiology
2. Pathogenesis
   (a) immunogenic
   (b) direct toxic
   (c) metabolic
   (d) other
3. Clinical patterns
   (a) exanthematic
   (b) urticaria and serum sickness
   (c) photosensitivity
   (d) eczematoid
   (e) purpuric
   (f) lichenoid
   (g) fixed drug eruption
   (h) other
4. Diagnosis
5. Treatment

A drug eruption is any unintended alteration of the skin or adjoining mucosae which is produced by a sytemically absorbed drug administered in normal doses. The incidence is difficult to assess. Transient and minor reactions may be attributed to other causes and, even when recognised, are unlikely to be reported. Drug eruptions are common, and are becoming more common. It is estimated that as many as 5 per cent of patients admitted to hospital suffer a cutaneous drug reaction.

Aetiology

Most drug eruptions are presumed to be allergic in nature, although an immunological mechanism is clearly demonstrable for only a few. Some proteins and carbohydrates used in therapy contain molecules which are large enough to be antigenic in themselves, but most drugs are small molecules which become antigenic only after conjugation with body

346

protein. When a drug is conjugated with carrier protein to form the complete antigen, the linkage appears generally to be through covalent bonds. For covalent bonding to occur, most drugs need to be metabolised to more reactive molecules which are the true haptens.

However, immunological reactivity to a drug does not necessarily result in clinically recognisable drug reaction. Conversely, drug reactions may be accompanied but not caused by immunological changes.

Allergic drug eruptions are characterised by an asymptomatic latent period, usually one to three weeks from first exposure to the drug. The latent period sometimes lasts for years, but, once sensitisation has occured, the eruption quickly follows absorption of even very small amounts of the drug.

There may be cross-sensitisation to chemically related drugs, but cross-reactions are somewhat unpredictable, partly because individuals may be sensitised to different components of the same molecule. Being the expression of an immune reaction, an allergic eruption is not specific for a particular drug, many drugs producing identical reactions. Conversely, the same drug may induce allergic reactions of more than one type, so that dissimilar eruptions may follow the same drug in different people and even in the same person at different times.

Pathogenesis

Although the details regarding most drug eruptions are not fully known, pathogenic mechanisms can be divided into four categories.

Immunogenic

■ The *type I* reaction occurs when circulating polyvalent antigen interacts with molecules of IgE bound to specific sites on the surface of mast cells and circulating basophils. The antigen bridging of IgE molecules triggers the release of histamine and other mediators, which in the dermis produce the characteristic weal type reaction. Penicillin is the classic drug invoking this mechanism.

■ The *type II* reaction, although imporant in some haematological disturbances, has not been related to cutaneous drug reactions.

■ The *type III* reaction follows the interaction of circulating antibody with circulating antigen. Antigen–antibody complexes are formed, and there may be complement activation. Experimentally, large complexes often precipitate within venules, with local activation of the complement cascade, platelet aggregation, release of vasoactive amines and infiltration by polymorphs. It is likely that similar mechanisms are involved in the pathogenesis of leucocytoclastic vasculitis, including that due to drugs. Complexes which are smaller are less likely to precipitate at the site of formation, but may be filtered off at sites of relative statis or greater permeability in the vascular bed. Drugs utilising the type III reaction are penicillin and sera. The serum sickness syndrome combines changes ascribed to circulating immune complexes and features of the type I reaction.

■ The *type IV* reaction follows interaction of specifically sensitised T-cells with the appropriate antigen. Soluble factors are released and T-cells transform into larger cells with the ability to damage target cells. The type IV reaction underlies allergic contact dermatitis, but is not normally involved in drug eruptions. However, patients who have been previously sensitised by skin contact with a drug used topically, may develop an eczematoid eruption after systemic administration of the same drug or a related drug with which it cross-reacts. This can be seen in patients allergic to ethylene diamine (the stabiliser in Kenacomb cream) who have asthma and react to aminophylline, which is a mixture of theophylline and ethylene diamine.

Direct toxic

Some drug eruptions appear to be a direct toxic effect. The cutaneous pigmentation resulting from gold therapy is dose-related and confined to light-exposed areas, which implies an alteration of melanocyte function by the metal in the skin. Patients treated for long periods with high doses of chlorpromazine may develop a slate-grey pigmentation of exposed skin, due to a stable complex of melanin with a metabolite of the drug. Aspirin and X-ray contrast media directly release histamine from mast cells but some people are more sensitive to this effect than others.

Metabolic

There are many drug reactions in which factors other than allergy are important. Genetically determined differences in drug metabolism are important in some systemic reactions. Adverse effects from isoniazid, dapsone and hydrallazine are more frequent in 'slow acetylators', and dapsone-induced haemolysis is more likely when cells are deficient in glucose-6-phosphate dehydrogenase. Whether similar mechanisms are relevant to a significant number of cutaneous reactions remains to be shown. There is evidence, however, that the factor which determines susceptibility to carcinogenesis after arsenic ingestion is an individual difference in absorption, storage or excretion of the element. The frequency of ampicillin eruptions in patients with infectious mononucleosis is difficult to explain on an immunological basis.

Other

The risk of developing allergic sensitivity to a drug is influenced by its route of administration, and by the age and sex of the individual. Altered T-cell reactivity may also influence the likelihood of sensitisation, but these are minor factors of little relevance to most patients.

The incidence of ampicillin eruptions approximates 5 per cent of those treated, but exceeds 50 per cent when the drug is given to patients with infectious mononucleosis, patients with lymphatic leukaemia, and those taking allopurinol for gout.

Clinical patterns

There are few cutaneous diseases which are never imitated by a drug eruption. The range of lesions produced by drugs is enormous, but in most cases the eruption conforms to one or a small number of well-defined patterns.

In about two-thirds of cases the rash is exanthematic or urticarial, and 90 per cent of all drug eruptions belong to one of the following groups:

Exanthematic	46%
Urticarial	23%
Photosensitive	5% to 10%
Fixed eruption	5% to 10%
Eczematoid	5% to 10%
Erythema multiforme	5% to 10%
Purpuric	1% to 5%
Lichenoid	1% to 5%
Pruritus alone	1% to 5%

■ *Exanthematic*. Patients never previously exposed usually develop the eruption from seven to fourteen days after beginning to take the drug. Those who are already sensitised are likely to exhibit the rash by the second or third day. There are many exceptions, but the eruption is generally brightly coloured, sudden in onset, widely and more or less symmetrically distributed. Constitutional symptoms are frequently absent, but there may be fever and other systemic features. Pruritus is common.

Individual lesions are macules, papules, or a combination of both, sometimes with an urticarial component. The colour may be pink, bright red, or purplish. Distribution is usually most dense over the trunk with variable involvement of other regions. In some patients, the rash bears a resemblance to rubella, measles, or scarlet fever. Progression to exfoliative dermatitis may occur, particularly when the eruption is due to gold salts.

Common causes include ampicillin, penicillin, trimethoprim-sulphamethoxazole, sulphonamides, barbiturates, carbamazepine, benzodiazepines, allopurinol, and gold salts.

■ *Urticaria and serum sickness*. Drug-induced urticaria usually occurs without systemic featurs, but may be accompanied by the fever, arthralgia, lymphadenopathy, leucopenia, and eosinophilia of serum sickness. Occasionally in extremely sensitive patients, a rapid onset of urticaria is the first expression of life-threatening anaphylaxis.

Common causes include penicillin, cephalosporins, aminoglycosides, sulphonamides, salicylates, phenylbutazone, barbiturates, quinine, dextrans, toxoids, and X-ray contrast media.

■ *Photosensitivity*. Light-sensitive drug reactions may be photo-allergic or phototoxic, but most drugs which are capable of inducing photo-allergy can also be phototoxic in high doses.

The photo-allergic reaction occurs in only a small proportion of people taking the drug and is preceded by a latent period during which sensitisation occurs. After sensitisation, only small quantities of the drug are sufficient to trigger an abnormal response to sunlight. The eruption is generally eczematoid and, although mainly restricted to light-exposed skin, does show some spread onto unexposed areas. Erythematous, exudative and lichenoid eruptions may occur, but are less common.

Photosensitivity may persist for a considerable time after withdrawal of the drug.

The phototoxic reaction is a direct chemical sensitisation to ultraviolet light, and is dose-related, both in respect of the quantity of drug and the intensity and duration of light-exposure. The eruption usually develops within 48 hours of drug absorption, with oedema, erythema, and sometimes blistering. The reaction is strictly confined to light-exposed skin, is of relatively brief duration, and closely resembles ordinary sunburn.

Common drug causes of photosensitivity include phenothiazines (especially chlorpromazine and promethazine), tetracyclines (particularly demethylchlortetracycline), psoralens, griseofulvin, nalidixic acid, chlordiazepoxide, tricyclic antidepressants (particularly protriptyline), thiazide diuretics, and sulphonamides.

■ *Eczematoid.* When contact sensitisation follows application of a drug to the skin, subsequent systemic administration of the same drug, or an analogue, may produce a generalised eczematoid eruption. Cutaneous sensitisation was so common with penicillin, sulphonamides and streptomycin that these agents have long been abandoned for use on the skin. Eczematoid eruptions are still encountered with antihistamines and other drugs which are used both topically and systemically. Contact sensitisation may be occupational in nurses, doctors, dentists, and veterinary surgeons.

In addition, eczematoid drug eruptions are an uncommon complication of treatment with gold salts, para-aminosalicylic acid, and methyldopa.

■ *Purpuric.* Drug-induced purpura may be a manifestation of toxic or allergic thrombocytopenia, or a pharmacological effect of anticoagulants. However, up to 1 per cent of patients taking oral anticoagulants may develop a characteristic pattern of painful purpuric necrosis, especially over the buttocks and upper thighs, during a transient, paradoxical, hypercoaguable state. People with deficiency of protein C are particularly prone to this effect.

Exanthematic and urticarial eruptions sometimes have a purpuric element, or petechiae may be added by scratching. Palpable purpura is a characteristic sign of cutaneous vasculitis, whether due to drugs or other causes. Macular purpura may be the only clinical feature of drug sensitivity and occurs in the absence of true vasculitis.

Common causes of purpuric drug eruptions include indomethacin, gold salts, frusemide, quinine, quinidine, sulphonamides, thiazide diuretics, phenylbutazone and methyldopa.

■ *Lichenoid.* Lichenoid papules are not too uncommon in patients with exanthematic drug eruptions. Less often, the whole eruption has a lichenoid appearance but lacks the typical distribution and mucosal lesions of lichen planus. On occasions, particularly with mepacrine, a drug eruption is clinically and histologically indistinguishable from lichen planus. The characteristic mucosal changes may be present and resolution of the cutaneous lesions may be followed by post-inflammatory pigmentation. Lichenoid drug eruptions are slow in onset and probably dose-related. The mechanisms involved are unknown.

Common causes include chloroquine and mepacrine, chlorpromazine and other phenothiazines, chlordiazepoxide, gold salts, thiazide diuretics, quinine, quinidine, para-aminosalicylic acid and azathioprine.

■ *Fixed drug eruption.* *(Colour plate 72)* The fixed drug eruption begins at one or more sites as a well-demarcated, oedematous plaque of dusky erythema. The oedema may be severe enough to cause blistering with secondary crusting and scaling. There is no great discomfort and there are no systemic features. Resolution of the acute phase leaves a brownish or slate grey pigmentation at the site. After recurrent acute episodes, the colour deepens, and may become black. Recurrences invariably affect the same sites, sometimes with the addition of new patches elsewhere.

Lesions range from a few millimetres to several centimetres in size. The mouth, genital and perianal region are frequent sites, but the eruption can occur anywhere on the surface. Pathogenesis of the fixed eruption is poorly understood.

Common causes include phenolphthalein, barbiturates, phenylbutazone, tetracyclines, sulphonamides, penicillin, dapsone, meprobamate, quinine and gold salts. Dyes used as colouring agents in cordials, sweets and capsules, and certain food additives have also been implicated.

■ *Other patterns.* Some drug eruptions closely resemble specific dermatoses such as lichen planus, cutaneous lupus erythematosus and acne. Compared with acne vulgaris, which typically shows a wide variety of lesions in differing stages of evolution, drug-induced acne is typically a monomorphic papulo-pustular eruption. Drugs responsible include the anti-epileptic drugs, anti-tuberculous medication, lithium, cyclosporin, glucocorticosteroids and anabolic steroids. A psoriasiform eruption may complicate therapy with lithium and β-adrenergic blocking agents, especially practolol, while chloroquine can aggravate psoriasis, sometimes to the point of generalised erythroderma. Penicillamine may induce lesions indistinguishable from perforating elastoma, pemphigus foliaceus and, rarely, pemphigus vulgaris. Iodides and bromides have a special tendency to cause vegetating, granulomatous nodules and plaques, usually multiple, on the face and limbs, much like lesions of chromoblastomycosis.

Drugs may exacerbate porphyria variegata and porphyria cutanea tarda, and drugs such as nalidixic acid and naproxen may reproduce cutaneous lesions of porphyria in patients with normal porphyrin levels. Gingival hyperplasia, hypertrichosis, hirsutism, gynaecomastia, erythema multiforme and toxic epidermal necrolysis are just some of the less specific reactions which are sometimes caused by drugs.

Diagnosis

▶ **Suspect a drug eruption**
In many patients the sudden onset of an itchy, roughly symmetrical, vivid erythematous rash within a few weeks of commencing a drug is at least very suggestive. However, there are no clinical features by which a drug eruption can be diagnosed with certainty, although the fixed eruption and a few other drug reactions are clinically characteristic.

351

▶ **Determine the most likely drug**

Even when a drug cause seems very likely, the patient is often taking several drugs, any one of which may be responsible. Ideally, in this situation, all non-essential drugs should be withdrawn and the others replaced by alternative, structurally unrelated, medication. However, this is usually not possible and in such a situation one should take two steps to help establish the causative agent. First, the length of time each drug has been taken should be established. As a rough rule, most drug eruptions occur within two weeks of commencing a medication, but this is not invariable. It is classic for penicillamine to have been taken for three or four months before pemphigus appears, and allopurinol may have been taken for years before it induces an exfoliative erythroderma.

Secondly, the clinical descriptive pattern of the rash should be established and a guide consulted to find the frequency with which each drug would be likely to cause an eruption with that morphology.

▶ **Withdraw the drug**

When the relevant drug has been discontinued, improvement is often apparent within a few days, and generally within a few weeks. Slowly excreted drugs, such as heavy metals or depot injections, take longer. Lack of improvement may be the result of inadvertent exposure to the drug or a related substance. The patient who is sensitive to quinine may be taking the drug unknowingly in tonic water.

▶ **Investigations**

■ *Biopsy*. There are no microscopic features which permit the confident diagnosis of a drug eruption. Early lesions are apt to show mild perivascular infiltrate of lymphocytes and histiocytes, but older lesions vary widely in appearance according to the clinical pattern.

Drug-induced lichen planus, when compared with naturally occurring lichen planus, may show subtle differences such as parakeratosis or plasma cells in the infiltrate, but at other times the histology may be identical. The histology of vasculitis, urticaria, erythema nodosum, and erythema multiforme are no different when caused by drugs. The histology of drug eruptions may be indistinguishable from viral exanthemata, secondary syphilis, and pityriasis rosea. Even with such clinically characteristic lesions as the fixed eruption, the histology does no more than confirm the probability of a drug cause.

■ *Immunological testing*. Eczematoid reactions can often be confirmed by patch-testing but skin tests are otherwise unhelpful and may be dangerous, by providing a challenge dose. Total oesinophil count and currently available in vitro tests such as the basophil degranulation test are of limited value.

■ *Deliberate challenge should be avoided.* With fixed drug eruptions, administration of the suspected drug does little harm and may confirm the diagnosis. With other drug eruptions, the 'challenge dose' is rarely justified because in some situations, especially erythema multiforme and urticaria, death may result. If a drug is really essential to the patient and cannot be safely replaced, it may be permissible, in hospital, to recommence with very small doses and gradually increase to therapeutic levels.

Treatment

■ *Prophylactic*. Drug therapy should always be preceded by enquiries about previous contact dermatitis or systemic drug reactions. Any incriminated drug is avoided, together with compounds of similar molecular structure. After treatment of adverse drug reactions or contact dermatitis, patients should be given the name of the substance which was held responsible and a written list of likely cross-reacting compounds. A patient sensitive to benzocaine is likely to have been sensitised also to procaine, sulphonamides, para-aminosalicylic acid and para-aminobenzoic acid.

When a choice is available, preference should be given to drugs with a lower potential for untoward reactions. This is particularly true when the patient has asthma or atopic dermatitis, or has a previous history of these disorders.

■ *Therapeutic*. The only effective treatment of lasting value is permanent avoidance of the drug concerned. When more than a single drug is being taken, all should be suspended unless life would be endangered by so doing. If the eruption is no more than uncomfortable and several drugs are being used it may be sufficient to discontinue those commenced in the four weeks before onset of the eruption. When the responsible drug is a heavy metal, chelating agents are sometimes prescribed, but these too may cause troublesome side-effects.

For mild type I reactions, antihistamines give symptomatic relief. However, antihistamines oppose the action of histamine by occupying the same receptors and this effect takes some time to become apparent. Therefore, with pharyngeal or laryngeal involvement or features of anaphylaxis where urgent treatment is required, use different non-occupied receptors by treating with parenteral adrenaline and cortisone as well as giving large parenteral doses of antihistamine. Intravenous injection of aminophylline may be necessary for bronchospasm, and tracheostomy for laryngeal obstruction. The rapid onset of urticaria soon after administration of a drug should warn of the possibility that other features of anaphylaxis may quickly follow.

Sometimes, even when there is no threat to life, symptoms from severe widespread drug eruptions may warrant treatment with the oral administration of corticosteroids. Provided there are no contra-indications, initial daily doses of 40 mg to 60 mg of prednisolone are generally sufficient to achieve suppression. The dose may be then reduced to 20 mg daily for 10 to 14 days. Topical therapy will vary according to the clinical pattern of the eruption.

25

Therapy

1. Topical
   (a) liquids
   (b) lotions, liniments
   (c) paints, tinctures
   (d) powders
   (e) creams
   (f) ointments
   (g) gels
   (h) pastes
2. Systemic
   (a) Corticosteroids
   (b) antibiotics, antiviral and
       antifungal drugs
   (c) retinoids
   (d) psoralens
   (e) sedatives, tranquillisers,
       antidepressants
   (f) antihistamines
   (g) antimalarials
   (h) cytotoxic drugs
   (i) anti-androgens
3. Surgical/physical
   (a) office surgery
   (b) skin biopsy
   (c) curettage
   (d) electrosurgery
   (e) cryotherapy
   (f) ionising radiation
   (g) laser surgery
   (h) ultraviolet light

The successful management of diseases of the skin, as of other organs, requires an accurate diagnosis. Secondary factors such as infection and trauma need to be assessed and treated. The patient should be asked about, and warned against, succumbing to the natural impulse to 'help' things along by self-treatment.

When a cutaneous disease has been produced by a specific agent, as with allergic contact dermatitis or a drug eruption, removal of the cause and simple measures to protect the skin are followed by a return to normal. For other diseases, such as impetigo and tinea, specific curative treatment is available. However, for many diseases of the skin, specific causes have not been found and treatment remains palliative. In the great majority of these disorders, good relief and often remission can be achieved with appropriate therapy.

Corticosteroids are potent, non-specific anti-inflammatory agents. They are effective in relieving so many diseases of the skin that the inexperienced prescriber may be tempted to take therapeutic shortcuts, bypassing the logical progression from diagnosis to treatment. When a dermatosis is self-limited, little harm may follow, although even self-limited disease may be altered and prolonged by ill-advised therapy. In dermatoses which are not self-limited, symptomatic treatment without a firm diagnosis is illogical and often harmful.

The skin is that part of the patient which he or she sees and touches, and which plays a large part in shaping the self-image. It is the part of the patient seen by friends and relatives, so that disfiguring skin changes exert a profound effect on the patient's ability to take part in many social activities without embarrassment. The atopic child is deeply influenced by the attitudes and comments of schoolmates, and sometimes by unconscious rejection by a parent. The psoriatic may well be improved by sun and surf, but this is not helpful if he or she is too embarrassed by the disease to bare the skin in public. The benefits of sympathetic reassurance and explanation to such patients are self-evident. Although there are few cutaneous diseases which are primarily emotional in origin, there are also few in which emotional factors do not become relevant.

The skin is also the part of the patient which is most easily visible and accessible to the physician, who should be constantly alert to the possibility of uncovering some inner mischief from its cutaneous manifestations. At the same time, it is obviously unnecessary to suspect an emotional upheaval or a systemic malfunction hidden beneath every minor blemish.

Topical therapy

Topical therapy is sometimes prescribed with curative intent (gamma benzene hexachloride for scabies), often aimed at providing symptomatic relief (corticosteroids for eczema) or, as happens when wet dressings are used on ulcers, designed to protect the skin while it heals itself.

As the skin alters during the development and healing of a dermatosis, the needs of the skin change and the appropriate application will therefore depend upon the phase of the disease. Obtaining the properties required of a topically applied preparation can be achieved not only by altering the perceived active ingredient, but also by changing the way it is delivered to the skin. Most applications used belong to one of the following groups.

1. Liquids	5. Creams
2. Lotions and liniments	6. Ointments
3. Paints and tinctures	7. Gels
4. Powders	8. Pastes

Liquids

The liquids are watery solutions which are brought into contact with the skin by wet dressings or by baths, where the area is soaked in a container of the solution.

Uses

■ *Soothing*. The evaporation of liquids will cool the skin and provide relief of itch and the local heat produced by acute inflammation.

■ *Drying* of moist oozing areas occurs within two to four days as a result of the evaporative effect.

■ *Cleansing* can be achieved gently by these substances which remove debris and previous applications.

■ *Protection* is obtaind by providing a sterile environment, removing debris that encourages infection and by drying exudate, which denies potential pathogens a suitable culture medium.

■ *Easy application* is sometimes an important consideration. Bathing is a method of delivery which avoids the pain that manual applications of creams or ointments would produce if used on tender skin. It also ensures that poorly accessible regions are reached and that large areas are treated with minimal effort.

Wet dressings

Layers of soft cotton material are soaked in the liquid and applied to the skin. The compress may be left in place for half-an-hour several times a day, but for acutely inflamed areas it is better to leave the pack in place continuously. The compress is kept moist by removing the outer layers for rewetting, leaving in place the layer next to the skin. Once in 24 hours, the innermost layer is also removed and replaced by clean material. Wet dressings obviously need to be moist, but no useful purpose is served by excess loading of the pack with liquid. The compresses are designed to allow continuous cooling by evaporation. They should not be covered by such impermeable materials as plastic sheeting, which reduce evaporative cooling, lead to maceration of the covered skin, and encourage the growth of bacteria. The following liquids are commonly used.

■ *Saline solution* has the advantage of being non-irritating, non-sensitizing, inexpensive and easy to prepare. A teaspoon of table salt is dissolved in a half litre of water.

■ *Chlorhexidine* aqueous solution 0.5 per cent is used when the area treated is already infected. It is effective against both Gram-positive and Gram-negative bacteria. At this concentration, irritation and sensitisation are rare.

■ *Potassium permanganate* solution, one in ten thousand, is antiseptic by virtue of its oxidising properties. However, this means it must be prepared freshly each time it is used. In practice, the patient prepares a solution of Condy's crystals to a light pink colour, avoiding undissolved crystals which may cause severe irritation. It is important that stronger concentrations be avoided; otherwise, the liquid is irritating and stains skin and nails. Permanganate may also stain enamel tubs and is therefore better avoided for baths.

■ *Aluminium acetate* solution is protective and mildly astringent. Burow's solution is usually prescribed and then diluted one in twenty with water.

■ *Silver nitrate* as 0.05 per cent aqueous solution, by its protein precipitating action, is particularly drying and is therefore useful for areas of persistent oozing areas which do not respond to the usual liquids. Systemic toxicity limits its use to small areas and short duration.

■ *Hydrogen peroxide* 5 per cent in water releases oxygen in large amounts, which makes it very effective in the treatment of anaerobic infections. Crusts and necrotic debris are also loosened and removed by its effervescent action.

Baths

Wet dressings are unsuitable for large areas, and for hands and feet it is better to immerse the part in a bowl of the liquid for 10 minutes every hour or two. For the genitocrural region and for extensive areas of involvement, baths are used.

The liquids used in wet dressings are also used in baths. However, a number of materials are used primarily in baths alone.

■ *Oatmeal* baths are moisturising and relieve the pruritus of dry irritable skin. About 0.25 kg of oatmeal is placed in a muslin bag or the foot of an old stocking and hung from the bath tap or placed so that water runs on to the bag as the bath is filling. The bag is then used as a bath sponge instead of soap. Proprietary preparations of 'colloidal oatmeal' are added directly to the bath.

■ *Bath oils* are water dispersible mineral oils that coat the skin and reduce the rate of water loss. They are therefore useful in patients with dry skin. Proprietary bath oils are convenient to use and appreciated by many patients, but are expensive and less effective than emollients applied directly to the skin. For children with atopic dermatitis, baths prepared with 50 g of aqueous cream in 50 litres of water provide an acceptable method of cleansing without the use of soap, and have some residual emollient effect.

■ *Tar baths* are useful in the treatment of psoriasis and chronic scaly dermatitis, and have mild antipruritic properties. Coal tars have more antipsoriatic activity than pine tars. Proprietary preparations stain the bath less than the traditional 50 mL of LPC in 90 litres of water.

Lotions

The traditional lotion is a suspension of an insoluble powder in water. The powder settles on standing, so the lotion must be shaken before use. To avoid the necessity for shaking, an emulsifying agent may be added to produce an emulsion-lotion. These are more convenient than the older shake-lotions and most proprietary lotions are of this type.

■ *Advantages*. Lotions are a convenient way of applying a thin, fairly uniform layer of powder on the skin. Evaporation produces some cooling, but the antipruritic effect of this cooling has been overrated. The antipruritic effect may be increased by incorporating 0.2 per cent menthol, 1 per cent camphor or 1 per cent phenol. However, preparations containing phenol should be applied to small areas only, as significant absorption may follow its use over large areas.

Lotions are useful vehicles for such active ingredients as 25 per cent benzyl benzoate in the treatment of scabies, or 1 per cent gamma benzene hexachloride for the treatment of head lice infestation.

Lotions have a drying effect and are suitable for early exudative lesions. A traditional lotion for this purpose is calamine lotion:

zinc oxide	5%
calamine	15%
glycerine	5%
water	to 100%

Lotions are applied two or three times daily, with the fingers or a cotton wool pad.

■ *Disadvantages*. The drying effect of lotions may cause discomfort and excessive desquamation if used too often or for too long. Powder tends to accumulate on the skin, producing an appearance unacceptable to some patients and necessitating removal by washing at least once daily. Even gentle washing can be irritating to acutely inflamed skin. Shake lotions are inconvenient to use, while the addition of emulsifiers and stabilisers introduces potentially sensitising chemicals.

Liniments

To avoid the drying effect of standard lotions, oil vehicles are sometimes used and the preparation is then called a 'liniment'. Liniments are little used today. An example is:

phenol	0.5%
camphor	0.5%
liquid paraffin	25.0%
lanette wax	2.5%
talc	6.5%
calamine	6.5%
water	to 100%

Paints and tinctures

These are rapidly drying liquid applications, particularly useful in skin folds such as the groins, natal cleft, beneath pendulous breasts, and between the toes. When the vehicle is alcohol, the preparation is referred to as a 'tincture'. When substances are dispensed in large volumes of alcohol, the preparations are sometimes referred to as alcoholic lotions rather than tinctures. Examples include salicylic acid, minoxidil, and clindamycin lotion.

Castellani's magenta paint remains a very useful, although messy, application for tinea cruris. Applied once daily for seven days, in half or full strength, the paint gives symptomatic relief and may obviate the necessity for griseofulvin. Magenta paint is also useful for small, weeping areas of dermatitis, a few days usually being sufficient to dry the surface. The paint stings when applied to inflamed skin and, if used for too long, may result in considerable irritation.

Aqueous solution of gentian violet is an effective application for candidiasis of flexural areas, especially on the napkin area of infants.

As 0.25 per cent paint, the gentian violet is applied twice daily for four or five days. Prolonged application and stronger solutions may result in superficial necrosis.

Many applications for warts are paints or tinctures that have added substances such as collodion or benzoin compound. These dry to leave a flexible film that acts to prolong contact with, and confine treatment to, the area of application. One such paint, well tolerated on most parts of the body, is:

salicylic acid	17%
lactic acid	17%
collodion	to 100%

A tincture commonly prescribed for genital and perianal warts is:

podophyllin	10%
benzoin compound	to 100%

The tincture is carefully applied to the wart and allowed to dry before coming into contact with adjoining skin surfaces. The concentration of podophyllin is gradually increased at weekly applications to a maximum of 50 per cent. Patients vary in their reaction to podophyllin. Most experience some discomfort a few hours after application and many are unable to tolerate concentrations of more than 25 per cent. It is better to paint only a few warts at the first consultation, as some patients react strongly, even to the 10 per cent concentration. If carelessly applied in large quantities, sufficient podophyllin may be absorbed through the skin to cause serious central nervous system toxicity. Restraint in the use of podophyllin is particularly important during pregnancy.

Powders

Powders which incorporate active ingredients have little place in contemporary therapy. The use of powders is now virtually confined to intertriginous areas, where inert materials of fine texture are lightly dusted to provide some separation of apposed skin surfaces. This increases evaporation and helps to prevent maceration. Talcum powder is just as effective as more expensive proprietary preparations and lacks the sensitising potential of components added to 'medicated' powders.

The skin should be clean and dry at the time of application. In the presence of moisture, powders easily aggregate into caked masses and, if the particles are not sufficiently fine, may abrade the surface.

Creams

These are now the most frequently prescribed application in medicine. They are easy to apply and remove, and can be modified to allow the incorporation of a wide range of active ingredients. Simple creams are a suspension of a powder in an emulsion of water and oil.

An emulsion is simply a more or less stable suspension of one liquid in another with which it is immiscible. One of the two liquids is aqueous, the other oily. One of the two is suspended in the other, the stability of the suspension depending on the emulsifying agent. The suspended liquid is referred to as the dispersed phase and the other as the continuous phase. If the continuous phase is water, the emulsion is an oil in water (O/W) emulsion. If the continuous phase is oil, the emulsion is a water in oil (W/O) emulsion. Emulsions should be diluted only by addition of the continuous phase, that is, an O/W emulsion can only be diluted by adding aqueous liquids and a W/O emulsion only by adding oily liquids. If aqueous liquids are added to a W/O emulsion, the emulsion may separate or 'crack'. The W/O types are referred to as oily creams or cold creams, and the O/W creams as vanishing creams.

The ability of creams to accept additives is also dependant upon the pH of the cream, which is mainly a function of the emulsifying agent. Aqueous cream is an anionic cream with which acid substances such as salicylic acid are miscible, whereas the addition of chlorhexidine, for example, will cause all the components of aqueous cream to separate into distinct layers. Sorbolene cream is non-ionic and can therefore be chosen as the base when one is uncertain about the compatibility of the additives.

It should be understood that many proprietary creams are finely balanced emulsions in which the properties of the emulsifying agent may be altered by adding further ingredients. The stability of the emulsion may be decreased and the penetration of ingredients from the cream into the skin markedly altered. Some emulsions will not tolerate calcium ions, others salicylic acid, and many are intolerant of marked temperature changes.

Creams have the disadvantage that moulds grow easily on them. All creams, therefore, have added antiseptics to prevent the growth of moulds during storage. The most commonly used preservatives are parahydroxybenzoates (parabens) and chlorocresol. Many of these additives are capable of inducing contact allergy. When dermatitis becomes worse after application of a cream, sensitisation to a preservative should be considered.

Creams are easy to apply and, because of evaporation, have a cooling effect. Penetration of active ingredients is more rapid than from ointments, so they are suitable bases for such active agents as hydrocortisone and gentamicin.

Because of their high water content, O/W creams are a little drying and an oily cream may be better when there is already a degree of xeroderma. However, being non-greasy and easily removed with water, O/W creams are preferred for the scalp and are considered more cosmetically acceptable than W/O creams.

Sorbolene cream and aqueous cream, because they have white soft paraffin and liquid paraffin as part of their components, are themselves useful emollients, but for more effective lubrication, extra paraffin may be added. For example:

liquid paraffin	20%
sorbolene cream	to 100%

For xeroderma, glycerine may be added, as in:

glycerine	10%
sorbolene cream	to 100%

Ointments

With the complexity of modern pharmaceutics, it is difficult to draw a sharp line between ointments and oily creams. However, an ointment may be defined as the suspension of a substance in an oily vehicle. There are numerous vehicles, but the paraffins are most frequently used. Ointments do not require the preservatives necessary for creams, so that sensitisation to the base is less common. However, lanolin is incorporated in some bases and may cause contact allergy.

Ointments retain their ingredients better than creams, and provide prolonged action rather than rapid penetration. They are greasy and most patients prefer a cream, but ointments are particularly useful for lubricating dry skin, as on the legs of the elderly or the dry chapped hands of housewives with chronic dermatitis.

A useful emollient handcream is:

bismuth subnitrate	2.5%
zinc oxide	2.5%
ung. aqua rosae	to 100%

A traditional ointment for the treatment of tinea is Whitfield's ointment:

salicylic acid	6%
benzoic acid	12%
emulsifying ointment	to 100%

Under Australian conditions, Whitfield's ointment is too occlusive and irritating for most patients, particularly when used in intertriginous areas.

For the treatment of psoriasis, dithranol is frequently incorporated into a greasy base and applied once daily as:

dithranol	0.1–0.8%
salicylic acid	1.0%
soft paraffin	to 100%

Ointments are applied thinly and evenly, usually three or four times daily.

■ *Advantages*. Greasy preparations spread better and are therefore cheaper to use than creams. They are most suitable for dry skin and have a well-sustained effect. They are also preferable for hyperkeratotic conditions and for use with plastic occlusion.

■ *Disadvantages*. Ointments are unsuitable for weeping or oozing surfaces, or for use in most dermatoses of intertriginous areas. They are somewhat macerating and, being immiscible with water, are more difficult to remove than creams. Many patients object to the greasy feel of ointments.

Gels

The gel provides a greaseless, water-miscible base, from which active ingredients are rubbed easily into the skin without leaving a residual tacky or oily sensation. Generally clear and colourless, gels are particularly useful for hair-bearing and intertriginous areas. They are accepted well by most patients, but those that contain solid alcohols may cause some stinging when used on raw or oozing surfaces.

Pastes

These are similar in composition to lotions, creams, and ointments but are more viscid. When a shake lotion is stiffened by the addition of more powder, a drying paste is formed. When more powder is added to an ointment, a greasy paste results.

Pastes are often used for the treatment of psoriasis, as they adhere well to the scaly surface, for example:

crude coal tar	3%
salicylic acid	3%
zinc paste	to 100%

or:

dithranol	0.2%
salicylic acid	1.0%
zinc paste	to 100%

Tar pastes are very useful for chronic dermatitis, particularly in the presence of lichenification, for example:

liquor picis carbonis	4%
Lassar's paste	to 100%

Pastes are best applied generously under gauze dressings and left in place for 12 hours or so. They are therefore often left on overnight. Under special circumstances, they may be left in place for days, as when Upton's paste is applied under an occlusive dressing in the treatment of plantar warts:

trichloracetic acid	one part
salicylic acid	six parts
glycerine	to a stiff paste

A simple protective application to reduce irritation from urine and faeces is Baltimore paste:

aluminium powder	20%
zinc oxide	40%
liquid paraffin	40%

■ *Advantages*. Water-miscible pastes allow normal evaporation from the skin and are therefore very useful in providing protection for the skin without causing the maceration which might result from an ointment or greasy paste.

■ *Disadvantages*. They are viscid and therefore difficult to apply and remove. They require dressings to protect clothing and to hold the paste in place. Active ingredients must be prescribed in higher concentrations than in ointments and creams.

How much to prescribe?

An experienced nurse, who applies an ointment thinly but evenly, uses about 20 g for a single application to the whole body surface of an average adult. With a cream, she may need 30 g. Patients inexperienced in application will use more. For one leg from the knee down, with four sparing applications daily, a patient will use 50 g to 60 g a week. Using four sparing applications daily to treat most of the trunk, a patient will need 300 g for a week of treatment.

Topical corticosteroids

The most commonly prescribed topical preparations, corticosteroids require an understanding of the factors influencing their effectiveness and toxicity for safe negotiation of the maze of topical steroid preparations available in Australia and thus for their prescription on a rational basis.

Potency

Achieved by manipulation of the steroid molecule, potency is enhanced even further due to the unique pharmacological properties of the topical route, which increases potency by many orders of magnitude compared with systemic administration.

■ *Hydroxylation* in the 11 position is essential for corticosteroid activity. The skin does not contain the appropriate enzyme, so all topically applied steroids are already hydroxylated.

■ *Fluorination* in the 9 position enhances both mineralocorticoid and glucocorticoid activity but insertion of a double bond between carbon atoms 1 and 2 abolishes most mineralocorticoid activity.

■ *Esterification* at the 17 position enhances penetration through cell membranes and receptor binding within the cytoplasm. Both of these effects enhance potency.

The long list of topical corticosteroids available in Australia can be loosely graded according to potency into four groups.

1. 'Weak' corticosteroids—for example:
    hydrocortisone 0.5%
    hydrocortisone acetate 1%
    alclometasone dipropionate 0.05%
2. 'Dilute' corticosteroids—for example:
    betamethasone valerate 0.02%
    triamcinolone acetonide 0.02%
3. 'Half-strength' corticosteroids—for example:
    betamethasone valerate 0.05%
    betamethasone dipropionate 0.05%
    triamcinolone acetonide 0.05%
    fluclorolone acetonide 0.025%
4. 'Full-strength' corticosteroids—for example:
    betamethasone valerate 0.1%
    flucinolone acetonide 0.025%
    halcinonide 0.1%

Penetration

Penetration can be further influenced by the base, added agents, occlusion and regional variations.

■ *Ointments*, as a general rule, bind the active agent less avidly than other vehicles and therefore achieve higher skin levels.

■ **Additives** may act as a penetrant to help take topical steroids through the skin. Although many of these exist, propylene glycol is the only one that is used in Australia.

■ **Occlusion** for anatomical reasons (as occurs in the axillae, groins and other large flexures), or with plastic occlusive dressings, will macerate the skin to produce a less effective barrier and so enhance penetration.

■ **Regional differences** can influence effectiveness. Reduced penetration through the thick keratin layer of the elbow, knees, palms and soles often makes these areas difficult to treat. Enhanced penetration over the genitalia, periorbital region, perianal and intertriginous areas predispose these regions to unwanted steroid-induced side-effects.

■ **Intralesional injection** is an alternate effective way of producing very high local concentration of steroid that is sometimes necessary when treating conditions such as lichen simplex, lichen planus, discoid lupus erythematosus, hypertrophic scar and alopecia areata. To avoid atrophy of the dermis and fat, the total injected dose of triamcinolone should not exceed 4 mg/cm^2.

Concentration

This may not necessarily be as important as first assumed.

■ **Optimal concentrations** exist above which very little extra benefit is obtained. For example, the most practical effective concentration of hydrocortisone is 1 per cent. Increasing the strength to 2.5 per cent merely promotes more rapid removal from the site of application with only a minor rise in tissue concentration.

■ **Dilute preparations** of the esterified fluorinated corticosteroids will still produce the unwanted side-effects attributable to 'strong' topical steroids if they are applied to the face and intertriginous zones. To avoid this problem, hydrocortisone should be used in these areas.

Adverse effects

Those attributable to systemic administration of corticosteroids are mostly avoided by topical use but unwanted toxic effects which are mainly local, can still occur.

■ **Systemic absorption** is an uncommon practical consideration, given the small amount applied in milligrams and the barrier effect of keratin, which limits penetration to a very small percentage of that applied. The risk is greatest when high concentrations of corticosteroid are applied to large areas with a defective epidermal barrier. In practice, the adverse effects of systemic absorption are most commonly seen during the neonatal period, when the ratio of surface area to body weight predisposes to this problem.

Percutaneous absorption may disturb the pituitary-adrenal axis and occasionally produces Cushing's syndrome, but when applied to adults with an intact epidermis, the risk is relatively small.

■ **Telangiectasia**. Dilatation of superficial vessels may complicate prolonged corticosteroid therapy, especially on the face and in the intertriginous zones.

■ **Peri-oral dermatitis** follows steroid therapy on the face. The effect is reversible but withdrawal of the application is initially followed by an exacerbation. This effect of topical steroids is very unlikely to occur with hydrocortisone acetate.

■ **Cutaneous atrophy**. Prolonged application causes thinning of treated skin, particularly with occlusive therapy or in the flexures. The atrophy is generally diffuse over the area, but may form linear striae. The dermis and epidermis may be affected either singly or together.

■ **Petechiae and ecchymoses**. Pinpoint or larger areas of bleeding into the skin may occur in the treated area and are really another indication of atrophy. Dermal atrophy decreases collagen support to tiny vessels which become more fragile and rupture with bleeding into the dermis.

■ **Follicular pustules**. These may be streptococcal, candida or non specific. The leg is the most common region affected and is more likely with occlusive bases such as ointments or pastes.

■ **Enhancement of fungal infections** that occur when topical steroids are mistakenly used as the only treatment characteristically presents as suppressed erythema over a very large zone of involvement. Tinea is typically the infection involved, but candida can also be subject to this effect.

However, if the appropriate antifungal treatment is used, concurrent topical steroid use will not slow improvement of fungal infections. Also, if the correct antibiotic is used to treat rashes secondarily infected with bacteria, topical steroid use will not slow resolution of these infections either.

■ **Worsening of non-infective rashes**. Rosacea and acne, although sometimes initially helped by topical steroid use, are eventually exacerbated as a result of prolonged corticosteroid application. Psoriasis will often undergo a flare when topical steroids are suddenly ceased and pustular psoriasis commonly results when this happens. Eczema complicated by the presence of secondary bacterial infection will fail to respond to corticosteroid application unless the infection is treated as well.

■ **Gluteal granulomas** have been seen in infants as a complication of therapy with fluorinated steroids over the napkin area. The lesions, which are bluish-red nodules, resolve within a few weeks of topical steroids being withdrawn.

■ **Glaucoma and cataracts**, although rare sequels of corticosteroid treatment of dermatoses involving the eyelids, may result from accidental contamination of the conjunctival sac.

Corticosteroids plus other substances

For the following reasons, it is best to avoid using preparations that contain corticosteroids mixed with other agents.

■ **Exact diagnosis** is often avoided because of the erroneous assumption that all possibilities have been covered.

■ **Sensitisation** is made more likely, often for very little gain.

■ **Chemical interaction** with the steroid to reduce its potency has been demonstrated when tars or salicylic acid are added to the preparation, and probably occurs with other substances as well.

■ **Inactivation** of the steroid frequently occurs when proprietary corticosteroid preparations are diluted by extemporaneous mixing with bases that are inappropriate.

Systemic therapy

1. Corticosteroids
2. Antibiotics
3. Retinoids
4. Psoralens
5. Sedatives, tranquillisers, antidepressants
6. Antihistamines
7. Antimalarials
8. Cytotoxic drugs
9. Anti-androgens

Corticosteroids

Treatment with systemic corticosteroids is a valuable and sometimes life-saving measure in a number of cutaneous diseases, but the advantages should be balanced against the possibility of adverse effects in every patient for whom such therapy is considered.

The dangers of water retention in patients with hypertension, cardiac failure and renal disease restricts the use of systemic corticosteroids to important indications in the presence of these disorders. There may be aggravation of peptic ulcer, sometimes with haemorrhage. Latent diabetes may be unmasked, and infections such as tuberculosis activated. Osteoporosis is common after prolonged treatment with systemic corticosteroids, and aseptic necrosis of bone may occur. Venous thrombosis and pulmonary embolism are serious and sometimes fatal complications, while psychological changes and convulsions are not rare. Electrolyte disturbances, myopathy, neuropathy, immunosuppression and diminished adrenocortical response on withdrawal are all serious consequences. Less important adverse effects include lipodystrophy, hypertrichosis, atrophic striae and steroid acne.

For patients on long-term therapy, minimising adrenal suppression is an important goal. This can be achieved if three guidelines are followed:

■ Suppress the adrenal gland only when it is already maximally suppressed as part of the physiological diurnal variation.

■ Maximise the time available for pituitary ACTH release by choosing a corticosteroid with very short chemical half-life.

■ Avoid frequent administration of the steroid. Use one that has a very long-lasting anti-inflammatory effect.

In practice, this means using oral prednisolone, initially aiming for a single morning dose, and then eventually achieving an alternate mornings regimen if the response allows it.

When contemplating the commencement of oral corticosteroid therapy, alternative possibilities should be considered for patients with known contra-indications. In addition, whenever possible, steroid use should be avoided when treating the following:

■ *Endogenous eczemas*. When nothing is being done to change the basic reasons, it is going to be difficult to cease treatment.

■ *Psoriasis* requires very large doses of steroids for control and because tachyphylaxis inevitably occurs, it is extremely difficult to wean patients off treatment. In addition, cessation of steroids produces a rebound flare that is often pustular.

■ *Erythema nodosum* and *chronic urticaria*. Although often persistent and a nuisance, these disorders produce symptoms that can be controlled with alternative medication. They eventually resolve spontaneously. Steroid therapy may exacerbate a hidden infection that is the underlying cause of the rash.

Indications in dermatology

■ *To preserve life*. This is the most valid reason for the administration of systemic corticosteroids. The situation arises with acute anaphylaxis and with disorders such as pemphigus vulgaris, bullous pemphigoid, severe vasculitis, lupus erythematosus, dermatomyositis, erythroderma, bullous erythema multiforme and, occasionally, with angioedema and epidermolysis bullosa in children.

■ *To treat severe inflammation* when the cause has been removed, and which responds well, requires only brief treatment and will not recur when steroids are ceased. Allergic contact dermatitis, where the cause is known and removed, is one such situation.

■ *Rapidly progressive diseases* whose course is halted and 'turned off' by steroids include pemphigus vulgaris, Sweet's disease and pyoderma gangrenosum.

Dose and route of administration

These factors will vary according to the disease being treated. Pulse therapy, as is sometimes used in the treatment of pemphigus vulgaris, utilises one gram of methylprednisolone given intravenously. Cardiac arrhythmias may occur with this method due to rapid shifts in potassium and therefore patients should be in hospital and monitored. Even when pulse therapy is not used, pemphigus vulgaris may require very large initial doses such as 240 mg of prednisolone per day whereas bullous pemphigoid usually needs 60 mg daily for control. Hydrocortisone 200 mg intravenously is commonly used to treat anaphylaxis. Allergic contact dermatitis and severe irritant dermatitis respond satisfactorily to a daily oral dose of 30 to 40 mg of prednisolone.

Antibiotics, antiviral and antifungal drugs

Infections of the skin are normally treated with antibiotics selected on the basis of culture and sensitivity, but this is not always the case.

- **Acute bacterial infections** are expected to respond quickly to a short course of antibiotics. Usually a swab is taken and treatment commenced without waiting for results of culture and sensitivity. If there is no response, the sensitivities can be consulted to decide on the correct treatment. The preculture initial antibiotic chosen is based upon the likely infecting organism and this in turn depends upon the condition being treated.

- **Impetiginised eczema** must be treated with antibiotics that are effective against staphylococci. Penicillin and amoxycillin are not appropriate.

- **Acute paronychia**, infected onycholysis and bacterial infection in intertriginous zones are more likely to yield Gram-negative bacteria.

- **Epidemic impetigo** can be treated on the basis of sensitivities known from treating other patients.

- **Chronic bacterial infections** that require lengthy antibiotic therapy should have the diagnosis confirmed by culture, and the appropriate antibiotic determined by in vitro sensitivity testing, before treatment is initiated. Similarly, knowledge of antibiotic sensitivity is essential before treating infections such as boils and hidradenitis suppurativa where repeated courses of antibiotics have been used unsuccessfully.

- **Non-bacterial infections.** Culture is not usually obtained when treating tinea with griseofulvin. Resistance is uncommon, the alternatives are limited and serious toxicity very rare. Similarly, culture is not obtained when treating non-infectious conditions such as rosacea, dermatitis herpetiformis and acne vulgaris with antibiotics.

- **Acyclovir** given early in the course in herpes simplex infection usually shortens duration and lessens severity of episodes. In those with six or more attacks per year, continual low dose suppressive therapy is usually preferable. When acyclovir is given early enough, the occurrence of erythema multiforme secondary to herpes simplex can be reliably prevented. The treatment of varicella and zoster requires much higher doses, and crystallisation in the urine, producing obstructive nephropathy (which is the main toxic effect of this drug), should be prevented by ensuring adequate hydration. Encephalopathy can be seen in those with poor renal function who are using high doses. So far, resistance of herpes simplex to acyclovir has not been a significant problem.

- **Long-term treatment**, when possible, should not use drugs where the risk of toxicity rises with increasing cumulative dose. Ketoconazole hepatotoxicity during treatment of tinea of the toenails and peripheral neuropathy induced by metronidazole used to treat rosacea are examples.

Retinoids

Etretinate and isotretinoin are synthetic derivatives of retinoic acid (vitamin A acid). In adequate doses (0.5 mg to 1.5 mg/kg/day of etretinate) they impede keratinisation, and promote differentiation and mucoid biosynthesis in the skin. The precise mechanism by which they ameliorate various disorders of keratinisation is not yet known, but is believed to be related to some such basic function as RNA transcription.

Etretinate, the aromatic derivative, is frequently effective in the management of patients with erythrodermic and pustular psoriasis, Darier's disease, pityriasis rubra pilaris and severe forms of ichthyosis. Isotretinoin is a powerful inhibitor of sebaceous gland secretion and has a dramatic, beneficial effect on the severe, nodulocystic variant of acne. There is experimental evidence to suggest a potential role for the retinoids in the treatment and prevention of epithelial tumours.

Retinoids are teratogenic and may be used by women of child-bearing age only when pregnancy can be prevented. Due to the prolonged half-life of its principal metabolite, etretinate therapy necessitates avoidance of pregnancy for two years after cessation of the drug. Isotretinoin is cleared more rapidly but the characteristic retinoid embryopathy may still occur if conception occurs sooner than one month after completion of isotretinoin therapy. Both drugs may induce an elevation of cholesterol and/or triglyceride which is dose-related. Raised intracranial pressure is an effect of retinoid treatment which is most likely to occur if tetracyclines are concurrently administered. Less worrying side-effects include the almost inevitable dryness at mucocutaneous junctions, epidermal fragility, pruritus and elevated plasma levels of hepatic transaminases.

Psoralens

The psoralens are a group of naturally occurring phototoxic compounds, originally used for the treatment of vitiligo. The two psoralens now available for prescription are 8-methoxypsoralen (methoxsalen) and trimethylpsoralen (trisoralen). Methoxsalen is generally used in conjunction with long-wavelength ultraviolet radiation (UV-A), and this combination (PUVA) has proved valuable in the management of some patients with psoriasis, vitiligo, mycosis fungoides, mastocytosis, lichen planus and a few light-induced disorders. The use of tripsoralen is largely restricted to patients with vitiligo.

This group of drugs is remarkably free of short-term side-effects but psoralens remain in the lens of the eye for almost one day and, unless prevented from reacting with UV-A by the wearing of glasses with special filters, may alter lens protein to form cataracts. Because their mode of action involves light-induced interaction with DNA, carcinogenesis is a possible long-term effect of treatment. The genital skin of males is particularly susceptible to the development of PUVA-induced squamous cell carcinoma unless shielded from light during treatment. The use of psoralens by patients who have been exposed to other carcinogens, such as therapeutic X-ray and arsenic mixtures, increases the risk of cutaneous squamous cell carcinoma occurring elsewhere. However, although the psoralens have been widely used in the treatment of vitiligo since the 1950s and on a wide scale for other disorders since the 1970s, their carcinogenic potential has still not been fully determined.

Sedatives, tranquillisers, antidepressants

An effective systemic antipruritic is yet to be found, but nitrazepam or one of the phenothiazine group of antihistamines may be of great assistance to the patient whose sleep is constantly disturbed by pruritus. Pompholyx, nummular dermatitis, lichen simplex and neurotic excoriations are frequently linked to emotional problems for which diazepam or chlordiazepoxide may be very useful. Nortriptyline, amitriptyline and imipramine assist in management of the reactive depression which so often complicates itchy, disfiguring dermatoses. Pimozide and trifluoperazine have a special place in the management of delusional states involving the skin, particularly parasitophobia in the elderly.

Suitable drug therapy often provides helpful support for the patient suffering from cutaneous disease, but no drug replaces reassurance and explanation. In many cases, instruction in relaxation techniques obviates the need for psychopharmacological agents.

Antihistamines

The traditional antihistamines (H_1-blocking agents) share a chemical core with histamine and are presumed to function by competing with histamine for cell receptors. They neither decrease the production of histamine, nor do they have a direct inactivating effect.

Antihistamines are invaluable for the treatment of urticaria and its variants, but otherwise have little place in the treatment of cutaneous disease. It is likely that much of the benefit claimed for these drugs in dermatoses other than urticaria and angioedema is due to their sedative effect. The H_1 antihistamines that do not cross the blood–brain barrier and are therefore non-sedating, are effective in the treatment of urticaria but do not relieve pruritus produced by other disorders. The combination of H_1 and H_2-blocking agents provides little extra benefit in either the treatment of urticaria or the symptomatic relief of pruritus.

The antihistamines displace histamine from receptors very slowly. Adrenaline rapidly reverses the physiological effects of histamine by utilising different receptors. Therefore, in the treatment of anaphylaxis, adrenaline is used in conjunction with the intravenous or intramuscular administration of an antihistamine. Intravenous injection of hydrocortisone is also usually used.

Antimalarials

Hydroxychloroquine and chloroquine have a definite place in the management of cutaneous lupus erythematosus. They are frequently helpful in arresting progress of the cutaneous lesions and appear to exert a steroid-sparing effect. They are useful in porphyria cutanea tarda, but their value in polymorphic light eruption is controversial.

The risk of adverse side-effects from antimalarials, especially chloroquine, is a serious one. The decision to embark on chloroquine therapy implies adequate supervision by the physician and regular examinations by an ophthalmologist during therapy.

Cytotoxic drugs

Direct cytotoxicity may be the mechanism of action when this group of drugs is used in hyperproliferative states such as psoriasis and lymphomas. Immunomodulation secondary to effects on immuno-functional cells could explain the benefits these drugs produce in lupus erythematosus, pemphigus vulgaris and some forms of vasculitis. Cyclosporin has specific effects on T lymphocyte function, but whether this is the reason it is helpful in psoriasis, atopic eczema and pyoderma gangrenosum is not known.

Although the doses used in dermatology are usually low in comparison to those used in chemotherapy of cancer and transplant rejection, it is false logic to believe that toxicity is avoided. Low dose cyclosporin causes the same profile of toxic effects as regular doses and renal dysfunction, in particular, is just as common. The low doses of methotrexate used to treat psoriasis do not prevent it producing hepatotoxic effects. Chronic use of drugs of this type may allow reactivation of an old focus of tuberculosis or the emergence of lymphomas. Cytotoxic drugs produce very severe acute toxicity if metabolism and excretion are interfered with and in patients with slightly impaired excretion, interaction with other drugs may produce fatal effects.

The use of methotrexate and other cytotoxic agents is rarely indicated in the management of psoriasis, and they should never be used without adequate investigation and follow-up.

Anti-androgens

In females, the androgen-dependent disorders such as acne and hirsutism may be treated with anti-androgenic agents. Spironolactone has mild anti-androgen activity and cyproterone acetate is even more potent. When using these agents, menstrual cycle irregularities usually occur. The concurrent use of contraceptive steroids not only regulates the menses but also prevents the tragedy of accidental exposure to these drugs during pregnancy, producing feminisation of a male foetus. Cyproterone acetate is used during days 5 to 15 of the menstrual cycle to allow withdrawal bleeding to simulate the normal menstrual pattern. Spironolactone is taken each day but sodium and potassium levels should be monitored.

In the past, oestrogens were used to produce effects that opposed those of androgens. The very high doses required produce unacceptable toxic effects and this treatment is no longer used.

Surgical and physical methods

1. Office surgery
2. The skin biopsy
3. Curettage
4. Electrosurgery
5. Cryotherapy
6. Ionising radiation
7. Laser surgery
8. Ultraviolet light

Office surgery

Excision of small cutaneous lesions is an everyday procedure for most general practitioners. Results can be considerably improved by attention to a few simple details.

For cutaneous anaesthesia, 1 to 2 per cent lignocaine is very satisfactory, and in the quantities which are used for office procedures is very rarely associated with serious adverse effects. The addition of adrenaline is optional, but should be avoided for the digits, particularly in elderly patients; even without adrenaline, the injection of an excessive quantity of local anaesthetic around a digit may be sufficient to compromise the blood supply to the peripheral part of the finger or toe. This obstruction by compression is much less likely when the block is administered close to the interdigital webs. In any case, not more than 6 mL to 8 mL of solution should be injected into the digit. Warming the lignocaine to body temperature does not lessen the anaesthesia but reduces the pain of injection.

The lines of excision should be planned, when possible, to follow the 'wrinkle lines' of the skin. These differ from Langer's lines, which were produced by puncturing cadaver skin and marked the direction of wound spread. By and large, wrinkle lines follow a line at right angles to the direction of muscle contraction beneath the site. In those areas, as on the face, where there are mixed directions of action of underlying muscle, the wrinkle pattern is often circular. In areas such as the ear where there is no underlying muscle, there are no wrinkle lines. The pattern of wrinkle lines may be established by compressing the skin between thumb and forefinger. If the skin just crumples, then this is not the direction of the lines. If there is a wrinkle line, then this defines the direction of the wound. When no wrinkles form, the patient may be asked to smile, frown or screw up his eyes.

When minor lesions are excised from the vermilion border of the lip, better cosmetic results follow incisions parallel to the junction of skin and vermilion border. In all wounds around the lips, care should be taken to produce exact realignment of the junction of skin and vermilion border. Marking this junction prior to injection of local anaesthetic is very helpful.

Excessive hair should be removed, but rough shaving increases the risk of wound infection. The site should be washed with a chlorhexidine or povidone-iodine surgical scrub, firmly enough to be effective but short of causing irritation to the skin. The area is then prepared by painting with an alcoholic solution of chlorhexidine, or another suitable skin prep. The planned lines of incision should be carefully marked with, for example, a gentian violet tincture.

The simplest and safest method of excision is the ellipse, with angles no wider than 15°–30°. When excision is oval, the scar is considerably longer than the lines traced by the scalpel, and 'dog-ears' tend to form at the ends of the suture line. Using an appropriate blade, generally #15 to #10, the incision should begin at the most dependent end, to avoid the lower area being obscured by blood falling from the upper end of the wound.

Dog-ears can generally be avoided by following the rule that the length: breadth ratio should not be less than 3:1. The tendency to dog-ears is reduced by suturing so that each stitch divides the length of the unsutured wound by half. The halving principle minimises the hump and where a dog-ear is small, subsequent healing will correct the bulge. When a larger dog-ear has been inadvertently created, it can be corrected by lifting the elevation with a hook or suture and making an incision at an angle less than 60° to the imagined continuation of the wound. The free edge of the wound is then pulled over the extended incision to determine the excess, which is then excised, leaving a hockey-stick line which is closed.

When the lesion removed is suspected of being neoplastic, it is helpful for the specimen to be colour-coded before fixation and transfer to the pathologist. If the tumour is colour-coded and a margin is found microscopically to be not clear of tumour, then the precise location in need of re-excision or careful observation is known.

In considering the causes of poor wound healing, considerable attention is paid to infection, but the common causes of failure are dead space and excessive tension on wound edges. Dead space is not a great problem in the type of minor cutaneous surgery which is performed as an office procedure, but wound tension is very relevant. Proper selection should exclude procedures which necessitate extensive undermining by those inexperienced in surgical techniques. If in doubt as to whether undermining is necessary, the wound edges may be gripped between finger and thumb. If the edges do not come together easily, then the skin should be separated from the subcutis for a centimetre or so on either side with scissors or scalpel. The wound edges should be carefully approximated to avoid inversion of the edges. One or two vertical mattress sutures, or a horizontal mattress suture with bolsters, assist wound closure without tension.

In addition, wound healing requires a dressing that provides: haemostasis, a moist layer for the epidermal cells to move over, a clean environment that is not susceptible to infection, and protection from trauma.

A contour filling firm dressing will aid in securing haemostasis. Absorbent material such as gauze will minimise collection of exudate, which not only removes away from the wound a potential culture medium for bacteria, but also prevents crust formation, which is important because depressed scars result when epidermal cells migrate on the moist layer beneath a crust. If there is much exudation, the absorbent layer of the dressing should be changed frequently to prevent it becoming infected. The use of an antibacterial ointment on the wound will provide the necessary moist layer for epidermal cell migration as well as preventing infection. A nonstick layer between the wound and the absorbent layer, and non-irritant hypoallergenic adhesive tape will help minimise trauma from the dressing itself.

Sutures are removed at the earliest time compatible with adequate healing, which varies not only with the site but also with the degree of tension and line of the wound. Experience is the best guide to the optimal time for removal of sutures, but mattress sutures should be removed by the fourth day. On the face, four days are usually sufficient for healing and early removal gives better cosmetic results.

Sutures are freed by cutting on one side with a sharp pair of fine scissors or triangular scalpel blade, and drawing the cut suture towards the wound for removal. The wound should be supported by butterfly adhesive strips for five to seven days after the sutures have been removed. On sites such as the shoulder, two weeks may be necessary and on mobile areas such as the hand, suture material such as nylon allows these long times to be achieved without discomfort.

For best results, cutaneous surgery requires the use of suitable instruments—small blades, iris scissors, small forceps with good apposition of the edges, a Gillies combined scissors and needle holder, and fine suture material. All lesions excised from the skin should be sent for histological examination.

The skin biopsy

Considerable judgment is needed in the selection of an appropriate site for biopsy. The particular lesion chosen should be one which is most likely to give histological evidence of the disease process. In many cases, this will be an early lesion which has not been altered by trauma or therapy. In others, more mature lesions provide better samples. In some diseases, more than one biopsy at different stages of the disease may be necessary to establish the diagnosis, and in some cases several biopsies may be needed from a single lesion to establish the extent of invasion or to exclude malignant change in, for example, an area of Bowen's disease.

Small lesions are best excised completely. The size of the biopsy from larger lesions varies, but should be of sufficient diameter and depth to provide a representative sample of the pathologic process.

The tissue removed should be handled gently with plain forceps to minimise distortion. Local anaesthetic should not be injected too close to the wound. On the face, and particularly around the eyes, a smaller ellipse will usually be excised. If using a biopsy punch, the skin can be held stretched at right angles to the wrinkle lines so that when the procedure is completed and the tension released, the resultant wound is an ellipse.

Curettage

A small, sharp-edged, spoon-shaped curette may be used to remove superficial benign cutaneous lesions. The technique is useful for molluscum contagiosum, solar and seborrhoeic keratoses, and may be combined with electrocautery or electrodesiccation.

In experienced hands, small basal cell carcinomas of the non-fibrosing type are suitable for removal by curettage and cautery, provided that the lesion is superficial and an adequate margin of apparently normal skin is removed. The technique is generally unsuitable for lesions on the nose, around the eyes, and on the legs below the knees. Curettings are examined histologically.

Curettage should not be used for lesions of a doubtful nature. Although permissible for such clinically distinctive benign tumours as an obvious seborrhoeic keratosis, the method is generally contra-indicated for pigmented lesions.

Electrosurgery

Electrosurgery involves the use of heat to destroy tissues.

■ *Electrofulguration* is the use of high frequency electrical current to 'spark' tissue. *Electrodesiccation* is the use of the same high frequency current through a terminal in contact with the tissue. With both methods a single electrode is used. The heat generated is fairly localised (electrofulguration is more superficial), does not spread very well through blood and has little haemostatic effect. These modalities are used for destroying superficial relatively non-vascular lesions such as seborrhoeic keratoses and warts. Utilising a thin flexible electrode inserted correctly down a hair follicle, gentle electrodesiccation can permanently destroy the matrix of cosmetically troublesome hairs.

■ *Electrocoagulation* which produces thrombosis of vessels and tissue destruction requires two electrodes and is utilised to destroy highly vascular lesions. A two-electrode circuit is also required to produce a cutting current.

■ *Electrocautery* utilises a needle tip or wire loop that is heated by the resistance to flow of electricity through it. There is extreme destruction of tissue and effective haemostasis. Control is difficult because too little heat causes tissue to adhere to the wire and too much heat produces unacceptable scarring.

Undiagnosed lesions, particularly when pigmented, should not be treated by electrosurgery because the method is destructive and material submitted for histology is not satisfactory. Despite the intense heat generated by these modalities, viruses such as hepatitis and HIV can be transmitted by non-sterilised electrodes.

It is important to note that some types of cardiac pacemaker may be inactivated by the high frequency current used for electrodesiccation.

Cryotherapy

Properly used for superficial lesions, freezing with carbon dioxide slush or liquid nitrogen produces localised destruction of the superficial epidermis with little or no subsequent scarring. It is widely used for superficial keratoses and, occasionally, for small superficial haemangiomas and warts.

Dermatologists sometimes use cryotherapy to treat selected basal cell carcinomas. The technique depends upon producing sufficiently low temperature of ample duration to adequate depth. Correct use requires cryoprobes, devices to limit the spread of applied cryogen, measurement of extent of freeze beyond the area of application, and recording of thaw times to confirm adequacy of treatment. Only liquid nitrogen spray produces sufficiently intense cold to treat deeper lesions. Cryotherapy is not advisable for basal cell carcinomas where depth cannot be defined with certainty; therefore unsuitable types include fibrosing basal cell carcinomas and those involving embryonal fusion planes such as the perinasal fold.

Ionising radiation

In the past, radium and its products were sometimes employed, but radiotherapy of cutaneous lesions is now virtually synonymous with superficial X-ray therapy. By varying the operating factors, X-rays can be made to penetrate deeply or be dissipated in the most superficial layers of the skin. Properly used, X-ray therapy is a valuable modality with a wide margin of safety. Depending on the site and type of tumour, X-ray therapy may be the most appropriate treatment for carcinoma of the skin, but is never used for melanoma. Radiotherapy is a useful palliative for cutaneous lesions of lymphoma or leukaemia, and is sometimes used in the treatment of Bowen's disease and kerato-acanthoma.

The introduction of oral isotretinoin has seen the abandonment of X-ray as a treatment for severe cystic acne, which was formerly the commonest non-cancerous skin condition treated with ionising radiation. As a consequence, X-ray therapy is nowadays virtually never used for non-malignant skin conditions.

Laser surgery

The laser beam is a stream of monochromatic radiation which is co-ordinated in phase, but which may be pulsed or continuous. The argon laser and the copper vapour laser produce wave lengths absorbed by haemoglobin. When these are used to treat vascular lesions, such as port-wine stains, red blood cells absorb this intense amount of energy and cells are created which are in an unstable state. This energy must be dissipated, which mainly occurs in the form of heat, causing vaporisation of the surrounding vessels. However, heat is the form of physical destruction that causes most scarring of the skin and therefore the laser dosage must be adjusted to that which is sufficient to produce vascular destruction yet also causes minimal conduction of heat into the surrounding skin. Usually this is calculated by first test-treating several small non-conspicuous areas with varying doses and then commencing treatment weeks later with the dose that produced clearing and no scarring when the area was assessed. However, this is far from ideal, because a vascular naevus does not always have uniform depth or density.

With most lasers the vascular naevi that respond best, in addition to being superficial, have a high concentration of red blood cells per unit area. Unfortunately, this is not the type of naevus that is usually seen in young children, but commonly occurs later in adult life, when the childhood-type naevi generally change from pink to a blue-red and from completely flat to having slightly thickened areas. Recent work with lasers that emit frequent bursts of light lasting only a few microseconds (flash pumped lasers) suggests that this type of laser may not only minimise conduction of heat, and therefore minimise scarring, but also, by producing a different type of vascular injury, be effectively used in the treatment of the flat pale pink telangiectatic naevi seen during early childhood.

The carbon dioxide laser emits a continuous beam of radiation within the infrared range. The CO_2 laser is not colour selective, but can be used to produce selective vaporisation of small volumes of tissue with minimal conduction of thermal energy into adjacent areas. Excisional CO_2 laser therapy has been used to treat a range of small vascular lesions in the skin, and for the removal of tattoos.

The unique properties of laser beams provide enormous potential for future application. The tunable dye laser allows alteration of the lasing medium so that the wavelengths of the beam can be adjusted to achieve maximum absorption in particular tissues. This allows dissipation of the radiation in the lesion being treated, with minimal damage to normal skin.

Ultraviolet light

Either as sunlight or from artificial sources, ultraviolet radiation is widely used in the management of many skin disorders.

UV-B is effective in the treatment of psoriasis, pityriasis rosea, pityriasis lichenoides, very early mycosis fungoides, and will commonly relieve the pruritus of renal failure. UV-A, in conjunction with psoralens, is useful therapy for vitiligo, psoriasis, mycosis fungoides, lichen planus and mastocytosis.

Treatment is usually commenced with the dose that produces minimal erythema and then each dose is incrementally increased to maintain faint redness.

Less commonly, ultraviolet light is used for diagnostic purposes. To detect substances that become contact allergens only following irradiation and interaction with skin components, photopatch testing is required. Confirmation of polymorphic light eruption and solar urticaria can be achieved using special exposure techniques.

Induced tolerance to ultraviolet light is a feature of some photosensitive disorders such as solar urticaria and polymorphic light eruption. By receiving deliberate exposure to gradually increasing, controlled amounts of the causative wave lengths during early spring, affected patients can often experience a less troublesome summer.

Index

Bold entries indicate main references.

Bold entries indicate main references.

Bold entries indicate main references.

Bold entries indicate main references.

Bold entries indicate main references.

Bold entries indicate main references.

Bold entries indicate main references.

Bold entries indicate main references.

Bold entries indicate main references.

Bold entries indicate main references.